THE BEST ALTERNATIVE MEDICINE

Dr. Kenneth R. Pelletier

Introduction by Dr. Andrew Weil

A Fireside Book
Published by Simon & Schuster
New York   London   Toronto   Sydney   Singapore

FIRESIDE
Rockefeller Center
1230 Avenue of the Americas
New York, NY 10020

Copyright © 2000 by Dr. Kenneth R. Pelletier, Inc.
All rights reserved, including the right of reproduction in whole or in part in any form.
First Fireside Edition 2002
FIRESIDE and colophon are registered trademarks of Simon & Schuster, Inc.
For information about special discounts for bulk purchases,
please contact Simon & Schuster Special Sales:
1-800-456-6798 or business@simonandschuster.com
Designed by Pagesetters Incorporated
Manufactured in the United States of America

10 9 8 7 6 5 4 3 2 1

The Library of Congress has cataloged the Simon & Schuster edition as follows:
Pelletier, Kenneth R.
    The best alternative medicine : What works? What does not?/
Kenneth R. Pelletier ; introduction by Andrew Weil.
        p.   cm.
    Includes bibliographical references and index.
    1. Alternative medicine.   I. Title.
    R733.P45   2000
    615'.5—dc21   99-26629
                                                                  CIP
ISBN 0-684-84207-6
    0-7432-0027-6 (Pbk)

ACKNOWLEDGMENTS

From the cover of *Time* magazine to the innovative research funded by the National Institutes of Health, there is a virtual explosion of recent interest in complementary, alternative, and integrative medicine. Rather like any "overnight" phenomenon, this area of research and clinical practice has been in gestation for decades in the United States and hundreds of years in indigenous healing traditions in every nation on earth. Conducting my research and writing this book would not have been possible without the genius, dedication, research and clinical funding, encouragement, and enduring friendship of so many colleagues over these last twenty-five years. Each person named here has made a major, significant contribution in sorting through the complexities of complementary and alternative medicine and integrating demonstrably effective interventions into conventional health care.

Acknowledging these individuals has given me the opportunity to reflect upon each person and their unique contributions and abiding perseverance. Although this enumeration is incomplete, it is surely heartfelt. First of all I would like to thank my longtime friend and colleague Dr. Andrew T. Weil for his forward to this book; I am truly honored by his reflections. From the onset I thank my colleagues at the Stanford University School of Medicine, including Dr. John W. Farquhar, Dr. William L. Haskell, Dr. Stephen P. Fortmann, Dr. John A. Astin, Dr. James F. Fries, Dr. David Spiegel, Dr. Christopher Gardner, Dr. Marcia Stefanick, Dr. Wes Alles, Dr. Abby King, Dr. C. Barr Taylor, Dr. Walter Bortz, Dr. Gene Spiller, Professor Alain Enthoven, Dr. Jeffrey Croke, Dr. Halsted Holman, Chris Scott, and Peter Van Etten, president and CEO of the UCSF/Stanford Health System. Paralleling the work of my Stanford colleagues are the individuals who made the writing and preparation of this book possible: Ms. Cindy Wood, Ms. Lauri Young, Ms. Adeline Hwang, Ms. Sandra Stahl, and Ms. Ellen DiNucci. For their consummate editing and writing skills, I am indeed indebted to both Ms. Kathy Goss and Cameron Stauth in the sculpting of the final manuscript.

Most important, I wish to thank Frederic W. Hills of Simon & Schuster for more encouragement, patience, and mentoring than I could have imagined. Also, a thanks to his able assistant, Ms. Priscilla Holmes for her work on the manuscript. At ICM, I want to thank my representatives, Ms. Lisa R. Bankoff and Ms. Suzanne Gluck, for securing such a renowned editor and publishing house.

Research requires funding, and that difficult task attains Herculean proportions in new areas such as complementary and integrative alternative medicine. For their vision and courage of commitment, I would like to acknowledge the National Institutes of Health, National Center for Complementary and Alternative Medicine (NCCAM), with particular respect for Dr. Wayne B. Jonas, Dr. Richard L. Nahin, Dr. Geoffrey Cheung, Dr. Carole Hudgings, and Dr. William Harlan. In the funding of the NCCAM, there are the pioneering efforts of Senator Tom Harkin, Senator Orrin Hatch, and Dr. Joe Jacobs. Funding from the NIH-NCCATA has allowed the creation of the Complementary and Alternative Medicine Program at Stanford (CAMPS).

Additional funding and support has permitted CAMPS to undertake further innovative research and establish a clinic, thanks to the generosity of the Fetzer Institute with Dr. Jeremy Waletzky and Robert F. Lehman, the Nathan Cummings Foundation with Charles Harpen and Ms. Andrea Kydd, Michael S. Currier, the Fresno Foundation with Ed Rontell, Colby and Lani Jones, Larry Biehl, and E. Lewis Reid.

Additionally, Michael Murphy, George Leonard, and Steve Donovan and the board of directors of the Esalen Institute generously donated to CAMPS the Esalen Archive of over twelve thousand hard-copy articles from an Esalen program funded by Laurance S. Rockefeller. Research funding has also been provided by Dr. Albert R. Martin and Ms. Bobbi Kimball of Blue Shield of California; Jay M. Gellert, Dr. Arthur M. Southam, and Dr. Antonio P. Legoretta of Health Net/FHS; Bain J. Farris of Anthem Blue Cross/Blue Shield; Dr. Des Cummings, Jr., of the Florida Hospital/Disney/Celebration collaboration; and the participating companies of the Stanford Corporate Health Program, including AT&T, American Airlines, ARCO, Anthem Blue Cross/Blue Shield, Bank of America, Health Net (FHS), Disney, IBM, Kaiser Permanente, Levi Strauss, Merck, Mercer, Motorola, San Mateo county, Rite Aid/PCS, Shaklee/Yamanouchi, United Behavioral Health, Medstat, and Xerox.

For each chapter of this book and for research projects in various domains, a number of professional experts provided literature searches and reviews, critiques of draft materials, and a wealth of knowledge, wisdom, and critical assessment of these complex areas of clinical and research knowledge. Within the areas of mind/body medicine, a particular acknowledgment goes to Dr. John A. Astin, Dr. Frederic Luskin, Ms. Katie Newell, and Dr. John Kabat-Zinn; in chiropractic, Dr. William Meeker; for acupuncture, Dr. Joseph M. Helms, Dr. Brian Berman, and Dr. Yuan-Chi Lin; nutrition and dietary supplements, Dr. Pamela M. Peeke, Dr. Christopher Gardner, and the late Dr. James H. Whittam; European herbals, Mark Blumenthal and Dr. Ted Kaptchuk; traditional Chinese medicine, Dr. Miki Shima and Dr. Subhuti Dharmananda; Ayurvedic, Dr. Shri K. Mishra; homeopathy, Dr. Jennifer Jacobs, Dr. Roger Morrison, and Dana Ullman; naturopathy, Dr. Carlo Calabrese; within the area of spirituality, Dr. Dick Tibbits and Dr. Larry Dossey; and for the insurance coverage of CAM, John Weeks and Ms. Ariane Marie. Individually and collectively, these scholars and clinicians contributed their best insights and critical orientation to those complex areas and I am hopeful that the results are a modest reflection of their dedication. Whatever insights reside in these chapters is due to their knowledge. Whatever deficiencies remain are solely due to my limitations.

With the funding of ten collaborative research centers, the NIH National Center in complementary and Alternative Medicine (NCCAM) has enabled a core group of researchers to meet, work together, and engage in the critique and mutual development of an array of increasingly sophisticated research. Details of these centers are included throughout the book and many of these colleagues have already been acknowledged, or will be in the final section of this introduction. For now, I wish to thank the following Center colleagues for many exciting and productive meetings: Dr. Leanna J. Standish, Dr. Brian M. Berman, Dr. Fredi Kronenberg, Dr. Thomas J. Kiresuk, Dr. William L. Meeker, Dr. Samuel C. Shiflett, Dr. Judith Stern, Dr. M. Eric Gershwin, Dr. Guy S. Parcel, Dr. Mary Ann Richardson, Dr. Steven F. Bolling, Dr. Sarah Warber, Dr. Nancy Schoenberger, Dr. Betsy B. Singh, Dr. Ann Gill Taylor, Ms. Christine Wade, Dr. Fayez K. Gishan, and Dr. Andrew Weil.

As I was writing this book, my wife, Elizabeth, was thrown from one of her horses and sustained severe injuries. While conventional medicine provided excellent diagnostics, it offered virtually nothing in terms of treatment. Fortunately, a skilled group of alternative medicine practitioners combined and coordinated their skills in a model of true health care that resulted in a full and complete recovery. For their insight, dedication, extraordinary professional skills, and loving care, we want to extend a heartfelt personal acknowledgement to Ms. Pat Scott, Ms. Diana Herold, Ms. Rhonda Hackett, Dr. Roger Morrison, Dr. Miki Shima, and Dr. Harry D. Friedman, who are among the true healers of our time.

Finally, let me conclude with an anecdote that Jane Goodall recounted to open a lecture at the State of the World Forum in the fall of 1996. Standing before a plenary of world leaders, she acknowledged her colleagues by noting a Texas aphorism: "When you see a turtle at the top of a telephone pole, you know it did not get there by itself!" For over twenty-five years, the field of complementary and alternative medicine has been painstakingly built upon the vision, courage, tenacity, and analytic skills of true pioneers.

Although this recitation of their names is incomplete, it is with deep honor, respect, and admiration that I am proud to acknowledge these individuals as colleagues, friends, and mentors: Dr. Andrew T. Weil, Dr. David Eisenberg, Dr. Herbert Benson, Dr. Hans Selye, Dr. C. Norman Shealey, Dr. Jonas Salk, Dr. Tom Ferguson, Norman Cousins, John E. Fetzer, Dr. Tracy Gaudette, Ms. Sue Fleischman, Dr. Richard Friedman, Dr. Redford B. Williams, Jach Pursel, Dr. Dean Ornish, Dr. Shirley Brown, Ram Dass, Jerry Green, Dr. Michael Carlston, Dr. Joan Borysenko, Dr. Michael Lerner, Roger S. Greaves, Dr. Rachel Naomi Remen, Dr. Martin L. Rossman, George Vithoulkas, Dr. Paul J. Rosch, Dr. Claude Rossel, Dr. Ray H. Rosenman, Dr. Steven E. Locke, Dr. Chandra Patel, Dr. Deepak Chopra, Dr. David Sobel, Dr. James S. Gordon, Ms. Joan L. Schleicher, Dr. Emmett E. Miller, Dr. Daniel Goleman, Dr. Judith Orloff, Dr. Irving Oyle, John Robbins, Dr. Bernie S. Siegel, Dr. Robert E. Kowalski, Dr. William Regelson, Dr. Bill Goldman, Dr. Anton Jayasuriya, Dr. Sadja Greenwood, Dr. Samuel Benjamin, Dr. W. Ross Adley, Dr. Robert O. Becker, Dr. David E. Bresler, Dr. Jeffrey Bland, Dr. Harry B. Demopoulos, Dr. Ken Dychtwald, Dr. Anthony E. Elite, Dr. Joel

Elkes, Dr. Harry D. Friedman, Jack Schwarz, Dr. Jessie C. Gruman, Dr. Malik Hasan, Dr. W. Brugh Joy, Dr. Richard A. Lippin, Dr. Gay Luce, Dr. George Solomon, Dr. Alvin R. Tarlov, Dr. Art Ulene, Dr. Donald M. Vickery, Ms. Faye Wattleton, Dr. David Watts, Arthur M. Young, Ms. Deborah Szekely, and Brendan O'Regan.

Each of these individuals has touched and inspired me as well as many, many others, and each of them personifies the vision of keeping your eye on the distant horizon while mapping your course one measured step at a time.

For Elizabeth

She is my North, my South, my East and West
My working week and my Sunday rest
My moon, my midnight, my talk, my song
I thought that love would last
for ever and a day
I was not wrong.

RESPECTFUL PARAPHRASE OF
W. H. AUDEN

CONTENTS

PART II

CAM THERAPIES FOR SPECIFIC CONDITIONS

THE BEST
ALTERNATIVE
MEDICINE

INTRODUCTION

Alternative medicine is now the fastest-growing sector of American health care. Despite continuing objections from the rearguard of the scientific establishment, many forward-looking doctors have begun to recognize the virtues of complementary medicine. As for the American consumer, millions are voting with their feet and their pocketbooks for treatments other than those conventional physicians are trained to provide. Alternative medicine is clearly moving into the mainstream. Moreover, what is happening in this country is happening around the world. In fact, some countries—notably Germany and China—are far ahead of us in recognizing the validity of alternative therapies and working to integrate them with conventional, Western medicine. In the United States, the National Institutes of Health has created the National Center for Complementary and Alternative Medicine (NCCAM) to study complementary and alternative medicine. Also, a special presidential commission was established in 1999 to study this subject. Clearly, this movement is not a fad but rather a global sociocultural trend with deep historical and intellectual roots.

In the United States the change began in the 1960s with loss of blind faith in technology. Up to that time our culture was captivated by a technological dream, the belief that science and technology would do away with all human ills, including poverty, illiteracy, disease, and, possibly, even death. Science and technology revolutionized medicine at the end of the nineteenth century, and throughout the first half of the twentieth century enabled us to make great strides in understanding human biology and intervening in cases of illness. Then in the 1960s came the realization that technology creates as many problems as it solves. In medicine, the created problem is expense—expense that has become unbearable as the new millennium approaches. All over the world health care systems are breaking down as the cost of standard medicine continues to increase.

The logical American response to this economic breakdown has been a corporate takeover of health care institutions by people whose only interest is getting what profit they can from a sinking system. This is managed care, and it is making the lives of many people—doctors and patients alike—miserable. Physicians resent their loss of autonomy and inability to practice medicine in the way they imagined it to be when they were idealistic students. Patients are increasingly angry about the impersonality of managed care and the lack of time they get to spend with physicians. This frustration is surely an immediate reason that so many of them are seeking alternatives.

But there are other, deeper reasons for the growing popularity of the ideas and practices described in this book. When medicine embraced technology hundreds of years ago, it turned its back on nature and on all of the simple, inexpensive ways of influencing health and disease that previous generations used, many of which are still current in other cultures. It also lost touch with the most basic precepts of its own historical tradition. After all, Hippocrates enjoined physicians first to do no harm and also to revere the healing power of nature. People all over the world are increasingly concerned about the harm inflicted by modern, technological medicine, especially adverse reactions to pharmaceutical drugs that are now so common. In deciding what to put into their bodies, they are more inclined to pay attention to the wisdom of nature and be wary of all that is artificial. They are also fascinated by mind/body interactions, interested in spirituality, and disillusioned with medicine that looks at human beings as physical bodies only.

I first met Ken Pelletier at a conference on "holistic" medicine in 1974. The holistic medical movement of those days was an early sign of the discontent that was building, although in the absence of the current economic crisis in medicine, it was easy for most physicians and medical administrators to ignore it or regard it as a fringe movement of little significance. However, both Ken Pelletier and I saw it differently and understood it to be the seed of something of great importance. Three years later, Ken published his landmark book, *Mind as Healer, Mind as Slayer,* which defined the emerging field of mind/body medicine, now a central focus of alternative medicine, and one that has great potential to challenge the underlying assumptions of the conventional system. It is also the alternative field backed by the greatest amount of research demonstrating efficacy in the largest number of conditions. Always drawing on mainstream science, Ken Pelletier's work continues to create the foundation for our understanding and applications of mind/body medicine.

Another major thrust of his work has been health promotion and disease management through the Stanford Corporate Health Program at the Stanford University School of Medicine, which aims to educate the purchasers of medical care about creative solutions for the unchecked rise in costs of benefits. One approach that Dr. Pelletier advocates is the management of disease as well as the promotion of wellness through attention to lifestyle. Another is the thoughtful integration of alternative therapies with conventional ones, relying on basic research as well as research in clinical and cost outcomes to make sure integration proceeds wisely toward an integrative medicine.

I am a strong advocate of integrative medicine, because I see it as the way of the future that will bring medicine back into balance, restoring its connection with nature, refocusing it on health and healing rather than on disease, and thus satisfying the needs of consumers. At the University of Arizona College of Medicine in Tucson I direct a new Program in Integrative Medicine, the first of its kind, which is now training physicians and developing new models of medical education. A number of other leading medical schools, Stanford among them, have indicated intentions of moving in this direction. Most patients who come to our clinic, like most patients going to alternative providers in general, are paying out-of-pocket. This limits the availability of integrative medicine to the affluent, and if it does not escape that limitation, it will not have the influence necessary to correct the course of medicine. If integrative medicine cannot be incorporated into the reality of managed care, it will remain a curiosity rather than a mainstream trend.

For many years I have regarded Ken Pelletier's pioneering work, and especially this book, to be essential to the development of the kind of medicine I would like to see. In these pages he dispassionately and objectively explains what treatments are actually effective, based on the best and most up-to-date domestic and international research on all the major areas of complementary and alternative medicine. In addition to his evaluations of the major therapies, he offers research-based recommendations for specific conditions and diseases. This is information that the consumer can trust, and it will be invaluable to educators, to physicians in practice, to insurers, to administrators and purchasers of health plans as well. It is an important work that will greatly further the movement toward a sound integrative medicine.

Andrew Weil, M.D.
Director, Program in Integrative Medicine
Clinical Professor of Internal Medicine
University of Arizona School of Medicine

When Health is absent,
wisdom cannot reveal itself,
art cannot become manifest,
strength cannot be exerted,
wealth becomes useless,
and reason is powerless.

HEROPHILUS
300 B.C.

I manifest for thee those hundred
thousand, thousand
shapes,
that clothe my mystery;
I show thee all my semblances
infinite,
rich,
divine,
my changeful lives,
my countless
forms.

BHAGAVAD GITA

PART I

MAJOR AREAS OF TREATMENT

CHAPTER I

THINK HORSES, NOT ZEBRAS

Throughout recorded history, every culture has had its own alternative medicines, from tropical Tahiti, Eskimos in the Arctic, American Indians, Mayans, and Gypsies to groups and sects throughout the ancient and modern world. Scientists reported in 1998 that the "Ice Man" discovered in 1991 at the foot of a retreating glacier where he had been buried for 5,300 years had used natural remedies. Since he had been dried by Alpine winds and then encased in ice, his body and belongings had been remarkably well preserved. Examination of his intestines noted eggs of *Trichuris trichiuria*, or whipworm, which is a parasite that causes abdominal pain and anemia. Researchers are quite certain that the Ice Man used a botanical product to treat this infection, since among his belongings they found two walnut-sized lumps tied to leather thongs. Analysis revealed them to be the fruit of *Piptoporous botulinis*, a plant containing oils that are toxic to parasites, as well as very strong laxative compounds that would cause expulsion of the dead and dying parasites and their eggs. In addition, he had what appeared to be several "tattoos" on his body. These were made by cutting into the skin with a sharp object, filling the incisions with herbs, and then cauterizing the wounds. Further investigation indicated that most of the lesions were situated over joints that had been damaged by arthritis. In addition to herbal medicine, the investigator speculated that he might have used these tattoos as a form of localized therapy for relief of muscle and joint pain. Surely, many forms of alternative medicine have been extant for thousands of years.

It is a humbling experience to thoughtfully examine the complex array of medical systems that CAM comprises. Certainly, this matrix of cultures, philosophies, traditions, and techniques is as subtle and complex as a rainbow.

Today, every medical student is taught the old aphorism, "Think horses, not zebras." It is an admonition to pay attention to what is evident about the patient, and to rule out obvious, common conditions before reaching a diagnosis of a rare condition.

This time-honored rule is profoundly valuable in evaluating the best possible treatments for the most common health problems that our society now faces.

Currently, the United States, and much of the rest of the world, is experiencing an epidemic of chronic and degenerative illnesses, such as cardiovascular disease, cancer, diabetes, arthritis, and depression. Very often, these illnesses are the result of obvious, common lifestyle risks, such as smoking, overeating, or being too sedentary. Frequently, such illnesses can be prevented, arrested, and even reversed when individuals stop making these lifestyle mistakes and rebuild their health with various conventional as well as alternative, complementary, or integrative therapies.

Research indicates that many forms of complementary and alternative medicine, or "CAM," are exceptionally effective at preventing and quelling the widespread chronic diseases that now plague much of the world. However, effective CAM therapies are often so deceptively simple that they may be overlooked. In effect, medical researchers and clinicians are failing to "think horses, not zebras." They are overlooking the obvious: Lifestyle factors cause a great many chronic diseases, and complementary and alternative medicine can have a powerfully positive impact upon those diseases.

However, proponents and practitioners of CAM frequently make an equally egregious intellectual error. They often tend to believe that virtually any form of CAM is superior to any form of conventional medicine. Some advocates of alternative medicine seem to adopt CAM as a veritable religion, and fail to see that CAM, like conventional medicine, has many limitations, and can also be reductionistic, as well as harmful, if used improperly.

This book challenges the polarized, dogmatic thinking that often surrounds the conflict between conventional medicine and CAM. Both of these medical traditions need to be evaluated objectively, using the best research available. Perhaps surprisingly, many conventional medical practices lack any real scientific basis. A 1990 report from the United States Office of Technology Assessment of the United States Congress concluded that upwards of 80 percent of conventional medicine lacked an adequate basis in research. During 1991, Dr. Richard Smith, editor of the *British Medical Journal,* examined twenty-one common medical practices and concluded that the evidence for seventeen out of twenty-one was "poor to none" in an editorial commentary on the necessity of research-based medicine. Most recently a review by Jeanette Ezzo and Dr. Brian M. Berman of the University of Maryland was undertaken under the auspices of the international Cochrane Collaboration that focuses on "evidence-based medicine" for both conventional and alternative medicine. Based on 159 reviews of conventional medical practices, the reviewers found that only 20.8 percent evidenced a positive effect on the treated group over the control group. For the vast majority of the conventional medical practices, the evidence ranged from 6.9 percent demonstrating harm to 24.5 percent resulting in no effect at all.

To avoid a double standard, all therapeutic interventions should be held to the same rigorous standards of evidence-based medicine. Essentially, the purpose of the book will be to rigorously evaluate the most common forms of CAM, based on the best scientific research, and to shed light upon: (1) What works; (2) What doesn't work; and (3) What is "in the works." It is very important to underscore that negative findings on "what does not work" will be very limited, out of necessity. This is due to the fact that negative research findings are not frequently published. Emphasis throughout will be predominantly on what CAM therapies work for which conditions, and for whom, based on the best available research evidence today.

Groucho Marx once quipped, "Be open-minded, but not so open-minded that your brains fall out." In the evaluation of complementary and alternative medicine, it often seems as if some clinicians' and researchers' brains have "fallen out." No other area of medical research generates such acrimonious and often unenlightening debate as does the area of complementary and alternative medicine. Debate over this subject is highly polarized, and highly politicized. In fact, both advocates and critics of CAM may decry this book's attempt to hold to a middle ground, and to sort fact from fiction. On every controversial issue, we hear accusations from one side or the other that the sky is falling. These extreme positions create mass confusion on vital issues, such as chemical and pesticide hazards, food additives, cancer therapy, silicone breast implants, and even on issues as mundane as the value of high-roughage cereals. There is a shortage of fact and a plethora of opinion.

As the debate rages on, however, we remain in the midst of an epidemic of inadequately treated chronic illness. Heart disease remains the major cause of disability and death, despite decades of major advances in treatment. Sixty million Americans have hypertension, forty million suffer from arthritis, and twenty-three million have chronic migraine headaches. A million Americans each year are diagnosed with cancer. Almost 40 percent, or nearly every other person you know, will eventually develop this terrifying disease. On the increase is the prevalence of asthma, multiple sclerosis, chronic fatigue, immune deficiency syndrome, HIV, and a host of other debilitating conditions. Compounding this dire litany is the fact that more than forty million Americans—the total population of thirteen states—have no medical insurance!

Nevertheless, treatments do exist that are extremely effective at preventing and ameliorating these maladies. Many of these therapies are deceptively simple.

For a moment, reflect on a "breakthrough" intervention now being supported by decades of research from the National Institutes of Health. This breakthrough has been acknowledged by the American Medical Association and the United States Surgeon General. It has the documented effect of reducing virtually all forms of illness. It helps patients prevent or recover from high blood pressure, diabetes, osteoporosis, breast cancer, arthritis, and chronic pain. It improves mental function, sleep, weight loss, and muscle mass, and extends life expectancy. Miracle drug? New product of advanced genetic engineering? Discovered in an arcane Chinese medical text? None of the above. It is . . . exercise! Exercise is more important for health than most of the more exotic forms of CAM, and a great many forms of conventional medicine. Think horses, not zebras.

In fact, many CAM modalities, including various forms of exercise, stress reduction, and optimal nutrition, have been embraced by conventional medicine in recent years.

Despite this growing collaboration, the atmosphere of the debate surrounding CAM is still often strident, shrill, and short of fact. In *Choices in Unconventional Cancer Therapies,* Dr. Michael Lerner states, "Critics have characteristically dismissed the alternative therapies as quackery . . . and have worked systematically and often effectively to . . . disbar or 'defrock' physicians, researchers and attorneys. Practitioners have faced legal prosecution, lengthy trials with high legal expenses, suspension or loss of their licenses to practice medicine, and sometimes jail terms. . . . Opposing the Quack Busters is a coalition of proponents of alternative cancer therapies. . . . While some members of the coalition are moderate in tone, others use harsh language and tactics. Opponents of alternative therapies have been seriously compared to Nazis. Conventional therapies such as surgery, radiotherapy, and chemotherapy are denounced as 'cut, burn, and poison.' . . . While for many years the Quack Buster coalition held the advantage in this vociferous conflict, a significant shift in the balance of societal forces has occurred in the last 10 years, so that conditions are now somewhat more favorable to the proponents of alternative therapies." Between the strident and polarized opinions is a vast middle ground where the issue of what does and does not work needs to be addressed by scientific research and clinical judgment, not by uninformed diatribes from both extremes.

One result of this vitriolic polarization is that patients, starkly aware that many conventional doctors disapprove of complementary and alternative medicine, often hide their use of CAM interventions from their conventional physicians. In the classic 1993 study of alternative medicine by Dr. David Eisenberg of the Harvard Medical School, less than 40 percent of patients who used alternative medicine told their doctors. In certain instances, this can have disastrous results, since some CAM modalities, such as use of certain herbal supplements, may interact negatively with medications.

What is needed in the ongoing debate over complementary and alternative medicine are more constructive yet critical voices similar to that of Dr. Wallace Sampson of the National Council for Reliable Health Information. Recently, Dr. Sampson founded a new journal entitled *The Scientific Review of Alternative Medicine,* which interjects a healthy note of skepticism into the alternative medicine debate. Through the NCRHI, such publications provide an invaluable service by sorting fact from fantasy through rigorous science and evidence-based medicine.

This book is intended to build such an evidence-based foundation.

WHAT IS CAM?

According to Dr. David Eisenberg of the Harvard Medical School, a widespread, accepted definition of CAM, which was used in his 1993 and 1997 studies, is "Those practices explicitly used for medical intervention, health promotion, or disease prevention which are not routinely taught at United States medical schools, nor routinely underwritten by third party payers within the existing United States health care system." Because medical schools and insurance companies are gradually accepting various CAM modalities, the practices included in this definition are constantly being revised.

In March of 1997, the National Center for Complementary and Alternative Medicine (NCCAM) formulated another definition: "CAM includes those medical systems, interventions, applications, theories or claims that are currently not part of the dominant (conventional) biomedical system. Classification of a practice as CAM may change, depending upon changing attitudes, scientific data, and experience." Given the rapidly evolving nature of CAM, this operational definition will be used throughout this book.

For this book, we will examine the following CAM modalities: Mind-Body medicine; dietary supplements, phyto- or plant-based nutrients, and hormones; traditional Chinese medicine; acupuncture; European herbals; naturopathy; homeopathy; chiropractic; Ayurvedic medicine; as well as spirituality and healing. These are currently the most predominant forms of CAM used by the largest number of people in the United States and abroad, according to several national and international surveys.

Many areas of alternative medicine are not addressed in this book, which predominantly focuses on those that are most common, according to national surveys. Bear in mind that the Office of Alternative Medicine has identified over six hundred specific terms describing an array of CAM practices. It is simply impossible in the confines of this book to address them all, including areas such as chelation, aromatherapy, multitudinous varieties of meditation, applications of bioelectromagnetic fields, and other promising areas of research and clinical practice. No matter what area is addressed, the right approach by a clinician or individual is one of well-informed, cautious involvement.

Research indicates that these various forms of CAM are now extremely popular in America, accounting for approximately 425 million visits to providers in 1990. It is important to note that this number exceeded the total number of visits to all United States primary care physicians for the same year, at only 330 million office contacts. Repeating his classic 1990 survey, Dr. David M. Eisenberg and his colleagues at the Harvard Medical School found that this number of visits increased by 47 percent from 1990 to 1997 for a total of 629 million visits. This 47 percent increase is in striking contrast to a much smaller increase in the number of primary care visits in 1997, to only 386 million. Generally, patients seek out CAM therapies mostly for prevention, and second for chronic, ongoing conditions, rather than life-threatening illnesses.

A 1998 national survey by Dr. John A. Astin of the Stanford University School of Medicine determined the general type of individual who uses CAM. Compared to the general population, CAM patients are better educated, have more health problems, have a greater belief in the healing power of the mind and spirit, had a "transformational experience" that changed their worldview, and participate more in environmentalism, feminism, esoteric spiritualism, and personal growth psychology. CAM patients tend most often to have the following health problems: back pain, obesity, anxiety, depression, insomnia, and chronic pain. They report that their primary reason for using CAM is that it relieves their symptoms better than conventional medicine. Most significant, the patients who use CAM do not express any greater dissatisfaction with conventional care than patients who do not use CAM! Only 5 percent of them rely primarily upon CAM. It was only this 5 percent that expressed greater dissatisfaction with conventional care.

Satisfaction of CAM patients with conventional care strongly suggests that there is, indeed, a fertile middle ground for patients and practitioners who wish to use both CAM and conventional care.

AN EXPLOSION OF INTEREST IN CAM

Amid the heated debate over CAM, one fact is certain: Consumers are not waiting for scientific experts to tell them that it is acceptable to use CAM. Pharmacies throughout the United States are experiencing a huge surge in the demand for alternative remedies. This is now the fastest growing segment of the over-the-counter market. From 1991 to 1996, this market doubled, to over $3.77 billion. It is projected to reach more than $6.5 billion by 2001, for an average growth rate of 12.5 percent.

Furthermore, in a 1996 study by Landmark Healthcare, over 70 percent of HMOs reported an increased request for CAM by their enrollees. Modalities most in demand were acupuncture (requested by 56 percent of patients), chiropractic (45 percent), massage (25 percent), acupressure and biofeedback (21 percent each), hypnotherapy (8 percent), and reflexology (4 percent). Perhaps even more telling is that 38 percent of the HMOs believed that offering alternative medicine would increase their enrollment.

A central reason that CAM is vaulting in popularity is simply that the general public demands the benefits of such CAM therapies. One of the most important and insightful articles in this regard was published in the *Journal of the American Medical Association* by Dr. J. Michael McGinnis, former director of the U.S. Office of Health Promotion and Disease Prevention, and Dr. William H. Foege, director of the Centers for Disease Control in Atlanta. Their 1993 article cited the usual "Ten Leading Causes of Death" in 1990, ranging from heart disease and cancer at the top to chronic liver disease and HIV infections at the bottom. These mortality statistics and supposed causes are so ubiquitously cited that they belie a more fundamental issue.

Upon closer examination, McGinnis and Foege contend that this familiar dire litany of mortality consists not of the actual causes of death but of the terminal diseases cited in a pathologist's report or autopsy. In fact, the actual "causes" from most impact to least are: tobacco (which caused approximately 400,000 deaths in 1990), diet and inactivity patterns, alcohol, certain infections, toxic agents, firearms, sexual behavior, motor vehicles, and finally, drug use, which was responsible for 20,000 deaths in 1990. This listing of the ten actual causes contributed to 1,060,000 deaths, or approximately 60 percent of all deaths in 1990.

From the somewhat different perspective of the benefits and liabili-

Causes of Death in the United States

Ten Leading Causes of Death*		Actual Causes of Death**	
Heart disease	720,058	Tobacco	400,000
Cancer	505,322	Diet/inactivity patterns	300,000
Cerebrovascular disease	144,088	Alcohol	100,000
Unintentional injuries	91,983	Certain infections	90,000
Chronic lung disease	86,679	Toxic agents	60,000
Pneumonia and influenza	79,513	Firearms	35,000
Diabetes	47,664	Sexual behavior	30,000
Suicide	30,906	Motor vehicles	25,000
Chronic liver disease	25,815	Drug use	20,000
HIV infection	25,188		
Total:	1,757,216		1,060,000

*Sources: National Center for Health Statistics, "Advance Report of Final Mortality Statistics, 1990," *Monthly Vital Statistics Report,* Vol. 41, No. 7.
**Source: J. M. McGinnis and W. H. Foege, "Actual Causes of Death in the United States," *Journal of the American Medical Association* (1993), 270:2207–2212.

ties of managed care, Dr. David Blumenthal succinctly stated this issue in the *New England Journal of Medicine,* noting that "In 1991, the Harvard Medical Practice Study showed that adverse events occur in 4% of hospitalizations, that 14% of these events are fatal, and that as many people are dying from preventable causes each year in the United States as would die if three jumbo jets crashed every two days." Translated into terms of aviation disasters, it is obvious that such incidents would not be tolerated, and immediate remedial actions would be undertaken. What is evident from such observations regarding the real causes of the major causes of death is that the vast majority are lifestyle-related and are unequivocally amenable to prevention—which would result in a dramatic decrease in the number of conditions requiring either conventional or CAM interventions.

Once again . . . think horses, not zebras!

At the Complementary and Alternative Medicine Program at Stanford (CAMPS), which is one of twelve university research centers funded by the National Institutes of Health Office of Alternative Medicine, which became the National Center for Complementary and Alternative Medicine (NCCAM) in October of 1998, we are examining the leading causes of disability in the elderly. Each NCCAM research program has a different focus. At Stanford, the orientation is on "Successful Aging," or the healthy end of the aging continuum, with an emphasis on arresting, preventing, and even reversing the supposedly inevitable declines associated with aging. Annual statistics from NIH indicate that the two primary sources of disability were cardiovascular diseases, and diseases or dysfunction of the musculoskeletal system including arthritis, osteoporosis, chronic joint pain, and lack of muscle strength, endurance, and flexibility. These two sources of disability can both be prevented or ameliorated with the various lifestyle programs and other interventions that are often a part of complementary and alternative medicine.

Among the usual consequences of aging are: decreased function of the kidneys, liver, and lungs; decreased elasticity of blood vessels; increased atherosclerosis; increased blood pressure; decreased cardiac output; poorer circulation; wrinkled skin; graying hair; loss of muscle mass and strength; increased osteoporosis; increased osteoarthritis; slower reaction time; loss of hearing; loss of taste and smell; diminished vision; declining hormonal levels; and impaired immunity. Elderly people also often suffer cognitive decline, loss of energy, and increased anxiety, and frequently experience a tendency toward paranoia, depression, and emotional instability.

With each passing day, the need for CAM interventions appears to be increasing, due to the aging of our society. In the United States, by the year 2025, one of every five Americans will be over sixty-five. Each year, more than 385,000 Americans turn sixty-five. In addition, the segment called the "oldest old," those eighty-five or older, is the most rapidly increasing. In 1990, there were only three million people in this age group, but by the year 2040, there will be fifteen to eighteen million. To illustrate this most dramatically, in the United States there is a daily increase of 1,050 individuals over age sixty-five!

This graying of our society presents a monumental challenge to our health care system. Ironically, some researchers fear that complementary and alternative medicine may actually contribute to this problem of widespread infirmity by extending lifespan. Greek mythology recounts that the beautiful goddess of the dawn, Eos, fell in love with a mortal warrior, Tithonius, and asked Zeus to grant her lover immortality. Zeus granted her wish, but Eos overlooked asking also for eternal youth. With each century, Tithonius became increasingly enfeebled, until finally, as an act of pity, the gods turned him into a cricket. Similarly, as we have learned to prolong life, some believe we have also created an increase in chronic disabilities. Although this is a frequently espoused fear, it is both alarmist and inaccurate.

The graying of planet Earth is a worldwide phenomenon, occurring in virtually every nation. By the year 2025, 20 percent of the United States population and 27 percent of Japan's population will be sixty-five or older. Such projections hold true for all of Europe, the United Kingdom, and Canada. Since aging is associated with an increase in chronic diseases and disabilities, these nations, like the United States, are facing an increased burden of illness.

This same trend is also striking the developing nations. Today, the most rapidly growing populations of elderly people are in China, India, the former Soviet Union, and Southeast Asia. In China, which already has more than twice the elderly people of any other nation, researchers expect the population of elderly to double by 2025. For Latin America and the Caribbean, by the year 2000, 7.2 percent of the population is expected to be over sixty-five. By the year 2025, approximately 68 percent of the world's elderly population will be living in developing nations.

Global aging will dramatically alter disease patterns. The following table illustrates the changing face of global infirmity.

Many of the conditions that lead to disability, frailty, and loss of independence in older persons are not readily preventable by conventional therapies such as pharmaceuticals or surgery. They are, for the most part,

The Changing Face of Global Infirmity
(in order of frequency)

1990	2020
1. Pneumonia	1. Heart disease
2. Diarrheal diseases	2. Severe depression
3. Diseases of the newborn	3. Traffic accidents
4. Severe depression	4. Stroke
5. Heart disease	5. Chronic lung disease
6. Stroke	6. Pneumonia
7. Tuberculosis	7. Tuberculosis
8. Measles	8. War
9. Traffic accidents	9. Diarrheal diseases
10. Birth defects	10. AIDS

preventable only by cessation of risky health behaviors, including poor nutrition, chronic stress, physical inactivity, smoking, inadequate sleep, substance abuse, and exposure to a toxic environment. Therefore, new approaches are needed to prevent the development and progression of these chronic diseases. Prevention of the major cause of death and disability, cardiovascular disease, is largely dependent on a person's own health habits.

Without any significant increase in the attempt to prevent disease, it is certain that the aging of our global society will soon overwhelm our ability to respond.

While most people would like to live to be a vital 100 years old or more, many people might not wish to accord that same privilege to the tens of millions of their peers. According to Dr. Wilma J. Nusselder at the University of Amsterdam, "While eliminating fatal disease leads to an increase in life expectancy, life expectancy with disability may increase as well. This represents an increased burden to society." Such projections constitute the potential dark side of CAM interventions. This can be likened to the Scrooge phenomenon in Charles Dickens's A Christmas Carol. When Scrooge first confronted the impending death of Tiny Tim, his response was that Tiny Tim should die soon, in order to "decrease the surplus population." This Scrooge phenomenon may prove to be a true prophecy.

From the Columbia University School of Medicine, Dr. Willard Gaylin notes in a recent essay that preventive medicine may ultimately drive up the cost of health care by enlarging the population of the elderly, infirm, hospitalized, and disabled. Further compounding this is our tendency to discover "new disease," such as "infertility," which was not considered to be a treatable disorder until recent years. Also, many people these days engage in elective medical procedures; for example, they do not choose to have knee or elbow surgery to continue work but to continue skiing or playing tennis. As Gaylin asks, "Should 'inability to play tennis' be classified as an insurable disease?" He observes that people will "pay anything to defend against the possibility of death," especially when the money does not come directly out of their own pockets.

However, it is eminently possible that CAM therapies will not contribute to increasingly widespread infirmity, but will instead be a pivotal boon to societal health.

At the Stanford University School of Medicine, Dr. James F. Fries argues that it is an equally plausible scenario that the increased life expectancy over the next twenty-five years will be characterized by health. As individuals live longer, healthier lives, they might not experience the usual long, slow decline in physical and mental functioning, but instead may enjoy optimal health right up to the onset of death in what he has termed the "compression of morbidity." From Fries's research, he indicates that the greatest expenses occur when relatively young individuals remain alive with a chronic disease for decades. By contrast, individuals who have the same disease at advanced age tend to die more quickly and actually incur fewer medical costs. Furthermore, these healthy elders may have second or third careers, and continue to generate income, taxes, and net benefits to society.

While CAM may possibly engender some problems by increasing longevity, it may also solve these same problems. Nevertheless, it must be recognized that, in all probability, the long-term effects of CAM will be neither all good nor all bad. Common sense cries out for objective evaluation of CAM rather than strident advocacy or stubborn disapprobation.

CREATION OF THE OFFICE OF ALTERNATIVE MEDICINE

Starting in 1992, the National Institutes of Health launched the first major attempt by the United States government to objectively sift CAM fact from CAM fiction, with the creation of the Office of Alternative Medicine (OAM) by the National Institutes of Health. In 1998, OAM was upgraded to a national center with the new designation as the National Center for Complementary and Alternative Medicine (NCCAM). Initially, the OAM was created to evaluate the effectiveness of seven broad categories or taxonomy of CAM interventions: (1) Diet, nutrition, and lifestyle changes; (2) MindBody interventions; (3) Alternative healing systems; (4) Bioelectromagnetic applications in medicine; (5) Manual healing methods; (6) Pharmacological and biological treatments; and (7) Herbal medicine. This taxonomy continues to evolve, and at the present time there are actually more than six hundred specific CAM therapies grouped under these seven rubrics.

NCCAM has become singularly important in researching CAM modalities, because many of these modalities do not invite research by major corporations, since many of the modalities and products that must be researched are not easily patented.

It is the sheer number of CAM therapies which serves to dismiss the tiresome but ubiquitous debate between CAM advocates and CAM adversaries. How is it even conceivable to be categorically "for" or "against" such a complex array of over six hundred therapeutic modalities? These are modalities that undoubtedly range from highly effective to overt quackery and, in some instances, are lethal. One particular variant of this advocacy theme is most often evident in the innumerable conferences, websites, and health gurus advocating various alternative practices. Whenever there is a statement or citation of a study, often of questionable quality, that "proves" the efficacy of a CAM practice that has been in widespread use for "hundreds or even thousands of years," there is a knowing smile and smug nod. However, that therapy may never have been proven. There are thousands of therapies in both conventional medicine (such as bloodletting) and CAM (such as Dr. Wilhelm Reich's orgone therapy) that historically have proven to be completely unfounded and even dangerous. There is no room for smug self-congratulations at either end of the continuum, for science is indeed a process that grinds slowly but exceedingly fine. Debate is the essence of the NCCAM mission, and of all the subsequent chapters of this book.

In 1992, eight initial CAM research grants were cofunded for a total of $1,875,000. These grants assessed problems related to cancer, premenstrual syndrome, perinatal care, and cardiac patient recovery. Alternative medical treatments that were examined included stress management, diet, exercise, therapeutic touch, biofeedback, and novel pharmacological approaches.

As its next major initiative in 1993, OAM issued its first grants of up to $30,000 each to fund exploratory pilot projects to identify promising areas of future research. Collaboration between orthodox research investigators and alternative medical practitioners was encouraged. The following table is a brief sample of the subjects for which these initial, small pilot grants were awarded.

In 1994, OAM funded an initial two centers for alternative medicine research, with a total budget of $1.68 million. One of the two centers was at Bastyr University, a school of naturopathic medicine in Seattle. At

National Institutes of Health Research on CAM
National Center for Complementary and Alternative Medicine (NCAAM)

Therapy	Condition
Acupuncture	Unipolar depression
Acupuncture	Osteoarthritis
Massage therapy	HIV-1
Electrochemical DC current	Cancer
Acupuncture and herbs	Cancer
Hypnosis	Chronic low back pain
Massage therapy	Postsurgical outcomes
Chinese herbal medicine	PMS
Music therapy	Adjustments after brain surgery
Energetic therapy	Basal cell carcinoma
Massage therapy	HIV-exposed infants
Hypnosis	Accelerated bone fracture healing
Dance/movement therapy	Cystic fibrosis
Chinese herbal therapy	Common warts
Imagery and relaxation	Immunity control
T'ai chi	Mind balance disorders
Guided imagery	Asthma
Imagery and relaxation	Breast cancer
Macrobiotic diet	Cancer
Acupuncture	Postoperative oral surgery pain
Ayurvedic herbals	Parkinson's disease
Biofeedback and relaxation	Diabetes
Therapeutic touch	Immune response to stress

Bastyr, the research focus was on CAM therapies for AIDS. A second center was at the Hennepin County Medical Center at the University of Minnesota Medical School, which focused on addictions. In addition to these two initial centers, a second round of grant reviews resulted in the funding of nine additional centers including Stanford, Harvard, and Columbia. Of the existing research centers, the CAM program at Stanford is focused on exploring the upper or healthy end of aging to determine what is optimal and possible rather than average.

Of greatest significance is that in October of 1998 the United States Congress elevated the OAM to the status of the National Center for Complementary and Alternative Medicine (NCCAM), with independent funding authority. Also, the new NCCAM budget for 1999 was set at $50 million, and two additional research centers were funded. One center is focused on cardiovascular disease at the University of Michigan under Dr. Steve Bolling, a cardio-thoracic surgeon. A second center was funded at the University of Arizona Medical School in Tucson with a focus on children's health under the direction of Dr. Fayez Ghisban, a well-known pediatric researcher, and Dr. Andrew T. Weil, who also serves as director of the Program in Integrative Medicine at the University of Arizona.

Since large-scale, long-term, or longitudinal randomized clinical trials, RCTs, are the gold standard of biomedical research, NCCAM has matured to the point of initiating several major studies starting in 1999 and concluding between 2002 and 2004. These include the shark carti-lage trial, one of the largest ever conducted of an alternative therapy with the NCAAM-funded center at the University of Texas in Houston with Dr. Marianne Richardson and Dr. Guy S. Parcel. This multicenter RCT will test a substance made by Aeterna Laboratories, a Quebec biotech company that also markets cosmetics and food supplements. Laboratory studies showed the substance, which the firm calls Neovostat, blocked blood-vessel development, suggesting it would block tumor growth, and that in small-scale human studies, those receiving a higher dose of Neovostat experienced less tumor progression and weight loss than did those taking lower doses. The trial will combine cartilage treatment or a placebo with a standard regimen of chemotherapy and/or radiation.

Other major RCTs include a study cosponsored by the National Insti-tute of Mental Health (NIMH) and NCCAM to determine the effec-tiveness of St. John's wort in curbing depression, a trial examining the effects of a complex nutritional regimen on pancreatic cancer, and another longitudinal RCT evaluating the efficacy of glucosamine for restructuring the joint damage due to arthritis.

As a matter of policy, NCCAM does not offer advice to individual patients. According to NCCAM, their policy is: "We do not treat patients in our office, nor do we conduct clinical trials. We cannot answer specific medical questions until we have definitive evidence from the research and clinical trials now taking place. The office cannot make referrals to individual practitioners, nor recommend any particular therapy for indi-vidual patients."

Overall, NCCAM and its research projects have received a positive response from the scientific and medical professions. That is largely due to the science orientation of the National Center of Complementary and Alternative Medicine. NCCAM's role is not advocacy, but scientific research and objective evaluation.

Generally, if not universally, the willingness of health and medical professionals to accept the scientific findings generated by NCCAM has been a credit to the profession. Innovation in any domain is often greeted with suspicion, if not overt hostility. In Machiavelli's classic book *The Prince*, he observed, "There is nothing more difficult to carry out, nor more doubtful of success, nor more dangerous to handle, than to initiate a new order of things."

In fact, since the inauguration of the NCCAM, there has been a noticeable shift in sentiment about CAM. From the cover of *Life* magazine in September of 1996, with its lead article "The Healing Revolution," to a recent front page of the *Harvard Medical Alumni Bulletin*, which featured several prominent CAM practitioners, including Dr. Andrew T. Weil, Dr. David Eisenberg, and Dr. James S. Gordon, it is evident that conventional researchers, physicians, and medical schools are undertaking a serious evaluation of CAM.

Recently, Senator Tom Harkin stated, "With or without the Office of Alternative Medicine (NCCAM), alternative therapies are here to stay and consumers will continue to use them." This is precisely why we need a constructive, objective evaluation of CAM. Whether or not conventional clinicians approve, more and more people are availing themselves of alternative therapies. These people deserve to know which therapies have been proven effective and which have not.

One pivotal impetus to the growing acceptance of CAM therapies by the public, and the American medical community, is the popularity of alternative medicine in many other countries. As globalization of commerce and science increases, American physicians are becoming ever more aware of the successes of CAM therapies in other countries.

CAM:
A GLOBAL PERSPECTIVE

A great many therapies that are considered experimental in America are in fact considered mainstream medicine abroad. This is true among countries that are equally advanced in science and medicine, including Germany, the United Kingdom, France, and Japan.

In 1992, the Swiss government allocated $4 million focused on sociological research concerning alternative medicine users. This amount was almost as much as the United States budgeted to fund all research on CAM for that same year. In Europe, homeopathic medicine and acupuncture are primarily practiced by medical doctors, who have often learned these methods in medical schools and hospitals. Obtaining these credentials in France requires a three-year advanced degree. In Germany, all medical students are tested for their knowledge of natural therapies on their medical boards. Within France, four out of five herbal remedies are prescribed by doctors, while in Germany, 77 percent of pain clinics use acupuncture. In Britain, more than 40 percent of general practitioners refer their patients to homeopathic doctors.

In these and other scientifically sophisticated countries, the fundamental approach to healing often differs notably from the American model, but still achieves considerable success.

French clinicians have a deep concern with the *terrain,* or the vitality of the inner field of the body. This belief skews emphasis away from antibiotics, which fit the American concept of disease as invader, toward tonics, vitamins, and "modifiers of the *terrain.*" Such an orientation favors treatments such as rest to restore the *terrain.* It makes the French leaders in fields that concentrate on shoring up the *terrain,* such as conventional immunotherapy for cancer. If the *terrain* is as important as, if not more important than, the disease, it becomes less important to fight the disease "aggressively," and more important to strengthen the *terrain.* While American therapeutic interventions are often described as "aggressive," the French much prefer *les médecines douces,* or "gentle therapies." Preference for gentle therapies leads the French into much wider use of nonallopathic medicines, such as those used in homeopathy. Also, the French use lower doses of conventional drugs. Furthermore, in French hospitals, fewer invasive procedures are used in intensive care units than in United States hospitals, with patients faring equally well in both countries.

In Germany, the rate of cardiac catheterization, a procedure used to help diagnose and treat heart trouble, is only 75 percent as high as that of the United States. Great Britain performs only one-third as many catheterizations as the United States. Similarly, the rate of coronary supply revascularization, or reestablishment of blood supply procedures, is much lower outside of the United States. Nonetheless, patients appear to fare equally well in these countries.

A study by Dr. Harlan M. Krumholz of the Yale University School of Medicine, indicated that in Ontario, Canada, the number of medical procedures performed after a heart attack was strikingly lower than the number performed in the United States. Within thirty days after admission for acute infarction, damage to cardiac tissue due to a blood clot, elderly patients in the United States underwent coronary angiography, examination of vessels using an X-ray producer, 5.2 times as often as patients in Ontario; angioplasty or PTCA, surgical reconstruction of blood vessels, 7.7 times as often; and bypass surgery, 7.8 times as often. Despite these differences, the one-year mortality rates in the United States and Ontario were virtually identical.

Germany is one of the greatest innovators in the field of CAM therapies, with strong traditions of naturopathic, herbal, homeopathic, and spiritual approaches to medical care. German patients have a wider choice of both mainstream and CAM therapies than patients in any other modern industrialized country.

For Europeans, many alternative therapies are so well accepted that it may no longer be appropriate to consider them alternative. Among the most popular prescription drugs sold in Germany and France is an extract of *Ginkgo biloba*. In Germany, the market for herbs is the most substantial for any Western country. Homeopathic remedies, Europe's most popular alternative therapy, are prescribed by 39 percent of French doctors and 20 percent of German doctors. More than 40 percent of British general practitioners refer patients to homeopathic doctors, and 45 percent of Dutch physicians consider these remedies to be effective. For the flu, the top-selling remedy in France is a homeopathic medicine, representing 50 percent of the market.

Throughout China, Western approaches are carefully integrated with traditional Chinese medicine concepts. Virtually every hospital has a traditional Chinese medicine department, and a four-step clinical protocol explicitly links the two traditions for a person's care.

It is abundantly clear that the United States has a great deal to learn from other technologically advanced, scientifically sophisticated societies. This learning, however, can be achieved only if the approaches used by international CAM practitioners, and the approaches used by American CAM practitioners, are subjected to rigorous scientific inquiry.

In September of 1998, the prestigious *New England Journal of Medicine* published several negative studies of alternative medicine. Concluding the articles was a very critical editorial by the editors, Dr. Marcia Angell and Dr. Jerome P. Kassirer. Despite this negative stance, the challenge posed by Drs. Angell and Kassirer is one which is of utmost importance: "There cannot be two kinds of medicine—conventional and alternative. There is only medicine that has been adequately tested and medicine that has not, medicine that works and medicine that may or may not work. Once a treatment has been tested rigorously, it no longer matters whether it was considered alternative at the outset. If it is found to be reasonably safe and effective, it will be accepted. But assertions, speculation, and testimonials do not substitute for evidence. Alternative treatments should be subjected to scientific testing no less rigorous than that required for conventional treatments." That is a commendable goal, but it is overlooking the well-documented fact that the vast majority of conventional care—and virtually all of surgery—is lacking in a scientific basis.

All CAM therapies, as well as all conventional therapies, must be held to equal scientific, medical, legal, and ethical standards of an "evidence-based" approach to health care. This is the only sure way to sort fact from fantasy.

SORTING FACT FROM FANTASY

As previously emphasized, the primary intent of this book is to evaluate CAM therapies scientifically, seeking to determine which ones work, which ones do not, and which ones are currently in the works that might be the most promising according to current research. There will also be information about new CAM modalities that are now being evaluated. Most important, the purpose is to empower every individual, whether patient or practitioner, to make more informed choices.

As we evaluate each of the major forms of complementary and alternative medicine, we will evaluate the research that supports each approach. We will hold this research to rigorous standards. In most cases, the research that will be most strongly emphasized will consist of randomized, double-blind, placebo-controlled studies. This type of study, abbreviated as RCT, is widely considered to be the most reliable measure of efficacy.

In an RCT, participants are randomly assigned to two groups. One group is given the substance or treatment being tested, and the other is given a chemically inert substance or sham treatment known as a placebo. In a double-blind study, neither doctor nor patient knows which individuals are receiving the real substance or treatment. To be declared effective, the real substance or treatment must significantly outperform the placebo.

However, not all RCTs are equally well designed. In evaluating the studies that comprise this book, many questions were posed: Were enough patients included to make the study meaningful? Are the results consistent with other research? Could the results be attributed to other factors? These questions, and many others, resulted in the elimination of many studies lacking scientific credibility.

In short, we approached every study with extreme caution. In many cases, we found that the studies cited in support of CAM, as well as conventional interventions, were inadequate.

However, to provide a baseline against which to measure CAM, it is important to point out that as much as 20 to 50 percent of conventional care, and virtually all surgery, has not been evaluated by RCTs. According to Dr. Richard Smith, editor of the *British Medical Journal,* "Only about 15% of medical interventions are supported by solid scientific evidence. . . . This is partly because only 1% of the articles in medical journals are scientifically sound, and partly because many treatments have never been assessed at all." Also, the United States Office of Technology Assessment reported in 1978 and again in 1990 that only an estimated 10 to 20 percent of all conventional medical interventions have been empirically proven. That figure still remains accurate today.

Similarly, certain medical practices have been tested by RCTs and become conventional, but are still a source of controversy. To cite just one instance, doctors have argued over the value of digitalis, a commonly used heart medication, for over two hundred years. Advocates support its use to treat congestive heart failure (CHF), but critics argue that digitalis is toxic and that its use should be curtailed. In 1997, the *New England Journal of Medicine* published a study of over seven thousand patients, which indicated that digitalis reduced CHF hospitalizations by 8 percent, but did not reduce CHF death. Furthermore, more patients taking digitalis died of lethal heart arrhythmias. This study may finally relegate digitalis to the ranks of a secondary preferred drug. Even so, digitalis is still widely used.

Well-conducted research is by no means the only foundation of many of the common practices of conventional medicine. A great many conventional procedures, as well as CAM procedures, have simply evolved in clinical practice over time. This clinical creation of procedures is somewhat like the formation of law, which is often created by following precedents of prior cases and is most exemplified in surgery. Generally, clinical care is designed by adapting general guidelines, research findings, and procedures to individual patients, one at a time. This constitutes the "art" of medicine.

Further complicating the matter is the fact that not all patients respond similarly to the same interventions. In the case of common strep throat, virtually all patients respond consistently to administration of penicillin. However, in the case of a chronic disease, which may have been caused by a host of factors, patients may respond differently to the same treatments. Chronic diseases tend to be highly variable and idiosyncratic.

Health care providers have varying degrees of clinical skill. Individual clinicians often achieve better results than research would indicate are possible. Remember that in the percentages reported in any study, there is always a small percentage of individuals who respond both much better and much worse than average.

In addition, individual clinicians often receive insights and inspirations from sources other than existing research. In 1796, Dr. Edward Jenner was inspired to invent the smallpox vaccination, using a cowpox lesion, by the writings of poets who extolled the pock-free complexions of milkmaids. This bold experiment ushered in a major new era in medicine.

Another major element in both research and clinical practice is the placebo effect. *Placebo* is Latin for "I will please," and is used to describe the range of effects created by the patient's belief that he or she is benefiting from a medical intervention. Placebo effects often obscure the true efficacy of a treatment. It is generally believed that about 35 percent of patients experience the placebo effect. Remember that this placebo response complicates research, but a much more positive note is that upwards of 35 percent of people improve without the interventions!

Placebo effects are especially confusing in many complementary and alternative medicine interventions, because some of these interventions actively seek to elicit the placebo effect. Many CAM clinicians believe that the mind has a potent healing power, and that it is in the patient's best interests to enlist that power. Therefore, they urge patients to have positive attitudes about their therapies, which often creates a placebo response.

Contrary to conventional wisdom, the placebo response is not just a factor in sham, inert treatments, but also is present in physically active treatments. Very often, the placebo effect actually heightens the response to effective drugs and even to surgical outcomes.

By the same token, when individuals have negative outlooks, it can actually dampen their responses to helpful, active treatments. This phenomenon is called the "nocebo effect."

Many conventional providers dismiss the placebo effect as a worthless and confusing response. This attitude, while perhaps understandable from a scientific perspective, is less than laudable in the context of healing. When patients approach a clinician for help, often in pain and fear, they have only one concern: getting well again. Thus, a dismissive attitude toward the placebo response may be unwarranted. Rather than dismiss the placebo, we need more insight into why 35 percent of people get better because they believe they will. Placebo may in fact be the most pervasive, most powerful influence for healing the greatest number of diseases, among the greatest number of people.

In response to all of these complexities, the medical research community has recently developed a new approach to research, called "evidence-based medicine." This approach pays due homage to the randomized, double-blind, controlled study, but does not rely solely upon RCTs. In addition to RCTs, this approach integrates clinical expertise, epidemiological studies, and occasionally even anecdotal evidence, with the best clinical research. This integration of research and other evidence requires a delicate and complex balance, and can occasionally be misleading. However, striking this balance appears to be necessary in order to comprehend the true nature of healing.

Throughout this book, we adopted evidence-based medicine as the basic model of inquiry. Evidence-based medicine provides a reasonable middle ground. In his widely influential book *Causal Relationships in Medicine: A Practical System for Critical Appraisal,* Dr. John M. Ellwood also advocates such an approach. He cites the fact that "only a small fraction of therapeutic decisions can be supported by the results of randomized trials." Nonetheless, evidence-based medicine does rely heavily on RCTs, and especially relies on the systematic review of numerous RCTs. Evidence-based medicine, for both conventional and CAM therapies, is internationally represented in the quality reviews of the Cochrane Collaboration in London. Heading up the sections of the Cochrane Collaboration focused on the CAM areas is Dr. Brian M. Berman of the University of Maryland School of Medicine. As of 1999, there were eleven reviews completed and nineteen CAM reviews in progress.

In compiling the research for this book, an exhaustive international literature search was conducted. This search included, but was not limited to, a complete review of computer databases including ABI, BIOSIS, ERIC, LEXIS/NEXIS, MAGS, MEDLINE, PAIS, PSYC, SOCA, the Internet's World Wide Web (www), and inquiries to the academic research centers currently funded by the National Institutes of Health under the National Center for Complementary and Alternative Medicine (NCCAM). Even with such a thorough search, there are many CAM articles that are not even listed in these databases. Some of these are high-quality studies. As a result, we will often be citing fewer studies than actually exist. Therefore, we will offer an extremely conservative estimate of the effectiveness of a given CAM therapy.

Additionally, there are over fifteen thousand hard-copy articles concerning CAM on file at the CAMPS offices in an archive donated by Michael Murphy and the board of the Esalen Institute. We also received information from an extraordinarily broad range of CAM authorities and critics both in the United States and abroad. This use of international research is relatively unusual. Within the United States, the Food and Drug Administration (FDA) considers predominantly United States–based research findings, a practice that some critics consider scientifically limiting.

Most important, the specific studies cited in each chapter are indicative and representative of the results, both positive and negative, of the findings for a given CAM practice. It is not possible to be definitive without being encyclopedic. Additional, more definitive resources can be identified through the references, books, and professional organizations cited throughout the chapters.

Of ultimate importance in this search was to discover which interventions might pose a risk to patients. Still, it is essential to place this issue of potential harm in the total context of all medical care, including conventional care. Each year, there are more than 100,000 deaths associated predominantly with prescription drugs, and some over-the-counter drugs. As of 1998, adverse reactions to drugs now constitute the fourth leading cause of death in the United States. Ironically, more than half of these drug deaths occur with hospitalized patients who were admitted for conditions not related to drugs. Even ostensibly innocuous drugs, such as acetaminophen and ibuprofen, can have serious side effects. Acetaminophen has been linked to several cases of sudden liver failure, and now bears a warning label. Ibuprofen can induce severe stomach or intestinal bleeding, which has been fatal in some cases. Conversely, according to the U.S. mortality statistics from 1981 to 1993, there has been only one verified report of death from vitamin and mineral supplementation. During the same time period, there were no deaths from commercial herbs.

However, this does not mean that all CAM interventions are without harm. In 1994, several deaths were attributed to the herb *ma huang*/ephedra. Furthermore, a British survey, conducted by the daily newspaper *The Guardian* and published in *Nature,* revealed that 15.8 percent of CAM patients experienced mild to moderate adverse reactions from manipulation therapy. With acupuncture, 12.5 percent reported symptom aggravation, mental effects, fatigue, pain, and needle trauma. Patients using homeopathy indicated a 9.8 percent symptom aggravation, mental effects, and digestive effects. For herbal medicine, 7.6 percent reported primarily digestive effects.

Thus, we see that many therapies, from both CAM and conventional medicine, offer risks as well as rewards. In this book, we will analyze those risks and rewards as rigorously and objectively as possible.

How to Use This Book

At the heart of this book is an emphasis on sorting fact from fiction by establishing the three categories of (1) What Works; (2) What Does Not Work; and (3) What Is in the Works. This approach is known as "triage," and is an essential concept underlying truly informed consent. Triage is derived from the French verb *trier,* which means to sort, sift, or cull. For most individuals, this sorting, or triage, is best known as popularized in the $M^*A^*S^*H$ television series. In the MASH unit, soldiers were triaged into three categories: those who could wait for treatment, those who needed immediate care, and those with mortal wounds who were beyond help. Today, the triage process has assumed a central role in the initial evaluation and classification of patients seeking emergency treatment, and also has become increasingly used in the managed care setting for determining access and granting authorization for acute care.

It is actually the earlier definition which will be used and applied in all subsequent chapters of this book. One of the original uses of the French *trier* was in the sorting of coffee beans by size, type, and quality. Throughout each subsequent chapter, focusing on one specific CAM therapy, the scientific evidence supporting or refuting the claims will be sorted into three categories of "What Works," "What Does Not Work" (which will be the most brief due to the lack of published negative results), and "What Is in the Works" at the present time. This third area of triage is surely the largest and fastest-growing domain. It is also where the greatest caution needs to be exercised, since there may be premature findings or claims that may or may not be verified by later research.

Each area of CAM that the book covers contains selected references to a number of studies. Virtually all of these studies have been evaluated carefully for design flaws and lack of objectivity. Nevertheless, readers should still subject each study to their own rigorous standards. Readers should ask themselves: Who is promoting the study; was a financial incentive involved? How was the study conducted; did it involve only men, or women, or certain age groups? Were the study conclusions definitive or were they ambiguous? How many people participated in the study? Finally: Are the clinical results really applicable in my own life?

Furthermore, in evaluating the findings in this book, readers should try to free themselves of preconceptions that may be based upon faulty information. According to the FDA, many consumers arrive at preconceptions because of misleading marketing ploys. These marketing ploys include: celebrity endorsements without supporting research; inadequate and vague labeling; claims that the product works by a secret formula; unorthodox promotion of the treatment (in the back pages of magazines, over the phone, by direct mail, in newspaper ads in the guise of news stories, or in infomercials); products that are effective for a wide range of disorders (such as cancer, arthritis, and sexual dysfunction); or claims of "all natural," "inexpensive," and "no side effects." In short, if it seems too good to be true, it is!

It is a cliché to say "check with your doctor" before undertaking a course of self-care, but that is particularly good advice for those entering the domain of complementary and alternative medicine. No amount of information in any book can, or should, be a substitute for the help of a qualified practitioner, who can adapt general scientific knowledge to your own unique history, circumstances, condition, and overall health status.

"Education" derives from the Latin word *educare*, which means "to lead out." Hopefully, the information in the following chapters will lead out into new intellectual territory, by helping readers to think critically about both conventional and CAM therapies.

No book alone can provide you with the full range of information you will need in order to make informed decisions about exactly what procedures to use. Your complete quest for information should incorporate each of the following elements of advice:

- Seek out reliable information not only in the following chapters, but also in the many other books and resources noted throughout this book.
- Identify an experienced clinician who can help you adapt the research information to your own particular circumstances. More and more hospitals, clinics, and professional organizations offer responsible CAM services. There is absolutely no need to seek such therapies from questionable practitioners. Ask your primary care doctor for a referral to a CAM practitioner. According to 1998 statistics, over 60 percent of conventional doctors have recommended alternative therapies to their patients at least once in the prior year.
- Inform your primary care provider that you are using CAM therapies. One recent article in *Annals of Internal Medicine* by Dr. David Eisenberg of the Harvard Medical School is particularly useful to give to your doctor if he or she has a negative opinion of CAM. While the article may not alter that opinion, it may at least provide the basis for a dialogue.
- With any conventional or CAM therapy, obtain clear, and preferably written, information on the number of anticipated treatments, cost, whether or not this will be covered by your insurance, any possible side effects, and all possible contraindications or reasons why a ther-

apy may not be effective for your particular condition. Most of all, ask how you and the clinician will determine that you are better.

• Keep a record or diary of the treatment, in order to keep all of your clinicians well informed of the course of your treatment. Chart changes in the frequency and severity of your symptoms on a scale of one to ten. If you experience unusual or adverse reactions, notify your therapist immediately.

Ultimately, the most critical criterion for any therapeutic intervention is the one used most frequently among doctors themselves: Would you make this recommendation for your spouse, children, parents, or best friend? If there is any hesitation in your mind, the answer should be no!

A map is not the same as the territory it represents. Any set of guidelines, even those based on the best available research, is only a modest beginning. Much of CAM is unknown territory. Ancient map makers once inscribed "Here dwell dragons" at the margins of their maps, beyond the charted domain. That same inscription applies to much of alternative medicine. Caution needs to be exercised. Furthermore, new knowledge will open up new territories to be explored.

Ultimately, the distinction between CAM and conventional practitioners will disappear. It will fuse into an integrative approach that draws upon all reliable and effective practices—to swing the vital balance between health and illness . . . and life and death.

CHAPTER 2

SOUND MIND, SOUND BODY

MindBody Medicine Comes of Age

Of all the CAM interventions, MindBody medicine is supported by the greatest body of scientific evidence for the greatest number of conditions for the largest number of people. It has also gained the widest acceptance within the conventional health care system.

MindBody medicine is hardly a new concept. Until approximately three hundred years ago, virtually all philosophy and medicine treated body and mind as an integral whole. Then came the Enlightenment of the eighteenth century, and under its mechanistic and reductionist scientific model, the studies of body and mind were separated.

This mechanistic and reductionistic model of conventional medicine received a great boost when it helped to end the infectious disease epidemics of the early twentieth century. Modern scientific biomedicine helped control many of the infectious diseases that were formerly our major killers, such as smallpox, tuberculosis, and cholera. However, even these diseases had already declined to a very low incidence prior to successful medical interventions. Declines were due predominately to public health measures, such as improved sanitation, safer water, improved housing, and more widely distributed food for better nutrition.

Currently, the diseases that are killing most people in the developed nations are no longer these infectious diseases, but chronic, degenerative diseases, such as heart disease, high blood pressure, cancer, and diabetes, for which there is no pharmacologic "magic bullet." These diseases are inextricably related to psychological, lifestyle, environmental, social, and even spiritual factors.

Research on aging has revealed that long-lived people generally manifest psychological, social, and lifestyle characteristics that contribute significantly to their "successful aging" and longevity. These characteristics include a positive attitude, a sense of purpose, social connectedness, appropriate use of both conventional and CAM therapies, and a physically active lifestyle. Recognizing the medical value of these characteristics has spurred interest in MindBody medicine.

Interest in MindBody medicine has also been stimulated by the introduction of Asian healing systems into mainstream American culture. Recently, Western researchers discovered that practitioners of yoga are able to regulate physical functions that were once considered beyond the reach of conscious control, such as electrical activity of the brain, body temperature, heart rate, and blood pressure. Incorporating some of these Asian healing systems, Western medical researchers discovered new ways to forestall and heal diseases that had long been considered an inevitable consequence of aging.

Of all the CAM therapies, MindBody medicine is of particular, central importance. Essential to all CAM therapies, but often overlooked, is that the intervention or cure does not exist "outside" of the individual, independent of "inside" changes in attitude, lifestyle, and orientation toward self and environment. Such an approach demands internal, psychological transformation and the active, ongoing involvement of the individual. Since MindBody approaches necessitate such an orientation, they constitute an integral, vital part of all CAM therapies. It is essential to underscore the perennial observation that over 80 percent of all medical symptoms are self-diagnosed, self-treated, and self-limiting without medical care.

MindBody medicine recognizes that healing is not always synonymous with complete cessation of all physical symptoms. Healing literally means "to make whole." From this perspective, illness can be viewed as an opportunity to reclaim wholeness and completeness, even in the face of ongoing disease. This can occur, however, only when the mind and body are integrated into a whole, healing force.

It is not simply "mind over matter," it is rather that mind matters!

THE BASIC PRINCIPLES OF MINDBODY MEDICINE

There are many forms of MindBody medicine, but they are governed by six basic principles:

1. Mind, body, and spirit are interrelated, not only with one another but also with the external environment. MindBody interventions help physically as well as mentally, and physical interventions help mentally as well as physically.
2. Stress and depression contribute powerfully to chronic disease. "Fight or flight" stress responses usually compromise immunity, and so does depression. Stress and depression can double mortality from certain illnesses.
3. Demonstrably, the mind affects the body through psychoneuroimmunology, a new medical discipline that monitors the physical effects of the mind mediated by the central nervous system, peptides, neuropeptides, and hormones. These biochemicals help regulate immunity.
4. Mental outlook has an impact on physical health. Health is improved by optimism and acceptance, and is diminished by anger, pessimism, and unrelenting, chronic stress.
5. Placebo effects can induce healing. They can have a profound influence on many physical characteristics, and are an important element in many MindBody interventions.
6. Social support enhances and sustains health. Friends, family, and supportive clinicians bolster both effective conventional and CAM therapies.

Clinicians and researchers acknowledge these basic principles after observing the effectiveness of various MindBody interventions. These researchers also surmised, after observing hundreds of studies of MindBody medicine, that there are several fundamental qualities that make MindBody therapy a potent medical approach. Among these approaches are:

- *Relaxation:* A growing body of evidence shows that psychosocial stress is an important factor in many medical conditions, from coronary heart disease to chronic pain to immune problems. By contrast, MindBody therapies create a relaxed state, which is the opposite of the stress response. Meditation, relaxation techniques, imagery, hypnosis, and movement therapies such as yoga and Qi Gong can produce a biologically regenerative, relaxed state.

- *Breathing:* Many MindBody therapies help patients to enter a state of relaxation, meditation, or hypnosis by paying attention to breathing. Breathing represents an important point of contact between mind and body, since respiration occupies a unique interaction between the voluntary and involuntary nervous systems. Shallow and irregular breathing reinforces stress, and can have negative physical consequences. Deep breathing, however, induces relaxation and promotes circulation.

- *Psychological growth:* Numerous forms of psychotherapy have proven helpful in dealing with serious physical illnesses. Cognitive behavioral approaches are also used to help achieve relaxation. Individuals learn to recognize stress triggers and to respond to them actively.

- *Exercise and movement:* Exercise and movement, which are used in many MindBody therapies, decrease the harmful effects of stress, and help prevent some of the diseases of aging, including coronary heart disease, diabetes, osteoporosis, arthritis, hypertension, vestibular dysfunction, and depression. Some Eastern exercise disciplines, such as yoga and tai chi, address body and mind as an integral system. These Eastern practices also generally involve breathing techniques and meditation, and are part of a philosophical system that stresses balance and wholeness. Gentle exercises such as yoga and tai chi are especially valuable for elderly patients who can't do strenuous, high-impact exercise. In addition, these Eastern forms of exercise induce relaxation and activate the calming parasympathetic

branch of the autonomic nervous system, which promotes healing.
- *Social support:* Social support is an important healing force in many MindBody therapies. Social support most often comes from family, friends, support groups, clinicians, caregivers, as well as animals, and even the taking care of plants! Emotional support from all of these sources has been repeatedly shown to help patients reduce their risk factors for recurrent illnesses, and to increase chances of recovery and survival. Social support will be discussed in more detail in the later chapter on spirituality.

While each of these influences is indeed powerful, it has been difficult for researchers to determine which ones are most powerful. This is due to the fact that several of these factors may be present in various forms of MindBody therapy. Further complicating the research is the fact that MindBody therapies are almost always used in conjunction with physical therapies. Even though MindBody medicine is the most accepted form of CAM by conventional practitioners, there is a need for more high-quality, randomized, controlled research trials in this area.

Placebo-controlled studies for MindBody therapies are difficult to design, because these therapies often deliberately employ the placebo response as part of their mechanism of healing. Therefore, in MindBody medicine, the rigorous requirements of placebo-controlled studies appear to be less relevant than outcome-based studies, which demonstrate success anecdotally. This type of outcome-based research can be extremely valuable in medical research. Outcome-based research on multifactorial approaches has been responsible for much of the success in the treatment of cardiovascular disease in the last decade.

Nonetheless, all of the outcome-based research, as well as the RCTs that are cited in this chapter, was held to rigorous standards. It is important to emphasize that the research literature in the MindBody medicine domain is literally voluminous. Studies cited here are a limited sampling of representative applications and outcomes. More than any other chapter, the studies cited here are representative but far, far from exhaustive in this complex and burgeoning therapeutic discipline.

Following are selected examples of the most widely used forms of MindBody medicine, with selected instances of research that either supports or disputes the efficacy of each approach.

MindBody Therapies

Meditation and Relaxation

Meditation has been practiced for thousands of years as a component of various spiritual and religious traditions. Meditation has also long been known to be beneficial for health. In the secular context, meditation is a self-directed practice that quiets the mind and relaxes the body.

During the 1960s, reports began reaching the West about yogis and practitioners of meditation in India and elsewhere who were able to achieve an extraordinary degree of control over supposedly involuntary bodily functions. Some of these masters of meditation were studied at medical research centers in the West, including the Harvard Medical School, the Menninger Foundation, and the University of California School of Medicine in San Francisco. Overall, this early research substantiated the reports of the meditators' remarkable abilities.

One of the most prominent meditation movements in the United States in the 1960s was Transcendental Meditation (TM), founded by Maharishi Mahesh Yogi and popularized by the Beatles. This practice consists of sitting and silently repeating a mantra, a common word or sound, twice a day for twenty minutes to achieve "restful alertness."

Five volumes of research on meditation, under the direction of Dr. David Orme-Johnson, compiled by the Maharishi International University, constitute the most comprehensive review of research in this field. It includes more than 500 original research, review, and theory papers by some 360 researchers at 200 universities and institutions.

In the late 1960s, Harvard researcher Dr. Herbert Benson and associates at the Harvard Medical School began to study TM. Benson's work showed that meditation brings about a healthful state of relaxation, in which the responsiveness of the sympathetic nervous system is decreased, thus creating reduced heart and respiration rate, decreased plasma cortisol levels, and increased alpha or "relaxed" brain waves.

Eventually, Benson developed a generic relaxation method, based on his observations of TM, which he called the "relaxation response." Relaxation response techniques have become very popular in Western culture and are used in many hospitals throughout the United States and abroad through a training program of Dr. Benson's Mind Body Medicine Institute.

There are now also other popular forms of meditation practiced in the United States, including "mindfulness meditation," developed clinically by Dr. Jon Kabat-Zinn at the University of Massachusetts Medical School, which entails maintaining awareness of bodily sensations and thoughts, without passing judgment on them. Mindfulness meditation is perhaps one of the most frequently used MindBody therapies in clinics and hospitals, including the Complementary Medicine Clinic, directed by Dr. David Spiegel, at the Stanford University Hospital.

WHAT WORKS

Presently, the largest body of research in MindBody medicine is in the area of meditation and relaxation, and many of the studies are on TM. Following are some of the relevant studies.

- In a randomized clinical trial conducted in Israel by Cooper in 1978, meditation significantly reduced both systolic (higher number) and diastolic (lower number) blood pressure.
- At the University of Massachusetts, Dr. Jon Kabat-Zinn conducted a study of patients with a variety of chronic diseases who engaged in an eight-week program of meditation. Participants in the program experienced less pain, anxiety, and depression than patients treated with conventional medications.
- Based on a 1987 study by Dr. David Orme-Johnson, meditators were found to utilize medical care services 30 to 87 percent less than non-meditators.
- From a study by Dr. Charles Alexander and Dr. Robert Schneider in 1996, meditation lowered the blood pressure of African Americans, a population at high risk for hypertension.
- Transcendental Meditation was used by Zamara in 1997 among 21 patients with coronary artery disease. After eight months, there was an improvement in circulation and improved exercise tolerance.
- At the Harvard Medical School, Dr. Margaret Caudill enrolled 109 chronic pain patients in a ten-session course of psychotherapy and relaxation techniques, and noted a 36 percent reduction in their use of clinics during the first year.
- One very significant study was reported by Dr. Joseph Blumenthal

and his colleagues at the Duke University School of Medicine in 1997. Using a stress management group plus muscle tension biofeedback with heart disease patients, the results were more effective than the usual care exercise group. Based on this stress management program, there were three fewer fatal heart attacks, three fewer bypass surgeries, and one less angioplasty. This savings of $70,000, or $2,100 per patient, resulted in an estimated return on investment of 7:1. Bear in mind that these cost savings were attained through the improvement of health, not the denial of care.

- Although yoga will be considered in a later chapter, it is often included among the meditation and relaxation therapies. In the November 1998 special issue of the *Journal of the American Medical Association,* one study reported that an eight-week yoga program was more effective than splints in treating carpal tunnel syndrome, according to a report from the University of Pennsylvania School of Medicine.

Nevertheless, meditation is overlooked by many health professionals. In 1991, the National Research Council issued a report on MindBody therapies. Its evaluation of meditation was quite negative, expressing concerns about weak experimental designs, failure to distinguish meditation from other sources of effects, and the absence of an explanatory mechanism. However, these negative conclusions were largely based on two previous reviews that had overlooked much of the relevant available research, and no one on the committee was personally experienced at researching or practicing any of the meditation techniques that they were reviewing.

Researchers are still uncovering clues about meditation's mechanism of action. It was recently proposed that meditation interrupts the vicious cycle that links chronic stress, disturbed serotonin metabolism, and disruptions in the hippocampus and pituitary of the brain. Other research indicates that meditation and relaxation may be able to intervene in a wide array of "disorders of arousal," which involve overstimulation of the brain's limbic system. Such excessive limbic activity, it is argued, may inhibit immune function. Other clues come from the field of psychoneuroimmunology, which has begun to explain the impact of stress on the immune system. Both the research evidence and elaboration of these biological mechanisms have been detailed in two of my earlier books, *Mind as Healer, Mind as Slayer* and *Sound Mind, Sound Body.*

Currently, approximately four hundred universities are offering training in behavioral medicine, including mindfulness meditation, and thousands of hospitals, clinics, and individual practitioners offer this treatment. From the Deaconess Hospital of the Harvard Medical School, Dr. Herbert Benson's Mind Body Medicine Institute has several thousand patient visits a year, carries out active research, and trains doctors, nurses, social workers, and psychologists. More than one million people in the United States have been taught Transcendental Meditation, and most of them reportedly continue to practice it regularly.

Still, many issues remain to be addressed. Researchers need to determine if one form of meditation works better than others. Most important, the spiritual aspects of meditation need to be addressed. Some extreme fundamentalist Christian groups have blocked attempts to apply meditation in health care. It would be helpful to determine the common elements between Christian prayer and Eastern meditation in order to bridge this chasm.

Furthermore, most meditation was originally designed not for medical purposes but for spiritual enlightenment. It would be interesting to determine if Western patients using meditation also gained spiritual benefits.

Cognitive Behavioral Therapy

Meditation may be thought of as a form of cognitive behavioral therapy which is a form of brief psychotherapy that seeks to change negative thought patterns and attitudes in order to change behavior. It is part of a discipline known as behavioral medicine, which constitutes a vast domain of research and clinical practice. Overall, a particular focus of behavioral medicine is to teach healthy, new behaviors. These new behaviors affect an individual's responses to stress.

Components of cognitive behavioral interventions include education, training in coping skills, training in motivation techniques, behavioral rehearsal, and group support.

Behavioral medicine meets the needs of two groups of patients who are often not fully served by conventional medicine: those patients who have physical problems, such as tension headaches, that are caused primarily by stress and mood disorders; and those individuals who have chronic conditions that are strongly affected by stress and other psychological factors. These conditions include headaches, heart disease, high blood pressure, asthma, chronic pain, arthritis, and chronic fatigue syndrome.

Numerous studies indicate that an estimated 50 to 84 percent of patients have physical symptoms that do not have a diagnosable physical cause, or etiology. Approximately 90 percent of these patients do not have an overt psychiatric disorder, but still suffer from anxiety and depression. These patients are sometimes referred to as the "worried well," or "somatizers," because they tend to exacerbate their symptoms with negative emotions and behaviors.

Following are a few of the voluminous studies indicating the positive value of behavioral medicine interventions:

- An innovative intervention by Dr. James J. Strain used brief psychotherapy to reduce the duration of hospitalization for hip fracture by an average of two days.
- One classic study by Dr. Nicholas Cummings documented that when patients who made frequent visits to medical clinics received short-term psychotherapy, their health care costs were reduced by 10 to 20 percent for several years.
- A 1993 study by Dr. Kate Lorig of the Stanford University School of Medicine found that arthritis patients who participated in a behavioral pain management program experienced an increase in self-efficacy, an average 20 percent decline in pain, and a 40 percent reduction in visits to their doctors. Starting in 2000, Dr. Lorig's work under the Stanford NCCAM-funded program will extend for pioneering work in a study of arthritis patients learning mindfulness meditation.
- An NIH panel reported in 1996 that use of behavioral and relaxation approaches in the treatment of chronic pain was superior to placebo in eight well-designed studies.
- During 1997, a study by Drs. Keefe and Caldwell found behavioral interventions to be a viable alternative to conventional treatment for arthritis pain.
- A team of researchers at the former Harvard Community Health Plan, headed by Dr. Caroline Hellman and Dr. Matthew Budd, found that cognitive behavioral interventions reduced physical and

psychological distress and utilization of health care services for patients suffering for a variety of chronic diseases.

For cognitive behavioral therapy, the future is most promising, since it seems to effectively reduce medical care costs, especially those of patients who do not have specific physical pathologies. These patients are often high utilizers of health care services. Thus, such therapies are being increasingly incorporated into conventional health care.

Social support is a significant part of many cognitive behavioral interventions. Therefore, future research is needed to determine whether cognitive behavioral therapy is more effective when it includes a support group.

Hypnosis

Hypnosis involves focusing awareness and turning attention to internal stimuli. It is a state of focused concentration in which the individual is highly responsive to suggestion. It does not necessarily produce a trance state. A hypnotic state is similar to other forms of deep relaxation, with reduced sympathetic nervous system activity, decreased blood pressure, slowed heart rate, and increased alpha and theta brain wave activity.

Introduced in the late eighteenth century by German physician Dr. Franz Anton Mesmer, hypnosis is now viewed as a way of gaining access to the deeper levels of the mind in order to bring about changes in thinking and behavior. Hypnotherapy is currently used in health care to modify feelings of pain, anxiety, and fear, and to gain acceptance of new behaviors. It is also used, by itself and in conjunction with other treatment, to produce analgesia in surgery, to control allergies, and to reduce stress.

Individuals vary greatly in their hypnotizability. An estimated 90 percent of people can be hypnotized, and 20 to 30 percent are ideally responsive to hypnotic suggestion. Applied properly, hypnosis is safe and powerful. Patients with serious psychiatric problems, however, are not appropriate candidates. Elderly people or those with neurological disorders seem to be less susceptible to hypnosis. Many studies of hypnosis have been based on research with students and other young subjects, and the results may not apply to the elderly.

In the treatment of chronic illness, hypnosis helps to alleviate anxiety, to decrease the need for medications, and to make medical procedures more comfortable. Hypnotherapy is also used to reduce or eliminate the need for anesthesia in surgery to control bleeding, to decrease nausea following surgery, to accelerate postsurgical healing, to alleviate morning sickness, to shorten labor, to reduce heart rate and blood pressure, to control dilation and constriction of blood vessels, and to correct cardiac arrhythmias. Hypnosis is also used to eliminate risk factors for heart disease, such as smoking and chronic overeating.

Hypnotherapy was recognized as a valid medical treatment by the American Medical Association in 1958, and today the American Society of Clinical Hypnosis has more than four thousand members, who must be licensed health professionals.

Following are studies that indicate the wide, efficacious use of hypnotherapy, as well as its limitations:

WHAT WORKS

- During 1989, Dr. Giuseppe de Benedittis of the University of Milan demonstrated that hypnosis had a positive effect on the relief of pain due to ischemic heart disease with those patients who had high hypnotic susceptibility.
- A 1991 study by Dr. Edwin J. Weinstein and Dr. Phillip K. Au found that hypnotized patients undergoing the painful procedure of angioplasty could keep the balloon used in this procedure inflated 25 percent longer than nonhypnotized patients, reducing the need for surgery.
- In fibromyalgia patients, eight sessions of hypnotism reduced muscle pain, fatigue, and sleep disturbance, according to Hanerdos in 1991.
- A 1993 study using hypnosis for smoking cessation by Dr. David Spiegel, an expert in hypnosis at Stanford University School of Medicine, evidenced a 23 percent success rate in quitting smoking.
- Most significantly, a study conducted in 1989, also by Dr. David Spiegel of Stanford, found that social support and group therapy doubled survival time for women with metastatic breast cancer.

WHAT DOES NOT WORK

- A study by Dr. Marcia Greenleaf in 1992 indicated that if only a single session of hypnotism was performed, it did not increase recovery rates in coronary bypass patients.
- Breast cancer patients enrolled in an eight-session course of hypnotism had less depression and produced more "natural killer" immune cells. However, results were not sustained at a three-month follow-up.

WHAT'S IN THE WORKS

Recently, NCCAM funded two pilot studies in 1997 on the use of hypnotherapy.

- One study, by Dr. Patricia Newton at Good Samaritan Hospital in Portland, Oregon, evaluated the use of hypnotic imagery in twenty-five breast cancer patients. Patients had eight sessions of hypnotic guided imagery, with suggestions of strengthened immune function. Following this intervention, measures of depression and confusion were reduced, positive states were increased, and the percentage of natural killer cells was significantly increased, although these results were not sustained at three-month follow-up. Results of this pilot study suggest that hypnotic imaging may help in producing physical and psychological changes that will help patients deal with breast cancer by reducing depressions and increasing coping skills. Because hypnosis was able to significantly increase natural killer cells, the results suggest that hypnotic imaging may be able to influence psychoneuroimmunological functioning.
- Another NCCAM-funded study by Dr. Helen Crawford of the Department of Psychology at Virginia Polytechnic Institute explored the effect of hypnotically suggested numbness to pain on electrodynamic functioning of the brain, and was able to distinguish two separate pain processes that were affected by this sort of numbness involving attention to pain and perception of pain.
- At the present time, Dr. David Spiegel is replicating his pioneering research while monitoring the immunological status of the women

participants. Such a study will determine more precise outcomes as well as a possible psychobiological mechanism to account for the findings.

To continue to increase in effectiveness, hypnotherapy needs to grapple with several questions. Researchers must try to understand why some patients are easier to hypnotize, and must find out whether receptiveness to hypnosis is an ability that can be taught.

Since hypnotism is usually an adjunctive therapy, researchers need to clarify its value as a stand-alone therapy. They need to find better ways to positively employ the trancelike state that most people experience on occasion in everyday life. Finally, they must also clarify the mechanism of hypnotism, to better understand how it might be beneficially applied.

Imagery and Visualization

Imagery is a flow of thoughts that includes sensory qualities from one or more of the senses. Imagery is often incorrectly referred to as "visualization" since it can include smell, touch, hearing, taste, proprioception, and motion as well as images.

Imagery is used in many MindBody therapies, including biofeedback, hypnosis, desensitization and aversion techniques, Autogenic Training, Gestalt therapy, Jacobson's Progressive Relaxation, Neurolinguistic Programming, and Rational Emotive Therapy. Furthermore, many meditation and relaxation techniques also involve imagining a sound, mantra, object, or environment. Imagery is also related to hypnosis, in that both elicit similar states of consciousness and have similar applications. In fact, research has found that there is a correlation between the ability to imagine imagery and the ability to be hypnotized.

Imagery has clinical applications in at least three major areas: diagnostic work, psychological rehearsal, and therapeutic interventions.

For diagnosis, a patient may be asked to describe his or her problem with images. This method can help clinicians reach a diagnosis, and can also help patients to become more aware of their deeper inner thoughts and emotions.

In psychological rehearsal, imagery is used to prepare patients for medical procedures, to relieve pain and anxiety, and to soothe side effects that are aggravated by anxiety. A patient is generally guided into a relaxed state and then led through a series of images in which the treatment, the recovery process, and the desired outcome are described in sensory terms. Often, this decreases the arousal of the stimulating, or sympathetic, branch of the autonomic nervous system, which helps reduce anxiety and perception of pain. After surgery, this technique can help patients to experience less pain by learning to relax the muscles around the incision site, to hasten the return of bowel function, or to prevent excessive blood loss by redirecting blood flow to other parts of the body.

Psychological rehearsal has yielded highly positive and often dramatic results, such as reduced pain and anxiety, shorter hospital stays, less need for medication, and decreased side effects. Unfortunately, though, many of the studies on psychological rehearsal do not describe the specific procedures that were used, and so it has not been possible to replicate much of this research.

For many therapeutic interventions, imagery has been applied in the management of a range of chronic diseases, including heart disease. It has been shown to be useful in reducing stress, managing pain, changing behaviors that constitute risk factors, reducing heart rate reactivity, reducing blood pressure, and decreasing resting heart rate. Through imagery, patients enter into an altered state of consciousness, similar to hypnosis, that can lower heart rate and reduce sympathetic nervous system reactivity.

- In a 1994 controlled experiment, Dr. Christopher Sharpley used biofeedback-assisted imagery to train healthy subjects to lower their heart rate reactivity while being exposed to a stressor. This effect was found to have been maintained when subjects were followed up twenty-eight weeks later. In the workplace, those who had received imagery training showed less stress reactivity than the controls.

- A well-known use of imagery has been in the adjunctive care of cancer patients. This application of imagery was pioneered in the early 1970s by radiation oncologist Dr. O. Carl Simonton and Stephanie Simonton, who began teaching the active use of adjunctive imagery to cancer patients. Patients were encouraged to imagine their immune system cells engulfing and devouring vulnerable cancer cells. However, there has not yet been a definitive study that demonstrates whether this works. Nevertheless, many patients have found it helpful, even if they were not cured, and have reported relief of anxiety and pain, better toleration of chemotherapy and radiation, and an increased sense of control.

- On March 10, 1999, Landmark issued an updated report which confirmed their earlier projections in documenting that 67 percent of 114 HMOs offered at least one form of CAM. Among the most common were chiropractic at 65 percent and acupuncture at 31 percent. Furthermore, whether or not they presently offer CAM services, an overwhelming 80 percent of the HMOs think that the integration of conventional and CAM services will grow closer in the future.

- Research shows that imagery produces specific physiological effects in the body. Studies have indicated that imagery, particularly visualization, can have a direct effect on the immune system. It appears to directly influence production of immune system cells, increasing lymphocyte and neutrophil counts, and levels of secretory immunoglobulin A. One study of elderly patients showed an increase in killer T-cells.

- Although not strictly an imagery study per se, one of the most intriguing findings was published by Dr. Joshua M. Smyth and his colleagues in *JAMA* on April 14, 1999. For their study, 112 patients wrote an essay over a three-day period expressing their thoughts and feelings about a traumatic experience. For those patients with asthma or rheumatoid arthritis, there were positive changes in their health at four months later as compared to a control group. These changes were beyond those attributed to their conventional medical care. Whether or not these positive changes will persist beyond four months or whether this intervention can be applied with other diseases will be the subject of future research.

In the management of chronic arthritic pain, imagery has been used to raise skin temperature, relax muscles at trigger points, and decrease sensitivity to pain.

Some research has indicated that the ability for mental imagery may decrease with age. It is not known whether this may place limits on the use of imagery with elderly patients.

WHAT'S IN THE WORKS

Several recent pilot studies in imagery have been funded by grants from the NCCAM:

- From Lenox Hill Hospital in New York City, Dr. James Halper undertook a study of asthma patients and found that the use of imagery helped a significant number of subjects discontinue their medication entirely as compared with controls, although imagery did not have the same degree of influence on pulmonary functions or asthma symptoms.
- At George Washington University, Dr. Mary Banks Gregerson studied the ability of relaxation combined with imagery to affect immune system function, with potential applications in the treatment of cancer and AIDS.
- From the University of Texas at Houston, Dr. Blair Justice evaluated the benefits of imagery and social support in a study of women with breast cancer. It was found in this preliminary study that imagery and support groups had a small to modest positive effect on coping, attitudes, and support, but not on immune function.
- At the University of Michigan, a research team led by Dr. Martin Stevens, a specialist in diabetic neuropathy, is investigating the effectiveness of Reiki in the management of chronic pain in patients with pain due to the neurological damage caused by diabetes. Reiki is a healing technique that channels the "Universal Life energy" to recipients by the laying on of hands. Practitioners are taught standard hand positions, but positions may vary widely depending upon the needs and requests of the participant.
- Most significant, in 1999, at the newly funded research center at the University of Arizona, there are ongoing studies consisting of relaxation, guided imagery, and chamomile tea for children with recurrent abdominal pain.

Although imagery clearly affects physical symptoms, the mechanisms through which it operates are not well understood. An advanced imaging technology, positron emission tomography (PET), indicates that when people imagine something, the same parts of the cerebral cortex are activated as when they actually experience it. Hence, vivid imagery may trigger messages from the cerebral cortex that are transmitted to the brain's limbic system, or emotional center, and thereby influence the endocrine system and the autonomic nervous system.

Imagery work presents a number of challenges for researchers. Longitudinal studies demonstrating the long-term impact of imagery on healthy and ill populations have not been conducted. Also, because imagery is often combined with other MindBody modalities, studies need to be designed that will help separate the effects of each approach.

It is important, in considering imagery, to discriminate between clinical significance and statistical significance. Insistence on a statistically significant result can conceal successful individual cases. There are methods to capture these individual results in order to determine which patients are most likely to benefit from imagery.

In addition, earlier work showing that imagery has a direct effect on biological function should be replicated and expanded with better-designed and -controlled studies.

Imagery has important potential in multifactorial therapies for cancer, AIDS, and autoimmune diseases. This potential should be further explored.

Biofeedback

Biofeedback therapy is a training technique using biological measurement instruments to help patients learn to consciously regulate autonomic, or "automatic," bodily functions, such as heart rate and blood pressure.

Most commonly, biofeedback involves measuring brain waves, muscle tension, skin temperature, electrical resistance of the skin, and respiration. With the development of increasingly sophisticated monitoring devices, and multiple channel computerized instrumentation, new possibilities have been opened. Now there are sensors that can monitor the activity of the bladder, esophageal motility, stomach acidity, and the rectal sphincter to treat incontinence.

There are now more than ten thousand biofeedback practitioners in the United States, two thousand of whom have received national certification. Research and clinical literature on biofeedback is voluminous. Biofeedback is now used to treat about 150 conditions, including asthma, substance abuse, headaches, cardiac arrhythmias, hypertension, Raynaud's disease, fecal and urinary incontinence, irritable bowel syndrome, muscle dysfunction, epilepsy, hot flashes, attention deficit disorder, chronic pain, and nausea and vomiting associated with chemotherapy.

Biofeedback appeals to many patients because it helps place them in charge of their own healing processes. Many people who are uneasy with other relaxation techniques find biofeedback more appealing, because it appears to take a more scientific approach. Research also suggests that biofeedback significantly decreases medical costs.

For some conditions, including Raynaud's syndrome and certain types of fecal and urinary incontinence, biofeedback is the treatment of choice. In other conditions, including tension headaches, migraine, irritable bowel, high blood pressure, asthma, and various neuromuscular problems, it is one of several possible treatment choices.

Biofeedback is especially valuable for stress-related conditions. Biofeedback devices are often used with deep breathing or visualization, to monitor these techniques' ability to reduce the stress response. Once a person learns to relax using biofeedback, they can eliminate the use of the specific instrument by relying upon breathing, visualization, or one of the many forms of meditation.

Following are summaries of a few well-designed, representative studies:

WHAT WORKS

- In a review of studies by Dr. Jeanne Achterberg for the NIH in 1992, biofeedback was found to be efficacious for over 150 conditions.
- During a 1996 study by Dr. Angel McGrady of the Medical College of Ohio, patients with insulin-dependent diabetes were able to improve blood sugar stability.
- From a 1997 study by Nakao in Japan, hypertension patients using biofeedback learned to reduce stress-related increases in blood pressure.
- Following a fifteen-month study of asthmatics by Dr. Erik Peper and colleagues at San Francisco State University, biofeedback patients suffered fewer attacks and used less medicine.

For a discipline that is barely three decades old, biofeedback has accumulated an impressive and growing body of supportive data. Many issues, however, remain to be explored. It is not yet known what other physiological responses can be modified through biofeedback. In addition, just as some people are more hypnotizable than others, it is possible that some people are better candidates for biofeedback than others.

Also, since it would be more cost-effective to provide biofeedback training in a group setting, research needs to explore whether biofeedback would be effective in this way.

Tai Chi

Tai chi is the most popular form of exercise in China. It developed as a "soft" martial art in the early 1200s. It is now a component of traditional Chinese medicine, and is practiced primarily for its health benefits.

Tai chi consists of a precise sequence of slow, graceful movements, accompanied by deep breathing and mental attention, to achieve balance between body and mind and to focus the *qi* (pronounced *chee*), or vital energy. A practitioner's weight is shifted while the body is kept stable and upright.

Because it can be practiced anywhere, by people of any age and physical ability, tai chi is an attractive exercise program for disabled or elderly people. Tai chi involves an energy expenditure equivalent to that of other low to moderate aerobic activities. Exercises can be completed in fifteen to twenty minutes and are ideally practiced twice a day.

As with much of the research on Asian MindBody disciplines, many studies of tai chi have flawed designs, often lacking controls. Only limited research has been done in the United States on tai chi, focusing mainly on its benefits as an exercise form rather than looking at its broader health, psychological, and spiritual dimensions.

Practitioners of tai chi report mood enhancement and physiological changes similar to those produced by other moderate forms of exercise. However, tai chi is uniquely beneficial for improving posture and balance, and it is in this area that some promising studies have been done in the United States and abroad. Because of this effect, tai chi may help prevent injuries from falling.

Significant studies include the following:

- One of the earliest studies, in 1982 by Dr. Lansheng Gong of the Shanghai Medical College, studied the electrocardiograms of one hundred tai chi practitioners and found benefits. However, he also noted that these beneficial effects did not seem attributable to the amount of physical exercise, and other mechanisms needed to be discovered.
- During 1992, a study by Dr. Putai Jin of LaTrobe University in Australia indicated that tai chi improved heart rate and blood pressure as much as brisk walking.
- Based on a 1992 study by Dr. Shuk-kuen Tse and Dr. Diana M. Bailey, tai chi helped improve balance among people who were largely sedentary.
- From a 1995 study by Dr. Jin-shin Lai and associates, elderly tai chi practitioners showed significantly improved cardiorespiratory function, compared to sedentary subjects. However, another study found that tai chi conferred no significant changes in blood pressure or heart rate.
- At Emory University, a study by Dr. Steven Wolf in 1996 found that elderly people in a tai chi training course reduced their risk of falling by 47.5 percent, compared to controls, who took a training course in balance.
- In a 1996 study by Dr. Leslie Wolfson of the University of Connecticut, tai chi was compared to balance training, strength training, and combined balance and strength training in people with an average age of eighty. Those who learned tai chi gained significantly more balance and strength than the other groups.

WHAT'S IN THE WORKS

At Stanford University School of Medicine, an ongoing study by Dr. Kate Lorig will determine the potential applicability of tai chi for patients suffering from arthritis and fibromyalgia. A second study by noted researcher Dr. William L. Haskell will evaluate the role of tai chi as compared to traditional Western exercise in improving the physical and psychological health of older men and women.

Well-designed research seems to be affirming that tai chi, as a form of exercise for elderly people, may prove a valuable part of health maintenance programs, both for preventing falls and for maintaining fitness.

Qi Gong

Qi Gong (pronounced *chee gong*) is another ancient Chinese exercise involving physical movements and breathing exercises. An element of traditional Chinese medicine, it is used to circulate internal *qi*, which, according to Chinese medicine, is the vital energy that flows through the body in a system of subtle channels known as meridians. Qi Gong is intended to direct the internal *qi*, and promote health.

There are two basic kinds of Qi Gong, internal and external. Internal Qi Gong is used for self-healing and health maintenance. It can be performed in any position, including standing, sitting, walking, or lying down. External Qi Gong is practiced by Qi Gong masters or Qi Gong doctors, and involves projecting the *qi* energy out of one's body to heal another.

In China, Qi Gong is used for disease prevention and therapy. Although the movements resemble those of tai chi, they do not flow smoothly from one to another, but consist of short sequences of movements that are repeated many times.

Qi Gong has been studied in China for its impact on arthritis and cancer, and for general health maintenance. Numerous papers on it have been presented at international conferences over the past twenty years. However, scientific literature on it is very limited in the United States and consists of very few high-quality RCTs.

Among conditions that reportedly benefit from Qi Gong are many health problems of elderly people, including high blood pressure, heart disease, ulcers, arthritis, and gastrointestinal ailments. It also appears to help immune function. Studies on Qi Gong have suggested that many age-related changes can be affected through its practice.

WHAT WORKS

Among the representative positive studies are:

- A twenty-year study in China by Wang, completed in 1993, reported benefits of lowered blood pressure. Patients using Qi Gong experienced a 50 percent decrease in death and illness from strokes.

- Research in China by Sheng-han in 1994 indicated that Qi Gong was able to alter such physiological reactions as EEGs, EMGs, respiratory movement, heart rate, skin potential, skin temperature, sympathetic nerve function, stomach and intestinal function, and metabolic rate.
- During a 1997 study by Dr. Wen-hsien Wu of the New Jersey Medical School, Qi Gong was helpful for patients with reflex sympathetic dystrophy, a debilitating disease of the autonomic nervous system that often resists medical intervention. For these patients, Qi Gong significantly reduced pain and anxiety.
- At Columbia University, Dr. Paul Zucker showed that patients using Qi Gong averaged a drop in blood pressure of 10 percent.
- In a hospital in Beijing, ninety-three patients with advanced cancer were treated with a combination of drugs and Qi Gong exercises, while a control group was treated with drugs alone. Eighty-one percent of the Qi Gong group showed an improvement in strength, 63 percent in appetite, and 33 percent were free from diarrhea, compared to improvements of 10 percent, 10 percent, and 6 percent, respectively, in the other group.

WHAT IS IN THE WORKS

Beginning in 1999 and running into the next century is one Qi Gong research project at the Center for Complementary and Alternative Medicine Research in Cardiovascular Disease at the University of Michigan. Under the direction of Dr. Amy Ai, who is a sociologist and doctor of traditional Chinese medicine, this research will investigate the rate of healing of graft wounds in patients undergoing coronary bypass surgery.

Thus both tai chi and Qi Gong, which ostensibly are mild forms of exercise, demonstrate far-reaching applications for the amelioration of numerous chronic disorders.

Music Therapy

Music therapy is a behavioral intervention that uses music to bring about changes in emotions, physiology, and behavior. Music has long been recognized to have beneficial effects on health and healing. However, even though it was used therapeutically as early as Greco-Roman times, music therapy did not become a profession until after World War II, when music was used in the rehabilitation of emotionally disturbed soldiers. Today there are over five thousand registered music therapists in the United States.

In addition to more melodic forms of music, chanting has also long been associated with healing. Chanting is an important element of the healing traditions of Tibetans, Catholics, Buddhists, Sikhs, and Native Americans. Furthermore, there appears to be a remarkable similarity in the chants of various cultures.

Though scientists recognize that certain sounds do have unique effects upon human physiology, it would be reductionistic to view the wondrous effects of music only in terms of neurophysiology. Music, especially when shared simultaneously by many music-makers and many listeners, has profound effects that reach far beyond the physical realm.

A number of hypotheses explain the physiological effects of music. One theory is that it activates the right hemisphere of the brain and improves communication between the two hemispheres. Also, music appears to temporarily occupy the physiological "gates of pain," located primarily in the spinal cord, through which pain must travel on its way to the brain. Furthermore, listening to music may release chemicals, such as endorphins, that affect mood and pain sensitivity.

Music therapy can consist of both listening to music and making music. Therapists use music for a number of purposes, including reduction of stress, anxiety, and social isolation; helping patients achieve deep relaxation; enhancing learning and creativity; and promoting self-awareness. Music therapy is widely used in hospitals, nursing homes, psychiatric facilities, and drug addiction treatment centers. It is also used in surgery to facilitate anesthesia, and in dentistry to reduce stress and discomfort.

WHAT WORKS

Following are results of several influential studies on music therapy:

- In the treatment of heart disease, music has been used as a pacemaker, helping hearts to achieve proper rhythms in two studies, by

Haas in 1980 and Bason in 1992. It also reduces anxiety in heart attack patients. However, there is a relative lack of RCTs on music therapy for heart disease. Furthermore, some studies show that music was no more effective than bed rest for heart patients.

- A 1993 RCT by Dr. Thomas Lord and Dr. Jane Garner of Alzheimer's patients indicated that music therapy enhanced memory of past events and improved mood.
- From a 1994 study by Dr. Karen Allen and Dr. Jim Blascovih, a *JAMA* article indicated that when music was used in operating rooms, patients had fewer postsurgical complications, with less pain and shorter hospital stays.
- Patients with chronic obstructive pulmonary disease showed significant gains in ability to endure exercise when music therapy was used, according to a 1995 study by Thornby at the New York University School of Medicine.
- Music therapy appears to be quite helpful for chronic pain. In one RCT by Dr. Lani Zimmerman and Dr. Bunny Pozehl in 1989, it reduced not only suffering but also the physical sensation of pain, leading researchers to believe it had directly affected sensory perception. In another study, it apparently raised the pain threshold of rheumatoid arthritis patients.
- A 1997 pilot study funded by NCCAM showed that patients with chronic brain damage responded to music therapy with less depression and more empathy for others. However, their cognitive abilities were unchanged.

Music therapy may prove to be a cost-effective intervention, and is surely growing in popularity. However, research needs to be done to determine the "optimal dosage" to identify the optimal length of time and choice of music. Well-designed studies are needed to confirm the physiological and psychological effects of music. In addition, because music has also been found to improve the performance of health care professionals such as surgeons and surgical nurses, research needs to be conducted on the negative effects of "noise pollution," which pervades our modern environment.

THE FUTURE OF MINDBODY MEDICINE

MindBody medicine has clearly moved out of the research laboratory and into mainstream clinical applications. There are many notable instances of this. One of the most frequently cited examples is Dr. Dean Ornish's program for reversing coronary heart disease through an approach that combines a vegetarian diet with yoga, meditation, and group support. This program has been successful not only in halting progression of heart disease but also in reversing it. Another major program is the Stanford Coronary Risk Intervention Program (SCRIP) developed by Dr. William L. Haskell and his colleagues at the Stanford University School of Medicine. SCRIP includes intensive lifestyle intervention plus medication. In this program, all risk factors were significantly reduced, and the number of clinical events such as bypass surgeries and hospitalizations was reduced by half.

During 1999 and extending into 2000, Dr. Haskell, Dr. John W. Farquhar, and their Stanford colleagues, including myself, have been applying a practical version of SCRIP in three innovative projects. These three projects include an intervention at one General Electric worksite of 1,500 predominantly nuclear engineers, a second variant with fifteen primary care physicians in an Independent Practice Association (IPA) and in Santa Clara County, California, and third, an intervention focused on the 8,000 employees and retirees of an entire county, San Mateo, in northern California based on the classic three- and then five-city interventions conducted by Dr. John W. Farquhar. Once these three studies have been completed, this sophisticated MindBody medicine intervention will have progressed from a basic, randomized clinical trial to real-world demonstration interventions, and ultimately will be incorporated into the benefits and reimbursement structure of major health care providers and insurance companies. Beyond the particulars of this coronary heart disease intervention, this rigorous, stepwise progression serves as an excellent model of evolving from basic research into practical, applied programs for managing a wide array of chronic diseases.

Employers are finding that it is worthwhile to include MindBody approaches in their benefit packages, and in workplace interventions. Among the Fortune 500, such leading companies as AT&T, American Airlines, Citibank, Hewlett-Packard, Xerox, ARCO, and LeviStrauss are but a few of the many that have incorporated health promotion, disease management, and some aspects of alternative medicine into their health and medical plans.

Hospitals and HMOs are increasingly including MindBody components in their managed care programs. The Stanford University Hospital opened a new Complementary Medicine Clinic, under the direction of Dr. David Spiegel, in April of 1998 with clinical services including mindfulness meditation, psychosocial support groups for cancer patients, biofeedback, acupuncture, massage, and a growing array of clinical services based on scientific evidence of efficacy. Also in California, Kaiser Permanente's Pain Management Program offers training in meditation and relaxation, cognitive behavioral therapy, exercise, and social interaction. In Nashua, New Hampshire, the Matthew Thornton Health Plan has a very successful Behavioral Medicine Pain Program for patients with fibromyalgia, arthritis, headaches, low back pain, and chronic cancer pain. Throughout the United States and abroad, MindBody medicine is being integrated into many hospital systems.

Managed care is increasingly forcing providers to focus on issues of cost-effectiveness. MindBody medicine fares particularly well in this regard. Among the findings to date are that various of the MindBody interventions discussed in this chapter have been documented to reduce outpatient visits to clinics by 7 to 15 percent; pediatric visits for acute illness declined 26 percent; acute asthma care was reduced by one visit per year; outpatients with a tendency to express psychological problems as physical symptoms (somatizers) had two fewer visits per year, resulting in a 33 percent reduction in their annual medical costs; arthritis patients have reduced office visits by as much as 43 percent; chronic pain clinic use declined 38 percent; C-section deliveries have been reduced by as much as 56 percent in a number of studies; and postsurgical days in the hospital have been decreased by as much as 1.5 days. Bear in mind that these reductions are in excessive or inappropriate care, which results in higher risks to patients, since in all of the above studies, the patients experienced equal or better outcomes with less medical care.

With the growing number of research projects utilizing RCTs, it is becoming apparent that MindBody interventions have minimal side effects, are suitable for self-care, afford patients a feeling of empowerment, and are cost-effective.

In the future, to bring MindBody medicine into greater alignment with the accepted biomedical model, further research is needed to clarify many basic issues, including the mechanisms by which these interventions operate, and which of the interventions are best suited for certain people and for specific conditions.

Finally, the long-term use of some of these techniques, especially meditation and the movement disciplines, has the potential to open up new areas of awareness in the individual. Transpersonal experiences that may arise from MindBody practices are by no means a trivial part of the healing process. MindBody therapies are helping to push back the frontiers of our scientific understanding, and are challenging traditional scientific disciplines to grow.

More than any other area of CAM interventions, MindBody medicine has the most extensive reasearch base that has clearly demonstrated the most positive impact on the broadest array of conditions for the largest number of people. MindBody medicine is so widely used by the public, and by the medical profession, that it may be considered to be more conventional than alternative. To be sure, there are many unanswered questions. Nonetheless, although infinite and perennial mysteries remain in the complex and subtle interaction between mind and matter, there can be no doubt that MindBody medicine has come of age.

CHAPTER 3

FOOD FOR THOUGHT

Dietary Supplements, Phytonutrients, and Hormones

Many of the dietary and nutritional beliefs that were formerly accepted only by the alternative health community have in the past few decades been embraced by conventional clinicians, researchers, nutritionists, and dietitians. However, many nutritional issues remain fraught with inconsistency and controversy. Moreover, as might be predicted in a market economy, a new wave of commercial interests has entered the field, offering a bewildering array of nutritional products, which may not be helpful, and may even be injurious to optimal health. Currently, many studies are calling into question the value of some of America's most frequently consumed supplements. Thus, with a few notable exceptions, foods, rather than pills, need to be recognized as our best sources of necessary nutrients.

Even so, it is widely accepted that the American diet that accompanied industrialization has been associated with an increased incidence of degenerative diseases, including cardiovascular disease and cancer, which together cause more than two-thirds of all deaths in the United States.

Factors contributing to the decline of the American diet include the increased processing of grains, which strips them of fiber and nutrients, the overconsumption of animal protein and fats, and the heavy use of refined sugars and starches. Our food also now contains increasing quantities of additives, pesticides, drugs, and toxins. Even our soil has been depleted. These factors appear to contribute significantly to chronic diseases.

By comparison, other countries with different diets suffer fewer degenerative diseases, particularly heart disease. In Mediterranean countries, the use of largely monounsaturated olive oil as the primary source of fat confers considerable protection against heart disease. For many nonindustrialized countries, and in many Asian countries, the low consumption of animal products also helps protect people from a variety of chronic diseases.

Therefore, in keeping with the theme of "think horses, not zebras," our first step in assessing the American diet should be to pay attention to the obvious task of eating healthier foods, rather than taking esoteric and often questionable supplements.

REASONABLE DIETARY GUIDELINES

Recognizing that the American diet was producing a health crisis of degenerative diseases, about thirty years ago the U.S. government began to address the issue of an optimal diet for the American people. As early as 1969, the Senate Select Committee on Nutrition, chaired by Senator George McGovern, held hearings, and in 1977 they issued their conclusions. Despite strong opposition from the powerful American food industry, the McGovern Committee came up with important new recommendations in the form of the United States Dietary Goals. They recommended reducing calorie intake, increasing the consumption of complex carbohydrates, reducing the consumption of refined sugars, reducing overall fat consumption, reducing saturated fat consumption and balancing it with polyunsaturated and monounsaturated fats, reducing cholesterol consumption, and limiting sodium intake.

These recommendations were met with strong protests from the cattle, egg, sugar, and food-processing industries, and even the American Medical Association. In the intervening years, though, the AMA altered its antagonistic position.

In the early 1990s, the U.S. Department of Agriculture introduced a new "Eating Right Pyramid," which further deemphasized meat and dairy products. However, in the face of a new wave of protests from the meat and dairy industries, the USDA pulled back promotion of the pyramid, provoking criticism from the American Cancer Society and other agencies.

Nonetheless, many nutrition advocates, including the Physicians Committee for Responsible Medicine (PCRM), believed that the food pyramid did not go far enough. PCRM proposed its own "new" four food groups, which consisted entirely of plant foods—whole grains, legumes, fruits, and vegetables. PCRM maintained that a diet centered on plant foods presents the least risk for causing heart disease, stroke, high blood pressure, obesity, colon cancer, breast cancer, and osteoporosis. Plant foods, they said, have tremendous advantages. Plant foods contain disease-fighting substances known as phytochemicals and are rich in other nutrients. They are also low in fat and high in fiber, which helps prevent cardiovascular disease and cancer and helps to remove dangerous toxins from the system.

Many people, however, prefer not to subsist solely on plant foods, but would rather add a small amount of lean meat, fish, and dairy products to their primarily vegetarian diets. This type of diet is generally referred to as a "plant-based" diet. Pure vegetarian diets can be very healthy, but many people find them to be excessively restrictive and run the risk of being protein deficient. Therefore, a plant-based diet strikes a healthy middle ground.

In October of 1997, the American Institute for Cancer Research released the first sweeping report on diet and cancer since the 1980s. The report was based upon an examination of 4,500 studies. The Institute's primary directive was to eat a plant-based diet, drink no alcohol, maintain a moderate weight throughout life, and get some exercise. According to Harvard's Dr. Walter C. Willett, one of the report's authors, "Ten to 15 years ago, the notion was that cancer was caused by too many bad things lurking in our food supply. . . . This report really turns things around and says, cancer comes, really, from not getting enough of the good things."

One of the Institute's most important recommendations is to eat five servings of fruits and vegetables each day, because fruits and vegetables are a potent way to protect the body against cancer. Additionally, the report also called for meat consumption of no more than three ounces daily, which is an amount equal to about the size of a deck of cards.

Research supporting this type of diet is powerful and voluminous. Many recent studies have shown that vegetarians are nearly 50 percent less likely to die from cancer than nonvegetarians. For example, Japanese women who follow Western-type diets that include meat are eight times likelier to develop breast cancer than Japanese women who eat a plant-based diet. Vegetarian diets also help prevent heart disease, since animal products are the main dietary source of saturated fat and the only source of cholesterol. Low-fat vegetarian diets, along with exercise, are also effective at controlling adult-onset diabetes.

In 1988, the American Dietetic Association issued a position paper endorsing vegetarian diets as "healthful and nutritionally adequate." According to the ADA, vegetarian diets provide adequate protein, although they generally provide less protein than nonvegetarian diets. This may actually be beneficial, as we will see later. Both vegetarians and nonvegetarians alike, said the ADA, may have difficulty meeting recommendations for iron intake. Also, vegetarians who don't eat eggs or dairy products may need to take additional vitamin B_{12}.

It was Dr. Denis Burkitt who first promulgated the value of fiber in the diet. More recently, he has commented that while developed countries have steadily increased their intake of meat and dairy products over the last two hundred years, our bodies have not adapted to these changes in diet, and have no more use for such foods than they did twenty thousand years ago.

However, though it may be tempting to make an across-the-board recommendation that all humans should eat nothing but plant-based diets, it is just such dogmatism that has long created discord and misunderstanding on the subject of nutrition. Thus, it is important to heed the advice of pioneering nutritionist Dr. Roger J. Williams, the discoverer of pantothenic acid and folic acid, who originated the principle of "biochemical individuality." Throughout his prolific writing, Dr. Williams pointed out that each person is biologically unique, and that there is no one diet that is suitable for all. Because we are all unique genetically, we require slight variations in our nutrient intake. For example, some people don't produce enough of the enzyme lactase to properly digest milk. Environmental and lifestyle influences also contribute to our uniqueness. Furthermore, eating contaminated foods may make some people more chemically sensitive than others. Similarly, stress can affect digestion and nutritional needs. Even strenuous exercise creates an added demand for protective nutrients. Because of all of these factors, it is wise for each person to develop his or her own unique nutritional program.

Under the NCCAM grant at the Stanford University School of Medicine, the research team of Dr. Christopher Gardner, Dr. John W. Farquhar, and Dr. John B. Cooke has undertaken a number of innovative studies focused on plant-based diets. One study of a commercial garlic supplement was consistent with other studies indicating that garlic had little or no effect in lowering LDL cholesterol. Studies are under way in 1999 and into 2000 on the effects of phytoestrogens and soy protein on cholesterol, bone density, and breast cancer in postmenopausal women. One of the most innovative studies is to compare a plant-based diet to the currently recommended avoidance of fat and cholesterol diet. This research is oriented to determining an "optimal" diet that is as concerned with what is in a diet, phytonutrients, as with what is left out. Innovative research such as this will yield reliable, clear guidelines to create an optimal diet based on science rather than on marketing.

Nonetheless, for most people, research now clearly shows that a plant-based diet offers the most protection against the most common degenerative diseases.

Value and Danger of Various Food Components

Fiber. Eating a plant-based diet provides high levels of fiber. Water-soluble fibers, such as gums and pectins, protect against heart disease and diabetes by binding in the gut with bile acids, which contain cholesterol, thus preventing the reabsorption of these bile acids. Water-soluble fibers also delay glucose absorption and gastric emptying, which stabilizes blood sugar levels. Water-insoluble fibers, celluloses and hemicelluloses, protect against colon cancer by absorbing water, increasing stool volume, and speeding the passage of stool through the bowel. They also dilute the concentration of toxic bile acids, which can contribute to cancer. Presently, Americans consume an average of ten to fifteen grams of fiber per day, but should eat about twenty-five to thirty-five grams.

Recently, some nutrition experts expressed concern that high fiber consumption might inhibit the absorption and availability of minerals such as calcium, zinc, and iron. However, population studies disproved this.

Antioxidants. Our bodies are constantly exposed to "free radicals," or highly reactive molecules that can damage the body and are associated with degenerative diseases.

Fruits and vegetables are rich in substances known as phytochemicals, some of which act as antioxidants, protecting us against free radicals. Many phytochemicals in our foods have not yet been identified. This is a powerful argument for the use of whole foods rather than supplements. Another argument for this is that fruits and vegetables absorb more free radicals than isolated free-radical-scavenging vitamins, such as C and E. For example, ¾ cup of cooked kale can neutralize as many free radicals as 500 mg of vitamin C, or 800 IU of vitamin E, even though kale contains only 40 mg of vitamin C and less than 10 IU of vitamin E.

Other important phytochemicals occur in rice, tea, and spices. Cruciferous vegetables, including cabbage, broccoli, cauliflower, and Brussels sprouts, contain phytochemicals that seem to be protective against cancer. Some phytochemicals also appear to be helpful for minor illnesses, such as colds.

Fats. Government guidelines say that we should consume no more than 30 percent of total daily calories as fat. Actually, optimal fat intake may be much lower, perhaps 15 to 20 percent, or even less. To reverse coronary heart disease, Dr. Dean Ornish cuts fat to a mere 10 percent of total calories, and cholesterol to 5 mg. Most recently, concern has been raised from research that such an extremely low-fat diet may increase triglycerides and lower HDL, which would actually have the effect of increasing heart disease risk for some individuals. This contrasts with the American Heart Association's recommendation of 30 percent of total calories as fat and 300 mg of cholesterol.

Besides increasing the risk of cardiovascular disease, a high-fat diet also increases the risk of cancer, obesity, and diverticulitis, which is an inflammation of the colon due to pockets of stagnant digested matter.

There are three kinds of dietary fats: saturated, polyunsaturated, and monounsaturated.

Saturated fats are primarily found in animal foods and in tropical oils, such as coconut and palm oil, which are solid at room temperature. These fats can be the most harmful, because they easily clog arteries.

Polyunsaturated fats are found in safflower, sunflower, corn, and fish oils. They contain both omega-6 and omega-3 essential fatty acids (EFAs). Theoretically, humans evolved on a diet that consisted of small and approximately equal amounts of omega-6 and omega-3 fatty acids, but now most people eat about twenty times more omega-6 than omega-3.

Omega-6 is useful in repairing injuries and causing blood to clot and blood vessels to constrict. Omega-3, however, inhibits blood clotting, relaxes smooth muscles in blood vessel walls, and protects against heart arrythmias, thereby reducing the risk of heart disease. Many foods are rich in omega-3 EFAs, including cold-water fish, such as salmon and mackerel, and flax and flaxseed oil. Smaller amounts of omega-3 fatty acids are contained in great northern, navy, kidney, and soybeans. Among oils, flaxseed oil and canola oil are high in omega-3 EFAs, and so are soy, pumpkin seed, evening primrose, borage seed, walnut, and black currant oils. Actually, the best source of omega-3 fatty acids is flaxseed oil. It contains 50 percent omega-3, compared to the 10 percent found in canola oil.

With the discovery of the relationship between cholesterol and heart disease, Americans were encouraged to switch from animal fats, such as butter, to polyunsaturated fats, including the oils we just discussed. Unfortunately, this solution presented another set of problems. When these oils undergo metabolism, they are highly susceptible to lipid peroxidation, or rancidity, which gives rise to harmful free radicals. Most researchers now believe that it is better to use monounsaturated fats, which not only reduce the risk of lipid peroxidation but also reduce LDL, or bad cholesterol, while maintaining high levels of HDL, or good cholesterol. Olive oil and canola oil are high in monounsaturated fats.

Margarine is a polyunsaturated oil that has undergone hydrogenation to make it solid at room temperature. However, hydrogenation creates man-made molecules called trans-fatty acids, which may interfere with metabolic functions. Thus, in the rush away from butter, many people may have ended up compromising their health.

Nonetheless, very recently, some researchers concluded that monounsaturated fats may not be any better than polyunsaturated fats, because monounsaturated fats may be only slightly less susceptible to oxidation than polyunsaturated fats.

Therefore, when all these complexities are weighed and sorted, the bottom-line recommendation: Cut back on all forms of fats, except omega-3!

Dairy Products. Nonfat milk is an excellent source of calcium, but dairy products may be harmful to many people. It may not even be natural for our species to consume dairy products, since the consumption of cow's milk is a relatively recent phenomenon among humans. Milk protein allergy occurs frequently among young children, and lactose intolerance is widespread throughout the world.

Milk sugar is broken down into two simple sugars, glucose and galactose. Galactose may not be easily metabolized, and may accumulate in certain tissues; this may contribute to cataracts. Whole-milk dairy products also carry the risk of contamination with fat-soluble pesticides, sulfa drugs, and antibiotics. Nonfat dairy products do not carry these contaminants.

Calcium can also be obtained from plant sources, including dark green, leafy vegetables, many beans, almonds, and some dried fruits.

People who do want to consume dairy products should use only skim or 1 percent milk and dairy products. Children under the age of two should consume whole milk, if they use cow's milk, although soy milk is an excellent alternative. For infants, breast milk is the wisest choice. Milk substitutes, such as soy, almond, rice, or goat's milk, are an option for anyone wanting to avoid dairy products. Goat's milk is metabolized differently from cow's milk and may be a useful substitute for individuals with lactose intolerance to cow's milk.

Protein. Proteins play many important roles in the body, helping in the repair and maintenance of tissues. Plant proteins lower cholesterol and may improve the function of arteries. Proteins also make up hormones, enzymes, and neurotransmitters.

However, most Americans appear to eat too much protein. Protein cannot be stored in the body, so protein that is not used for body maintenance is converted to carbohydrate. During the process, the nitrogen-containing molecules that are left are processed by the liver into urea, which is excreted by the kidneys. Therefore, too much protein in the diet may overwork the kidneys and lead to sclerosis and reduced kidney function. High levels of protein in the diet also cause the body to lose calcium by increasing calcium excretion in the urine. Animal protein causes more calcium loss than vegetable protein.

Americans, on average, consume approximately twice the government's recommended level of protein. Even athletes do not need protein in excess of the RDA, which is 51 grams per 150 pounds of body weight. There is no evidence that protein supplements or high-protein foods are helpful in athletic training, and the old idea of the high-protein training diet has been discarded by most experts.

Recent evidence has shown that vegetarians do not need to engage in complex "protein combining" in order to receive complete protein, containing all of protein's amino acid "building blocks." This practice sometimes results in excessive protein intake.

If your diet contains animal products, it is likely that your protein intake already exceeds the RDA. Since excess protein in general, and particularly excessive animal protein, is associated with increased risk of bone loss, atherosclerosis, kidney stone formation, and impaired kidney function, it is a good idea to reduce or eliminate animal foods from the diet.

THE DEBATE OVER SUPPLEMENTS

Thousands of books and papers have been written about vitamins, and have created many controversies. To address these general controversies, we will focus on two specific antioxidant vitamins, vitamin E and beta-carotene, which have been of great interest to researchers in recent years. These vitamins are good examples of the complexity of the diet-versus-supplement question. They also illustrate the point that there is no easy answer to the question of whether it is possible to obtain all nutrients necessary for optimal health from the diet alone.

To better comprehend the controversy over vitamins, we must first consider the amounts of vitamins that the government deems appropriate for daily consumption. These amounts are referred to as the Recommended Daily Allowances, or RDAs. In the case of vitamin E, for example, the RDA is 12 to 15 IU. However, some proponents of supplements recommend that people take more than 1,000 IU daily!

To understand this conflict on vitamin dosages, it is important to know that the RDAs, which are revised every ten years, are the amounts of nutrients that are needed to help large population groups avoid deficiency diseases. The RDA for vitamin C is based partly on how much is needed to avoid scurvy. However, the RDAs may not be adequate to ensure optimal health. Some experts believe that the RDAs are too low, and allow minor nutritional deficiencies to occur, producing subtle symptoms that may appear to be part of the natural aging process. Thus nervousness, mental exhaustion, insomnia, improper immune function, and muscle weakness may be early warning signs of borderline deficiencies and may respond to supplementation and improvements in diet.

While diet remains the best source of meeting the RDAs for various nutrients, it may be impossible for individuals to obtain adequate quantities of some vitamins and minerals from food alone. Thus, some individuals may benefit from taking supplements. Furthermore, according to the principle of biochemical individuality, each person has unique nutritional requirements, and some may need supplements more than others.

As the following summary of research suggests, individual needs for vitamin E may vary greatly and are accentuated by those individuals who may feel they "need" vitamin E for as yet unproven benefits, such as the prevention of heart disease.

Consider the following well-documented research on vitamin E:

- A 1997 Finnish study, reported in *Consumer Reports*, indicated that smokers who took 50 IU of vitamin E daily had less risk of angina.
- From a 1977 study conducted in Atlanta of postangioplasty patients, those taking 1,200 IU of vitamin E daily had much less risk of reclogging of arteries.
- A recent Harvard study of 135,000 health professionals found that those who took daily vitamin E supplements had one-fourth to one-third less coronary risk than those who didn't.
- The major 1996 Cambridge Heart Antioxidant Study, reported by Stephens in 1996, found that vitamin E significantly reduced risk of nonfatal heart attacks.

It is difficult to receive high dosages of vitamin E without supplements. The richest sources are vegetable and seed oils, but these oils are high in fat. To get even 15 IU, the RDA for men, it would take 248 slices of whole wheat bread, 16 dozen eggs, or 20 pounds of bacon. Moreover, to protect against heart disease or cancer, dosage levels may need to be twenty to thirty times greater than the RDAs.

As of 1996, Dr. Kenneth Cooper, noted author and founder of the Cooper Institute, recommended 400 IU daily, and he recommended higher doses for those who engage in heavy exercise, who weigh more than two hundred pounds, or who are in other high-risk categories.

However, more than 400 IU of E a day may increase the risk of hemorrhagic stroke. People who take medications that inhibit blood clotting should not take vitamin E supplements without checking with their doctor.

One additional problem with vitamin E supplements is that they are generally in the form of alpha tocopherol, despite the fact that other tocopherols, which are found in foods, may be equally important. For example, gamma tocopherol, found in soybeans, nuts, and grains, protects against nitrogen oxides, which are free radicals that can cause DNA damage and inflammation. Nitrogen oxides are not particularly affected by alpha tocopherol. In fact, taking large amounts of alpha tocopherol increases elimination of gamma tocopherol from the body. This, again, is an argument for ingesting vitamins in foods rather than supplements.

Another important nutrient that may be better to ingest in whole foods is beta-carotene. As a supplement, it may even present health hazards for certain individuals. Beta-carotene is a precursor of vitamin A, a vitamin that can accumulate in fat cells and have toxic effects. When taken at ten times the RDA, vitamin A has been associated with birth defects.

Beta-carotene, which can be transformed into vitamin A after it enters the body, is a member of a group of substances known as carotenoids, which are the pigments in brightly colored red, orange, and yellow plants. Humans cannot synthesize carotenoids, so they must be derived from diet. However, they are not well absorbed. Carotenoids may help to protect LDL cholesterol from oxidation, thereby inhibiting atherosclerosis and heart attacks. Carotenoids also neutralize free radicals, reducing cellular damage. Different carotenoids have different antioxidant activity.

A summary of some important, representative research reveals:

- According to the Coronary Primary Prevention Study, conducted by Dr. Dexter Morris, low blood levels of carotenoids are associated with cancer and coronary disease. However, only a few high-quality RCTs have been performed.

- A 1996 study by Dr. Kenneth Cooper, reported in *JAMA*, found that 80,000 IU daily for 4.3 years did not affect heart disease or cancer but did lower overall mortality by 40 percent. This suggests a protective effect when beta-carotene is taken over a long period.
- In a 1997 Finnish study, male smokers taking beta-carotene actually had 18 percent more lung cancer. Another study, reported in 1996 by the National Cancer Institute, indicated a 28 percent increase in lung cancer in smokers, ex-smokers, and asbestos workers taking beta-carotene. A follow-up study, though, found increased risk only in people who smoked and also drank alcohol, or who smoked heavily. Another study found neither harm nor benefit.

One cautious conclusion we can draw is that heavy smokers and heavy alcohol drinkers should not use beta-carotene supplements. In general, it is best to get beta-carotene and other carotenoids in their natural form. It is too early to rule out beta-carotene supplementation entirely for people who are not heavy smokers or drinkers.

There are other reasons to be cautious about taking only beta-carotene since the other carotenoids are also known to have protective effects. Actually, the carotenoid lycopene, which gives tomatoes their red color, is ten times more potent than beta-carotene as an antioxidant, and apparently lowers rates of prostate cancer. A six-year study found that men of southern European ancestry were the most likely to eat tomato-based products, and the least likely to develop prostate cancer.

Sources of beta-carotene include yellow, orange, and green vegetables and fruits, such as apricots, broccoli, cantaloupe, carrots, mangoes, papayas, spinach, sweet potatoes, and turnip greens.

One final cautionary note is that the fat substitute olestra, according to some reports, dramatically interferes with the body's ability to absorb carotenoids. Since we need to get carotenoids as much as possible from the diet, olestra should be avoided.

These two much-heralded nutrients offer great promise in disease prevention. However, neither is a panacea, provident of perfect protection. In fact, for some people, these nutrients are distinctly problematic, particularly when ingested as supplements.

Surely, the same general principle holds true for many other common supplements. They can confer tremendous advantages but may not be as harmless as most people assume, and should be used cautiously.

SUPPLEMENTS:
WHAT WORKS AND WHAT DOES NOT WORK

Recently, the Third National Health and Nutrition Examination Survey showed that supplement use among adults ranges from about 36 to 51 percent. Furthermore, about 48 percent of children ages three to five take supplements. Currently, there are about six hundred supplement manufacturers in the United States, producing approximately four thousand products, with total annual sales of at least $4 billion and rising rapidly. Surveys indicate that consumers most often take supplements for disease prevention, boosting immunity, increasing energy, improving fitness, increasing alertness and mental activity, reducing stress, and treating medical problems.

For some time, the U.S. government has been concerned that consumers may be taking supplements for reasons that are not justified by scientific research. However, consumers are, for the most part, protected from unsafe products, because the government can remove supplements from the market if they present a significant or unreasonable risk of illness if used as recommended on the label.

Until recently, the literature used by distributors of dietary supplements was not allowed to contain health claims. A 1994 federal law changed this, and now publications that are reprinted in their entirety, and are not misleading, may be used in retail settings. Restrictions on labels are even more stringent; only a limited number of health claims is permitted on labels. Only four of these claims have been approved, including those dealing with the relationship between dietary calcium and osteoporosis; between folate and neural tube defects; between soluble fiber from whole oats and coronary heart disease; and between sugar alcohols and dental caries. Thus, the government remains conservative in its attitude toward supplements.

Among the supplements currently on the market are a number of controversial substances whose health benefits have not been definitively proven by RCTs. Some of the new substances have been popularized by special interest groups, such as bodybuilders, and by the lay press. Published research on such substances may lie outside mainstream medical literature.

Following is an analysis of some of the most popular of these substances. This analysis attempts to objectively assess the best existing research.

Selenium. Selenium is a trace mineral that has been the subject of extensive research and controversy. Found in brown rice, seafood, enriched white rice, whole wheat flour, and Brazil nuts, it is a powerful antioxidant, and is also a component of glutathione peroxidase, an antioxidant enzyme that helps to protect against free radical damage.

Much of the world's soil is deficient in selenium, which leads to low selenium intake. According to epidemiological studies, this accounts for an increased risk in certain regions of many kinds of cancer, including breast and colon cancer, and increased heart disease in certain regions. For example, people in selenium-depleted north-central China suffer some of the world's highest rates of esophageal and stomach cancer. However, these rates declined when some inhabitants were given selenium and vitamin E.

People need very little selenium to protect their health. For men, the RDA is 70 mcg (micrograms, or millionths of a gram), and for women it is 55 mcg. Many authorities now advise 200 to 400 mcg per day. However, 700 to 800 mcg a day may be toxic. Chronic ingestion of 5,000 mcg a day has been reported to result in fingernail changes, hair loss, nausea, abdominal pain, diarrhea, nerve problems, fatigue, and irritability. Because vitamin E enhances the effects of selenium, it can increase this possible toxicity.

Among the claims made for selenium are that it protects against cancer, improves immunity, protects against oxidative stress, prevents and treats AIDS-related pathology, and treats infertility. In actuality, though, RCTs present rather sketchy evidence of most of these claims.

- *High blood pressure in pregnancy.* According to a 1994 Chinese study by Han, pregnant women at risk for high blood pressure showed reduction and prevention of hypertension.
- *Cancer.* In 1996, an eight-year study by Dr. Larry C. Clarke at the University of Arizona revealed significant reductions in cancer mor-

tality among people taking 200·mcg daily. However, an analysis of Dutch cancer patients indicated that cancer patients did not have low levels of selenium in their bodies. Thus, selenium's role in cancer is unproven.

- *HIV.* A 1996 study of HIV patients by Delmas-Beauvieux showed that those receiving selenium had higher glutathione peroxidase activity, suggesting increased immune function.

Other conditions that showed an inconclusive reaction to selenium were myotonic dystrophy, asthma, and infertility. Also, selenium showed no ability to reduce oxidative stress in children with cystic fibrosis.

People with special antioxidant needs may benefit from moderate selenium supplementation, but most claims about selenium remain unproven.

Chromium. Chromium is necessary for insulin to function properly in the human body. Insulin not only helps to metabolize sugars, but is also involved in the body's use of protein and fats. Borderline chromium deficiency may help to trigger adult-onset diabetes, but is not the underlying cause of diabetes, so chromium cannot cure the disease.

A majority of the American population takes in less than the RDA of chromium. Estimates are that 50 percent of the American population has a marginal or serious chromium deficiency, especially the elderly, pregnant women, and athletes. Therefore, supplementation with 50 to 200 mcg may be prudent.

Chromium supplementation does present some dangers. Excess dietary chromium may accumulate in the tissues and cause chromosome damage, which may contribute to cancer. Daily supplementation of 200 mcg or more of chromium picolinate, an organic form of chromium, has been linked to iron deficiencies because chromium competes with iron for transport and distribution. Trivalent chromium, the form found in the diet, has very low toxicity and a great margin of safety, but hexavalent chromium is toxic, and long-term occupational exposure can lead to skin problems, perforated nasal septum, and lung cancer.

Among the claims made for chromium are that it promotes an increase in lean body mass, increases strength during resistance training, stabilizes blood sugar levels, and lowers cholesterol. Following is an examination of these claims.

- *Strength and lean body mass.* A 1989 study by Dr. Kenneth Cooper reported that football players were able to increase their muscle mass after taking 1.6 mg of chromium picolinate for two weeks, with total body fat decreasing from about 16 to 12 percent. This is a relatively high intake of chromium picolinate; some athletes take as little as 600 mcg a day (which is still equivalent to the dosage level that has produced chromosome damage in animals).

  However, two recent studies have contradicted the findings of this 1989 study. In a 1996 study reported in the *American Journal of Clinical Nutrition,* muscle mass increased with resistance training, regardless of chromium supplementation. In a 1994 University of Massachusetts study, the strength and body fat of athletes was unaffected by the supplementation.

  In a recent review of the clinical literature, Dr. Pamela Peeke, a National Institutes of Health researcher, failed to establish any beneficial effects of chromium supplementation on lean body mass and enhancement of strength. It appears as if the beneficial effects of chromium supplementation may occur only in individuals with impaired chromium status.

- *Weight loss.* Despite the negative findings of research on athletes, chromium supplementation was found in a recent study to help overweight people lose body fat and improve the ratio of lean to fat tissue. In a 1996 study by Dr. Gilbert R. Kaats, chromium supplementation at both 200 and 400 mcg daily resulted in significant fat loss.

- *Glucose tolerance.* Equivocal findings exist in studies that examine whether chromium helps to normalize blood sugar levels. Chromium supplementation can improve or normalize impaired glucose tolerance, but normal glucose tolerance is not further improved with chromium supplementation, according to studies by Anderson in 1991 and Abraham in 1992.

- *Blood lipids.* Some researchers have found no improvement in blood lipids with chromium supplementation, while others, including Press in 1990, have obtained more positive results. Many nutritional factors influence lipid metabolism, and it may be that only certain cases are related to a low chromium status because of impairment of glucose tolerance. These cases would be expected to improve with chromium supplementation.

In conclusion, because chromium deficiency seems to be widespread in the U.S. diet, individuals with impaired glucose tolerance or lipid metabolism may benefit from chromium supplementation, especially if testing shows low blood levels of chromium. For other people, it is probably wiser to rely on nutritional sources.

Chromium can be obtained in the diet from whole grains, brewer's yeast, wheat germ, liver, broccoli, prunes, nuts, cheese, and fortified cereals. One form of yeast, known as chromium-enriched yeast, has an even higher chromium content than brewer's yeast. Both of these forms of yeast contain GTF (glucose tolerance factor) chromium, which is much better absorbed by the body than the other forms.

Coenzyme Q_{10}. Coenzyme Q_{10}, also known as ubiquinone, acts like a vitamin in the body and works as a catalyst in chemical reactions, even though it is not actually an enzyme. It is found in every cell in the body. It has also shown potential as an antioxidant, helping to protect against free radicals. Its primary function in the body is to help convert food into energy.

Studies have suggested that coenzyme Q_{10} might be useful in protecting against tissue damage in heart disease, deterioration of the retina, breast cancer, and other illnesses. However, there have not yet been many large, well-designed studies on coenzyme Q_{10}.

Claims that have been made for coenzyme Q_{10} include that it slows aging by supporting immune functioning, prevents heart disease through its antioxidant action, and improves physical performance. No adverse effects have been reported.

- *Protection against tissue reperfusion, or restoration of blood flow, injury.* Coenzyme Q_{10} has shown promising results in protecting against injury from reperfusion, or rapid restoration of blood flow, to tissues after the blood supply has been stopped, as in heart attack or cardiac surgery. In a 1994 clinical trial in Italy by Chello, forty coronary artery bypass surgery patients who received 150 mg of Q_{10} a day for seven days before the operation showed less evidence of damage and a lower incidence of ventricular arrhythmias during the recovery period. However, when used just twelve hours before surgeries, Q_{10} showed no positive effect. Therefore, this application will remain a "gray area" until more large-scale studies are done.

- *Congestive heart failure.* Coenzyme Q_{10} has proven beneficial in patients with congestive heart failure. In a 1993 Italian study by Lampertico, supplementation produced improvement in a number of indicators of heart and lung function. However, the study had problems both in design and in the brevity of the treatment period. In another 1993 Italian RCT, this one by Morisco, patients using coenzyme Q_{10} required less hospitalization for worsening heart failure, and episodes of pulmonary edema or cardiac asthma were significantly reduced. Research in this area is still in the early stages, and it remains uncertain.

- *Muscle dystrophies.* Coenzyme Q_{10} was shown in two successful, small double-blind trials, both by Folkers in 1995, to improve physical performance in patients with a variety of muscular dystrophies and neurogenic atrophies. In both studies, definite improvement in physical performance was found in the patients receiving coenzyme Q_{10}. However, these were very small studies, performed by an ardent supporter of the nutrient.

- *Sports performance.* There have been claims that coenzyme Q_{10} can improve sports performance, but the evidence has largely been negative. In a 1991 study by Braun, triathletes and cyclists were not found to perform better after taking 100 mg a day of Q_{10} for four to eight weeks.

- *Cancer.* Coenzyme Q_{10}'s antioxidant activity has led to suggestions that it might be beneficial in the treatment of cancer. In one 1994 study by Lockwood, none of the patients in the supplemented group died, versus the predicted or expected mortality of four; none had further metastases; and six showed apparent partial remission. However, because a number of antioxidants were used, the results cannot be attributed to Q_{10} alone. Thus far, nothing definitive has been proven.

- *Gum disease.* In a study cited by Cooper in 1996, Japanese researchers reported in 1994 that coenzyme Q_{10} was used successfully in adult periodontitis, both as a treatment in itself and in combination with standard nonsurgical treatment. However, in 1995, researchers disputed this success in the *British Dental Journal*.

In conclusion, although research on coenzyme Q_{10} has yielded positive findings in some areas, its most promising applications appear to be in medical situations where the supervision of a physician is required. It has not been demonstrated that coenzyme Q_{10} is appropriate for use as a daily nutritional supplement among healthy people.

It is preferable to get coenzyme Q_{10} from food sources, which include spinach, sardines, and peanuts. However, some of these foods are high in fat.

Superoxide Dismutase (SOD). Superoxide dismutase, or SOD, is an extremely potent antioxidant that protects cells against damage from free radicals. It is one of the three main antioxidant enzymes found in our cells.

Human clinical studies of SOD are still at a very early stage, but some researchers claim it slows the aging process and has potential in treating Alzheimer's disease.

SOD supplements are sold in oral form, but consumers should be aware that oral SOD products are completely destroyed in the gut. Benefits of SOD come from injectable forms.

- *Skin problems and postradiation damage.* Although research is limited, a promising application of SOD is for severe skin diseases and radiation damage either from prolonged sun exposure or due to radiation treatment. One researcher, Michelson, has found SOD useful in treating various skin disorders, including a very severe case of scleroderma, an autoimmune disease. He also treated severe postradiation damage with two injections weekly for three months, with substantial improvement evident in two weeks. French and Japanese researchers have also reported positive results in treating scleroderma.
- *Arthritis.* SOD injections are used in Europe to treat musculoskeletal inflammation and osteoarthritis. Bovine SOD, injected into the joint, has been found beneficial in controlled double-blind studies in treating osteoarthritis of the knee. However, treatment of rheumatoid arthritis has been disappointing, according to Flohe in 1988.
- *Reperfusion or restoration of blood flow damage.* As with coenzyme Q_{10}, SOD is being investigated for its ability to protect against free radical damage, reducing injury to the brain and other organs caused by reperfusion, oxygen deprivation, drops in blood pressure, and increased cranial pressure after trauma.

  Based on a 1993 study by Marzi of patients with multiple injuries,

SOD helped to mitigate cardiovascular and lung failure, and reduced intensive care treatment and inflammation.

In a 1993 study of patients with severe head injuries, Muizelaar found that far fewer patients on high dosages of SOD died or lapsed into a vegetative state. Lower dosages did not help.

While SOD has shown exciting potential in this specialized medical application, results are not yet conclusive.

- *Anti-aging.* Despite claims, there is no evidence that SOD delays aging in humans. However, in animals, when both SOD and catalase are increased, maximum life span is significantly increased, according to a 1994 literature review by Warner.

Overall, SOD research is intriguing, but there is no form of SOD available to the public that will raise levels of SOD in the cells. It is much too early to recommend any use of SOD as an oral supplement, although it may have applications in specific medical treatments.

L-carnitine. L-carnitine is a substance that is essential for good health and for the regulation of fat oxidation in the body. Fatty acids are the main sources for energy production in the heart and the skeletal muscles, and these organs are especially vulnerable to L-carnitine deficiency. Symptoms of deficiency include muscle weakness, severe confusion, and angina.

Certain groups of people are at particular risk for L-carnitine deficiency, including kidney failure patients on hemodialysis, patients with liver failure, and patients receiving total parenteral (IV) nutrition. Some healthy individuals also have increased needs for dietary L-carnitine, including strict vegetarians, premature infants, pregnant women, and nursing mothers.

Dietary sources of L-carnitine are red meat, especially lamb and beef, and dairy products. There is little or no L-carnitine in vegetables, fruits, and cereals. How much L-carnitine is needed in the diet for optimal health is not known.

L-carnitine supplements are available in both the DL form and the L form. Only the L-carnitine form should be used, since the DL form has been shown to cause a muscle weakness syndrome in some individuals. Large doses of L-carnitine may cause diarrhea. Supplements may vary in purity.

Among the claims made for L-carnitine are that it increases blood flow and enhances energy production during exercise. Athletes and body-builders often use it.

- *Cardiovascular protection.* A number of well-designed clinical studies have shown that L-carnitine supplementation does have protective effects with heart patients. According to Bartels, Singh, and others, it appears to reduce angina and ischemia, and can significantly improve exercise duration. In patients with suspected myocardial infarction, it reduces infarction size, angina, cardiac death, and nonfatal infarction.
- *Exercise performance.* Evidence for improved exercise performance among athletes is not as convincing. In a 1997 review by Dr. Pamela Peeke, researchers found no controlled studies indicating improved physical performance in athletes. Two studies, one by Otto in 1987 and the other by Kasper in 1994, found that it did not produce an improvement for competitive runners.
- *Lipid metabolism.* Clinical studies are inconclusive on whether carnitine supplementation enhances the oxidation of fatty acids. A 1993 study by Natali found that L-carnitine did not influence lipid metabolism at rest, but did during exercise. However, two other studies found no effect, as reported by Decombaz in 1993 and Oyono-Enguelle in 1988.

While L-carnitine supplementation may help with deficiency states, there is little evidence that it helps healthy people.

Creatine. Creatine is an energy-producing substance that works as an energy storehouse and recharges the energy molecule adenosine triphosphate. Creatine is often used by bodybuilders and other athletes in high-intensity, explosive sports.

Dietary sources are meat and fish, though cooking can destroy it. Vegetarians are not able to get a presynthesized, concentrated form of creatine from their diet.

- *Supplementation increases muscle creatine.* In a 1995 study by Gordon of congestive heart failure patients, researchers found that creatine supplements did increase creatine phosphate in skeletal muscle, but only in patients whose total creatine level was relatively low to begin with. In this group, supplementation significantly increased strength and endurance.

- *Sports performance.* Creatine supplementation will not improve performance in endurance types of exercise, such as long-distance running, but does significantly improve performance in short-duration, high-intensity exercise. In a 1994 study of athletes by Birch in England, cellular energy production was higher and more efficient. A 1993 study by Dr. Paul Greenhaff found that creatine supplementation significantly increased performance of subjects doing maximal knee extensor exercise. According to Burke in 1996, a group of elite swimmers who received creatine supplementation showed no significant improvement. From a 1996 study of runners by Redondo, no statistically significant effect on sprint velocity was found.

Although creatine has no well-documented negative effects, supplementation does not seem necessary for daily maintenance of optimum health. However, it may help for specific power sports and bodybuilding. Athletes considering creatine supplementation for such purposes should consult with a sports medicine specialist.

DHEA. DHEA stands for dehydroepiandrosterone, a hormone that was first discovered in 1934. Its significance has been somewhat of a mystery ever since. Claims made for DHEA include that it prevents or slows the aging process, promotes weight loss, prevents or alleviates Alzheimer's disease, and combats AIDS, lupus, and some cancers. More than ten thousand scientific papers have been written about DHEA, and two international conferences have been held on DHEA research.

DHEA is the most abundant steroid hormone in our bodies. It is mainly produced in the adrenal glands, and also in the brain and skin. In the body, DHEA is converted in both men and women into estrogen, testosterone, and other steroid hormones. Production of DHEA peaks at about age thirty, and then gradually declines, reaching about 5 to 15 percent of the peak level at about age sixty. DHEA levels also drop during illness.

Research has shown that low DHEA levels in the blood are associated with heart disease, breast cancer, and a decline in immune competence. Most of the information about DHEA at present comes from animal studies, test tube experiments, and human population studies. Human clinical research is currently limited, with no long-term trials. It is not known at this point whether the effects of DHEA are due to the hormone itself or to the sex hormones and other steroids that the body produces, nor is it known which organs DHEA affects.

DHEA was found in one study to produce liver cancer in fourteen out of sixteen rats. While this does not necessarily mean that it would produce cancer in humans, if such a response were to occur in human research, DHEA would probably be banned by the FDA. Other studies have shown that DHEA supplementation can lead to increased insulin resistance, unwanted hair growth, and a drop in levels of "good" HDL. It must be remembered that DHEA is a hormone, and replacing any hormone that declines normally with aging must be carefully researched.

- *Aging.* Human studies on the effect of DHEA replacement on the aging process look promising, but it is too early to draw definite conclusions. In a 1994 study by Morales at the University of California at San Diego, people ages forty to seventy who took DHEA reported a substantial increase in physical and psychological well-being. However, HDL levels declined slightly in women.
- *Weight control.* Clinical research by Dr. William Regelson in 1996, done only on animals, showed that DHEA promoted weight loss in overweight animals even when they ate their usual diet. A 1991 human population study by Dr. Elizabeth Barrett-Connor found that lower DHEA levels in the blood were associated with increased body mass and impaired glucose tolerance.
- *Menopausal symptoms.* DHEA may help replace hormones in postmenopausal women, and thus protect against cancer, osteoporosis, and cardiac disease. Research is still preliminary, but in Europe, DHEA products are being marketed for menopause-related depression, and are being used in conjunction with estrogen to treat hot flashes and other menopausal symptoms. In a Canadian study by Dr. Pierre Diamond of twenty postmenopausal women, DHEA yielded reductions in blood insulin and glucose levels. Weight remained the same, but there was an improvement in the body muscle–to-fat ratio, an increase in bone density, a drop in blood cholesterol, and an improvement in vaginal atrophy and secretions.

    Studies by Casson in 1993 and 1995 also suggest that DHEA may help postmenopausal women, affording protection against heart disease by reducing blood lipid levels.

- *Heart disease.* DHEA may help to protect against heart disease in people besides postmenopausal women. A 1995 study by Herrington, reported at the New York Academy of Sciences, found significantly lower blood levels of DHEA in men who had blocked arteries. Another study reported at the conference showed DHEA supplementation reduced platelet aggregation, or the tendency of blood cells to stick together. Excessive platelet aggregation is another risk factor for cardiovascular disease.
- *Immune problems.* Researchers have reported that DHEA activated immune system functioning. In a 1993 study by Casson, 25 mg daily improved immune regulating response in postmenopausal women.

    There is some suggestion that autoimmune disorders also respond. In a 1995 study by Dr. Ronald van Vollenhoven of the Stanford University School of Medicine, twenty-five female lupus patients who received 200 mg of DHEA showed improvement in their symptoms, had more energy, and were able to reduce their prednisone dosage.

In conclusion, while popular literature enthusiastically endorses the use of DHEA, it is too early to recommend routine supplementation. Anyone considering DHEA supplementation should have their DHEA levels checked to make sure that they are low. Serum levels of steroids should be monitored medically while taking DHEA supplements. DHEA is not fat soluble, so any fat in a meal will block absorption of the supplement. Letting DHEA absorb under the tongue is one way to bypass the intestinal tract, but some people object to the taste. Since blood levels of DHEA are highest in the morning, supplemental DHEA should be taken in the morning, to follow the body's natural rhythm.

Because DHEA is converted into steroid hormones, it is not known what its impact might be on cancers that are sensitive to hormones. There is some evidence that DHEA exacerbates breast cancer, and possibly prostate cancer. If any kind of cancer is present, DHEA supplementation should not be undertaken without medical approval.

Melatonin. Melatonin is one of the new "miracle" hormones being widely promoted today. It is produced by the pineal gland, which begins to shrink at about age twenty, with an accompanying steady decrease in melatonin production of about 1 percent a year. Calcification of the pineal gland occurs in many people over sixty.

Melatonin helps regulate the body's sleep cycle. Light suppresses melatonin production, and dark stimulates it, inducing drowsiness. Older people with sleep problems often have low levels of melatonin.

Melatonin is popular as an aid for sleep, jet lag, and insomnia caused by working at night. It has also been claimed that melatonin is a powerful antioxidant that helps with aging and immunity, and reduces the risk of cancer and heart disease.

Research on melatonin is still in the preliminary stages, with most of the work having been done in animal studies or small studies of human subjects, often not completely controlled.

- *Sleep disorders.* A number of small studies indicate that melatonin helps people sleep and thus improves daytime alertness and well-being. Researchers usually give 2 mg at bedtime for sleep, but some individuals need as little as 0.5 mg. Other people, however, are stimulated by melatonin, or have nightmares or hangovers. Also, a 1997 paper by the National Sleep Foundation claimed it may harm the reproductive system.

- *Phase shift regulation.* Some small studies of night-shift workers have shown that melatonin helps people adjust to phase shifts. However, in studies by Folkard and Dawson, the use of bright light was generally more effective than melatonin in producing adaptation to changed sleep time. Studies of phase shift regulation remain inconclusive, since the groups studied have been quite small, and since the results were not always in favor of melatonin.

- *Jet lag.* Larger studies of airline crews and travelers found that melatonin helped adjustment to jet lag. Optimal timing of melatonin doses to prevent jet lag was different in different studies. In a 1993 study by Petrie, 5 mg doses were begun on arrival at the destination and continued for five days. In an earlier study by Petrie, jet lag was reduced by taking 5 mg of melatonin three days before the flight, during the flight, and once a day for three days after arrival.

- *Cancer treatment.* In a 1996 Italian study by Dr. Paoli Lissoni, thirty patients with brain tumors received either radiation therapy alone or radiation plus melatonin. Survival was higher in patients receiving the melatonin. Also, side effects of cancer immunotherapy were reduced with melatonin. From another study of thirty patients with gastrointestinal cancer, immune functioning after surgery was improved by melatonin and immunotherapy.

• *Protection of tissues.* Melatonin's protective effect against potentially harmful drugs and radiation may be due in part to its antioxidant properties. It is a potent scavenger of the hydroxyl radical, perhaps the most active of all the free radicals. In this capacity, melatonin is said to help retard the aging process. It is also believed to stimulate the production of glutathione peroxidase, which plays an important role in neutralizing free radicals. Also, it has been hypothesized by Reiter in 1995 that the waning of melatonin levels acts as a switch for programmed aging of the cells.

In the final analysis, the research on melatonin remains inconclusive. In addition, there are some warnings and contraindications that need to be observed. Some studies suggest that melatonin can deepen or induce depression and exacerbate allergies. Melatonin counteracts the effects of cortisone, so patients taking cortisone should avoid it. Also, some preliminary data suggest that melatonin may cause constriction of blood vessels, may inhibit fertility, may suppress the male sexual drive, and may produce hypothermia and retinal damage. As with any powerful hormone, melatonin should not be taken by pregnant women.

Another concern is the purity of the product. Quality of this hormone is not currently regulated by the FDA, and some products are inferior.

While melatonin does seem to have exciting potential, it is much too early to recommend taking such a powerful substance as an over-the-counter supplement. Anyone considering taking it for sleep or jet lag should receive medical clearance.

Testosterone. Testosterone is the primary male sex hormone. It is produced in both men and women, and is responsible for promoting sexual desire in both sexes. Levels of testosterone decline with aging, though the decline is not as sharp and dramatic as the decline of estrogen in women at menopause. Impotence in older men is due in some cases to declining testosterone levels. If testosterone deficiencies are found in men with impotence, injections of testosterone can sometimes help to overcome the problem.

When testosterone was first identified in the 1930s, it was hailed as a miracle substance that could slow aging. It was used to restore libido and mental and physical energy among older adults. When it was discovered that large doses could promote prostate cancer, its use declined. Currently, though, it is being used increasingly to treat aging men with slight reductions in testosterone levels.

Some women, too, are receiving testosterone replacement therapy after menopause. Women normally produce small amounts of testosterone, just as men produce small quantities of estrogen. In younger women, testosterone levels rise just before ovulation, producing a surge in libido. By age forty, testosterone levels in women have declined to only half their value at age twenty, partly owing to the decline in DHEA, the hormone used by the body to make testosterone.

- *Strength and muscle mass.* Bodybuilders and other athletes, both men and women, have been using testosterone and other anabolic, or muscle building, steroids to build muscle and lean body mass. Unfortunately, the high doses of steroids used by athletes have been linked to heart disease, stroke, cardiomyopathy, and possibly cancer. Other adverse effects include liver toxicity, decreases in plasma testosterone, atrophy of the testes, prostate enlargement, impotence, decreased sperm count, breast enlargement in men, increased injury of muscles and tendons, increased serum cholesterol, and decreased HDL. Psychological side effects can include euphoria, aggressiveness, irritability, nervous tension, changes in libido, mania, and psychosis. Female athletes have less-well-documented side effects, including irreversible lowering of the voice, increased libido, menstrual disturbances, aggressiveness, acne, increased body hair, and clitoral enlargement.
- *Arthritis.* Testosterone has been studied as a treatment for rheumatoid arthritis, with equivocal results. In a 1996 study by Booji, it caused improvement in rheumatoid arthritis symptoms. However, in a 1996 study by Hall, there was no significant effect on the disease.

Testosterone is not available as a dietary supplement. It is available only by prescription and is relatively expensive, at fifty to one hundred dollars a month. Besides injections, testosterone is now available in a new patch that can be worn on any part of the body, making it easier to use.

It was formerly available in the United States only by injection, or by a patch worn on the scrotum. In Europe, testosterone is available in pills, but these have not been approved for use in the United States.

To summarize, testosterone is appropriate for severe testosterone deficiency, and for older men, and perhaps women, whose low testosterone levels have caused loss of libido. However, even in small doses, it can encourage prostate tumors. Testosterone also increases the risk of stroke.

Testosterone is a very powerful hormone that can have very serious side effects, and should only be used under appropriate medical supervision.

CREATING A PERSONALIZED NUTRITIONAL PROGRAM

Biochemical individuality means that we all have slightly different dietary needs, based on our genetic endowment, exercise level, metabolic function, state of health, geographic location, and other factors. To sort out what this means in terms of diet and supplement choices, professional help is available from a number of disciplines.

Before making radical changes in your diet or lifestyle, remember that in order to maintain new health behaviors, these changes need to be supported by many sources, such as family and friends. Enlist the cooperation and encouragement of family and friends, and reinforce your decisions by reading material that underscores the benefits of the changes you are planning. If you are making significant changes in your diet, such as adopting a more plant-based or vegetarian diet, make every effort to ensure that your new diet is appealing to all your senses and includes a variety of colors, tastes, and aromas. This not only whets the appetite, it also helps to ensure that your diet will provide all the protective nutrients your body requires. Even a weight-loss regimen need not produce a feeling of deprivation. A slimming diet rich in grains, legumes, fresh fruits, and vegetables can be very satisfying and appealing to the senses.

It is wise to consult with your doctor or nutritionist before undertaking any supplementation beyond the use of antioxidant vitamins such as C, E, the B vitamins, and calcium/magnesium for women who require calcium throughout their lives as one deterrent to osteoporosis. Maintaining a balanced ratio of calcium to magnesium can also be delicate. Trained professionals are able to evaluate whether any medications or health conditions would contraindicate the use of the more controversial substances discussed above.

Many of the more controversial supplements have had intriguing claims made for their anti-aging and longevity properties, and research has begun to document the potential value of some of these substances for restoring and preserving youthful vigor. However, no nutrient, supplement, or magic bullet can take the place of a balanced, well-rounded diet and a lifestyle conducive to optimal health. Regular exercise, social engagement and support, good stress management practices, a feeling of optimism, and a sense of purpose in life are all just as important as any supplements you might take in assuring you a long and healthy life. Positive mental attitude grows out of and reinforces good dietary practices. Each positive lifestyle habit you cultivate magnifies and multiplies itself throughout every aspect of your life. When you know that you have made dietary changes that will be beneficial for you, your feeling of self-worth and empowerment will improve along with your level of physical well-being. Even older adults with chronic diseases have a better prospect for survival and for less troublesome symptoms when they know that they have control over those areas in their lives where they can exercise choice.

CHAPTER 4

TRADITIONAL CHINESE MEDICINE

Three Thousand Years of Evolution

Traditional Chinese medicine (TCM) is the contemporary version of the three-thousand-year-old medical practice of China. TCM is a complete theoretical and therapeutic system, and includes a variety of carefully formulated techniques, such as acupuncture, herbal medicine, massage, Qi Gong, and nutrition.

Presently, about one-quarter of the world's population uses TCM. In various forms, TCM has spread to Japan, Korea, Southeast Asia, Europe, and the Americas. In the United States, some twelve million people currently go to TCM practitioners. Out of the estimated $14 billion a year that Americans spend on alternative medicine, TCM accounts for $1 billion, 75 percent of which goes for acupuncture.

Developing out of shamanic and tribal origins, Chinese medicine evolved with Chinese culture. Early written accounts of TCM, dating from 180 B.C., describe herbs that are still used extensively. At about 100 B.C., the doctrines of TCM were codified in a series of classic texts, including *The Yellow Emperor's Classic of Internal Medicine*. Subsequent practitioners expanded on these texts.

By the time of the 1949 Communist revolution, China had been significantly Westernized, and TCM was not widely relied upon. However, faced with severe public health crises, the Communist regime reintroduced TCM, purging it of ineffective measures and pragmatically developing interventions that worked. Chinese TCM medical colleges updated their curricula, and researchers were sent into the Chinese countryside to interview traditional peasant healers. This led to the widespread introduction of many new remedies.

Today, practitioners of TCM in China are trained in well-organized schools and practice TCM in conjunction with Western medicine. Similarly, many conventional Japanese physicians also now prescribe traditional herbal formulas.

Chinese medicine was originally introduced into the United States during the 1700s by French-trained European practitioners. In the 1800s, Asian immigrants brought Chinese medicine with them to America. In the 1970s, with the normalization of United States–Chinese relations, new enthusiasm for TCM was created, especially for acupuncture. Currently, about fifty colleges of acupuncture and TCM exist in America and have licensed about ten thousand practitioners. Chinese medicine has been embraced by many American CAM practitioners, including a number of naturopathic and chiropractic physicians who employ elements of TCM in their eclectic mix of interventions.

Even when applied by Western doctors, though, TCM differs markedly from Western medicine in its philosophy and practice. With historical roots in Taoism, Confucianism, and Buddhism, TCM emphasizes the wholeness of body, mind, and spirit, and the unity of the individual with the natural environment. In contrast, the Western rational tradition tends to separate body, mind, and spirit, and to discount the importance of a patient's physical as well as psychosocial environment.

TCM does not conceptualize diseases as they are understood in the West. Whereas Western medicine focuses on the diagnosis and treatment of specific diseases, TCM focuses on the patient, identifying patterns of disharmony and imbalance that may ultimately lead to disease. Rather than addressing individual organ systems and the symptoms that arise in them, the TCM practitioner looks at the interplay among the symptoms and among the organs, defining a comprehensive syndrome that represents the state of the whole person. Thus, in TCM, people who have similar symptoms may be diagnosed as having completely different syndromes.

Central to Chinese medicine is the concept of *qi* (pronounced *chee*), which is the vital energy, or life force, that animates all living beings and the entire universe. According to Chinese medicine, *qi* travels through a system of energy channels, or meridians, which flow along the surface of the body and through the internal organs. In Chinese medicine, a balanced, harmonious flow of *qi* naturally creates a state of health. Illness results when *qi* is blocked or unbalanced. Thus, TCM emphasizes prevention and health promotion, rather than disease intervention.

Of central importance to TCM is the polarity of *yin* and *yang*, the feminine and masculine entities. Yin is associated with the feminine, passive, dark, and inner qualities, and yang with the masculine, active, light, and outer qualities. Yin and yang must be in balance for health to be present. Yin and yang influence and evolve into one another, so that by acting on the yang, TCM can change the yin, and vice versa. Acupuncture, as one modality of TCM, seeks to balance yin and yang by influencing the flow of *qi* energy through the body.

Another way of viewing the relationship between yin and yang is by considering the Five Elements, which represent successive phases in the transformation of yin and yang, in an eternal cycle. These Five Elements are fire, earth, metal, water, and wood. According to the Five Element theory, each of these elements (or different expressions of the balance of yin and yang) are reflected by specific seasons of the year, and by specific organs of the body. For example, water is the elemental energy state of extreme yin, and predominates during the winter, when the energy of nature is withdrawn. Within the body, water is associated with the kidney as a solid, or yin, organ, and with the bladder as a yang, or hollow, organ.

Patterns of disharmony within the individual are also described in terms of the Eight Principles, or four pairs of complementary opposites. These four opposites are interior-exterior, cold-hot, deficiency-excess, and yin-yang.

Overall, TCM views health and illness in very different terms from Western medicine. However, even though TCM clinicians employ a vastly different healing system, they often achieve results that are similar to those achieved by Western doctors.

The Methods Used in TCM

Diagnosis

For diagnosis, TCM practitioners closely observe the patient's outward appearance; they listen to the voice and breath, and note the smell of the breath, skin, and secretions. They question the patient closely about current complaints, family health history, personal health history, and lifestyle. Through touch (or palpation) they examine the skin, muscles, pulse, joints, and *qi*-based diagnostic points.

However, unlike Western medicine, in which the pulse is taken simply to determine the heart rate, taking the pulse in Chinese medicine is a complex and subtle procedure. Pulses are felt at six locations and three depths on each wrist, and are believed to have twenty-eight qualities. As one instance, a slow or tense pulse points to a cold syndrome, and a weak or thin pulse indicates deficiency. Pulses help the practitioner to determine the condition of *qi*.

In TCM, the tongue is believed to be another mirror of the body, so TCM practitioners observe its color, texture, thickness, indentations, and coating.

Based on all this information, the practitioner notes the patient's pattern of disharmony. He or she then applies some or all of the following modalities.

- *Acupuncture,* which is the primary TCM intervention used in the United States today.
- *Moxibustion,* in which acupuncture points are stimulated with heat.
- *Cupping,* in which a warm, hollow jar is placed on the skin to increase circulation.
- *Massage and manipulation,* in which fingertip or hand pressure is applied to the acupuncture points.
- *Herbal medicine,* which is the dominant TCM intervention in China.
- *Qi Gong,* which is an ancient system of exercise that integrates movement, breath, and meditation to help the flow of *qi.*

- *Diet and nutrition,* in which an individualized diet is based on the patient's constitution and pattern of illness.

Frequently, each one of these modalities is used in a comprehensive, synergistic program that balances the body's energy systems and stimulates vitality and immunity.

Chinese Herbal Medicine

Because herbal medicine is the most dominant TCM intervention worldwide, we will examine it in some depth. It is important to note that although we have attempted wherever possible to provide dosages, indications, contraindications, and cautions in Part II, it is essential, before using TCM or any other herbals, for patients to review the research and work with a certified TCM clinician. TCM herbals are very potent.

In purchasing any herbals, including TCM, it is imperative to identify a quality manufacturer, preferably one in or subject to U.S. regulatory oversight. Underscoring this point is a study reported in late 1998 in the *New England Journal of Medicine.* For the development of a computer database of Asian patent medicines, the California Department of Health Services, Food and Drug Branch, studied 260 such preparations collected from California retail herbal stores. Using gas chromatography, mass spectrometry, and atomic absorption methods, the department found that at least 83 of the 260, or 32 percent, contained undeclared pharmaceuticals or heavy metals, while 23 of the 260 had more than one contaminant. Although the majority of the products were tested as accurately labeled and safe, the large percentage of contaminated herbals requires the utmost caution.

About 85 percent of Chinese herbs are derived from plants, about 12 percent are from animals, and about 3 percent come from minerals. TCM herbal materials are generally processed in much the same way as Western herbal medicines. The active part of the plant is separated from the rest of the plant and is cleaned, freed of toxins, dried, and prepared for use. These herbs are then employed in the following forms:

Crude herbs are boiled to make herbal decoctions or strong teas. This is the preferred method of administering herbs among native Chinese practitioners.

Dried decoctions. For convenience, herbal teas can also be made from dried powder. These powders are imported to America from Taiwan, and are also manufactured in the United States by Taiwanese companies.

Patent medicines. Herbs are often combined in complex formulas, known as patent medicines. Patent medicine pills are relatively inexpensive, and are convenient. Some also contain Western drugs. However, there is no American quality control over imported products.

American pills and extracts. Several American companies now make Chinese herbal formulas. Most notably, the Sun Ten Laboratories in Irvine, California, produce herbal supplements to the same standards found among pharmaceutical manufacturers. They tend to be more expensive, but are more uniform in quality, are accurately labeled, and do not contain Western drugs. However, little clinical research has been done on these preparations.

TCM herbs are not prescribed on the basis of their chemistry, as we would understand it in the West. Instead, they are used to introduce certain influences into the body, in order to balance and harmonize the patient's vital energy. This energy is considered to be the primary healing force in TCM.

Chinese herbs are also prescribed on the basis of the Five Elements. Each of the elemental qualities is associated with a characteristic flavor. Wood, for example, is associated with a sour taste. Furthermore, medicinal herbs are also said to have the four natures of hot, cold, warm, and cool. Additionally, a fifth characteristic is identified as bland, which mediates between the others. California acupuncturist Al Stone, in his well-documented acupuncture site on the Internet, has offered an insightful example of how herbs are prescribed. In the case of an arthritis patient whose symptoms are aggravated by damp weather, the TCM interpretation would be that there has been an invasion of cold and damp into the acupuncture meridians and they are lodged in the joints. An herb used to treat this condition might be one that grows in a cold, damp climate, such as sea vine bark. Although this treatment might sound nonrational by the standards of Western medicine, it can, like a great many TCM herbal treatments, be quite effective.

TCM herbs seem to be particularly effective when used in combinations, or formulas. A formula often consists of the principal herb, or King herb; the associate, or Minister; the adjuvant, or Assistant; and the guiding herb, or Messenger. A King herb focuses on the main symptoms and dominates the formula. A Minister herb strengthens the effect of the King herb. An Assistant herb has a variety of different actions, including the treatment of less important symptoms, and the reduction of the toxicity or irritating properties of the King herb. A Messenger herb coordinates the effects of the other herbs, and delivers the herbs to a particular site in the body.

Clearly, Chinese herbal medicine operates on an entirely different principle from the reductionist approach of Western biomedicine, including Western herbalism. Modern Western medicine generally seeks to find a single active agent to address a specific complaint, whereas TCM herbal preparations employ a combination of medicinal substances with complementary qualities. With combinations of herbs, the overall impact of the formula is less drastic, and is intended primarily to harmonize the function of the organs and the *qi*.

There are 5,767 TCM herbs, but only about 235 are commonly used. In Japan, the national health insurance system recognizes 148 TCM formulas and 118 herbs.

Following are some of the TCM herbs that are commonly used in the United States today.

- *Ginseng (Panax ginseng, ren shen).* Ginseng root is highly valued as an adaptogen, which helps the body adapt to change, and thus prevent stress-related illness.
- *Tang kuei (Angelica sinensis). Tang kuei* is considered an excellent herb for women, but in complex formulas can be used by men to nourish the blood, improve circulation, calm nervous tension, and relieve pain.
- *Ma huang (Ephedra sinensis). Ma huang* is used as a stimulant; it opens the breathing passages, relieves lung congestion, and enhances weight loss. Its alkaloid components, ephedrine and pseudoephedrine, have both been made into modern drugs.
- *Licorice (Glycyrrhiza uralensis; gan cao).* This root is used to neutralize toxins, relieve inflammation, enhance digestion, and to treat hepatitis, sore throat, muscle spasm, and other ailments. It is present in about one-third of all Chinese herbal prescriptions, and is thought to enhance the effectiveness of many herbal formulas.

Excessive consumption over an extended period can cause a sodium-potassium imbalance, with symptoms of fluid retention or rapid heartbeat.

- *Ginger (Zingiber officinale; sheng jiang).* Spicy ginger root is beneficial to digestion, neutralizes toxins in foods, increases circulation to the limbs, clears the lungs, and soothes nausea.
- *Cinnamon (Cinnamomum cassia; kuei pi).* Cinnamon is used to warm the body, invigorate circulation, and harmonize upper and lower body energy. In large quantities, it can irritate the liver, and should not be used by people with inflammatory liver disease.
- *Coptis (Coptis chinensis; huang lian).* Rich in alkaloids, it combats infection and calms the nerves. One of its active ingredients, berberine, has broad antimicrobial activity. Coptis is closely related to the bitter American herb goldenseal.
- *Peony (Paeonia albiflora; pai shao).* Peony root is used to regulate the blood. It regulates blood vessels, reduces platelet stickiness, and helps promote circulation. Peony is also often used to help balance the female hormonal system.
- *Bupleurum (Bupleurum chinense).* One of the most frequently used herbs in Japanese herbal medicine, it has been used in Japan for treating liver disease, skin ailments, arthritis, menopausal symptoms, corticosteroid withdrawal, ulcers, and mental disorders.
- *Astragalus (Astragalus membranaceus; huang ch'i).* Probably the most commonly used herb today in China, it normalizes immune functions and has applications in immune deficiencies, autoimmune disease, and allergies. It is also beneficial to digestion, and to the skin, and is included in many formulas to promote the function of other herbs. Also it has been used in the treatment of AIDS and hepatitis.
- *Salvia (Salvia miltiorrhiza; dan shen).* Salvia is used in coronary artery disease, and in other cases where there has been damage to body tissues, including after a stroke or a traumatic injury. It is also used for chronic inflammation, infection, and degenerative diseases. Additionally, it promotes circulation in the capillary beds, reduces blood pressure and cholesterol, and helps liver function.

Many modern pharmaceuticals have been derived from TCM herbs. GBE, an extract of *Ginkgo biloba,* is used to treat cerebral insufficiency. Tanshinone IIA, isolated from salvia, is a coronary vasodilator. Sodium ferulate, derived from *tang kuei,* is an antiplatelet agent. Quercitin, derived from a variety of herbs, has anti-ischemic effects. Antiepilepsirine, derived from *Piper nigrum,* is a potent anticonvulsant. Huperzine A, from *Huperzia serrata,* is used to treat myasthenia gravis and senile dementia. What was considered alternative is now conventional! This, of course, indicates that these herbs do, indeed, have potent qualities and play a vital role in the future of integrative medicine.

For acute ailments, Chinese herbs might need to be taken for only one or two days, but for chronic problems, they can be taken for many months, or even years. It is unusual in the West to use herbs for such a long period of time, since they tend to be thought of as short-term treatments, like drugs. However, because herbs have milder effects than the drugs that are manufactured from them, long-term use usually doesn't cause side effects. In fact, the ingredients of these herbs are generally eliminated from the system in about four hours.

Also, the potentially toxic qualities of herbs are usually balanced by other herbs. In addition, toxic herbs are usually refined, to eliminate their harmful effects. Contaminants may be present in some TCM formulas in the form of Western drugs, perhaps toxic metals, and fecal matter. Generally, crude Chinese herbs are as safe as those used in Western herbal medicine. Even so, pregnant women and nursing mothers should be cautious about Chinese herbs, and people taking other medicines should be alert for drug interactions. For utmost safety, anyone taking TCM herbs should discuss this use with his or her physician.

MEDICAL USE OF TCM

Traditional Chinese medicine is an integral part of the health care system of China, helping to provide affordable health care for China's 1.3 billion people. TCM is also proving an effective complement to modern Western medicine in China.

In the United States, acupuncture is the most popular component of TCM. However, American schools of acupuncture are adding courses in Chinese herbal medicine, massage, and diet and nutrition, to reflect the full range of TCM interventions.

Growth of TCM in the United States is limited in part by a lack of adequate insurance coverage. Although acupuncture is frequently covered, herbal medicines often are not covered. Until more studies are done, it is unlikely that insurance companies will cover TCM herbs, and this will undoubtedly stunt the growth of Chinese herbal use in America.

However, despite lack of insurance coverage, there is an ethnic Chinese population who regularly patronize TCM practitioners, many of whom are essentially practicing underground. A recent survey of Chinese Americans revealed that first- and second-generation Chinese immigrants tend to use Chinese therapies at a rate of 44 and 42 percent, respectively. In New York's Chinatown, rheumatism is the complaint for which Chinese Americans most frequently seek TCM treatment. Chinese Americans in San Francisco's Chinatown most often use TCM for the treatment of rheumatism, bruises, and sprains.

In the United States, TCM may be a reasonable first choice of treatment for people who are marginalized by the present health care system. Those without health insurance may find TCM more affordable than insurance. A monthly TCM office visit and a month's supply of herbs averages about $120, while a group insurance plan averages about $160. For people who distrust conventional medicine, TCM offers a possible alternative, especially since it is currently licensed in thirty-four states. For people who don't regularly see doctors, going to a TCM practitioner could help reveal a medical problem, and help avoid a trip to an emergency room, which is often where sick people go when they don't have a family doctor.

In conventional medical facilities where TCM is offered, TCM may be the most reasonable first approach for certain conditions. If the patient has a condition that is not life-threatening and does not require a detailed medical diagnosis, then TCM might be tried first. This type of condition might include back pain, physical stress, PMS, mild digestive problems, minor infections, colds, flu, bronchitis, or sinusitis. Treatment with TCM generally produces positive changes within one to three months. If the problem persists, conventional care could be applied.

For the treatment of more serious diseases, TCM can be used in conjunction with Western medicine. This combined approach could help to reduce the amount of drug therapy, to help avoid surgery, and to enhance the outcome of conventional therapies.

A number of clinical trials indicate the value of TCM. Decisions about using TCM, however, should not be based solely on whether clinical trials support TCM use for particular illnesses. Such evidence is now generally lacking, and unnecessarily limits the application of TCM. Even the well-designed research that does exist can only offer examples of limited ways in which TCM can be used, without proving the efficacy of the system as a whole.

Another situation in which TCM can be appropriately used is in the treatment of terminal patients. Chinese medicine can help make these patients more comfortable and reduce their need for drugs.

In the United States, some practitioners are successfully integrating Western medicine and TCM, and currently at the Center for Integrated Medicine in Houston, Dr. Christina Stemmler, formerly of Duke University, uses both TCM and various Western modalities.

However, other doctors in the United States are practicing a hybrid form of Chinese medicine, in which they administer Chinese herbs as homeopathic preparations, herbal tinctures, or other low-dosage preparations, which is not part of the traditional practice of TCM. Such remedies have not yet been proven effective, so consumers should be cautious.

When used in conjunction with Western medicine, TCM herbal medicine has become a popular approach in the United States for addressing certain life-threatening diseases, particularly cancer and AIDS.

Writing in *Choices in Healing,* Dr. Michael Lerner has observed that TCM is the most popular nonconventional treatment used by Western cancer patients. TCM has no treatments that are used solely for cancer, but offers many formulas that help with various symptoms of cancer, including edema and pain. In addition, approximately 120 species of Chinese herbs are sometimes used to adjunctively treat cancer. Although the TCM view of cancer causation is quite different from the Western view, many TCM herbal formulas contain ingredients that have been proven pharmacologically active in treating cancer. TCM herbal therapies have already led to the development of a number of anticancer drugs, such as indirubin, derived from *dang gui lu hui wan,* and irisquinone, derived from *Iris lacteapallasii.*

WHAT WORKS

Based on the reliable TCM clinical research, the findings indicate:

- One widely used Chinese herbal remedy that has shown promise in cancer treatment is Juzentaihoto, or JT-48 or JTT. Traditionally used in anemia, loss of appetite, and extreme exhaustion, this herbal remedy is proving helpful for cancer when it is used in combination with chemotherapy and radiation. It also helps to prevent leukemia in cancer patients who are undergoing chemotherapy, according to Yamada in 1989.

- In a controlled clinical trial at the National Cancer Center Hospital in Tokyo, patients with advanced metastatic breast cancer were given chemotherapy and endocrine therapy alone, or in combination with Juzentaihoto. After thirty-eight months, the survival rate was significantly higher in the group receiving the Chinese herbal remedy. Herbal patients also showed improved quality of life, and were protected from the suppression of bone marrow, which is associated with chemotherapy.

- At the University of Texas, Chen found that an extract of the Chinese herb astragalus increased the anticancer activity of killer cells. When people with cancer took astragalus, they required only one-tenth as much toxic chemotherapy.

- In Chinese cancer hospitals, chemotherapy and radiation are often combined with TCM herbs, thus permitting lower doses of chemotherapy.

- Among people with HIV and AIDS, acupuncture and Chinese herbs are also considered the most promising unconventional approach. TCM reduces side effects of conventional medications and increases their efficacy.

Unfortunately, several problems have hampered research on TCM and AIDS. In a study by Dr. Donald Abrams in San Francisco, TCM clinicians were reluctant to apply a uniform herbal treatment, instead of one that was individualized. Furthermore, the FDA required lengthy testing of the herbs that were used in the study, despite the fact that they were already available in health food stores. In another study by Abrams, the TCM herbs that were tested were used at a dosage that was too low by TCM standards. In another, similarly ill-conceived study, researchers at San Francisco General Hospital tested the TCM herb *tang kuei* for treating menopausal symptoms and concluded that it had no effect. However, although the study employed sound methodology with reasonable dosage, it ignored the fact that *tang kuei* is not used alone for treating menopause in China, but is included as a minor constituent. Apparently the study was undertaken on the basis of reports that women in San Francisco were attempting to use the herb to treat menopausal symptoms. In this case, the application of the reductionist Western medical model reduced the research to meaninglessness.

These problems indicate the clash of philosophies between TCM and Western medicine, as well as the politicization that often clouds research.

Despite these research difficulties, however, many Western clinicians remain convinced of TCM's efficacy. According to Dr. Christina Stemmler, Chinese medicine, including acupuncture, is at least as good as Western medicine, if not better, for quickly resolving 90 percent of the common health problems that most patients suffer, without producing the cascade of side effects caused by Western drugs.

Prevention is another strength of Chinese medicine, since it can help to identify warning signals and reverse underlying problems before disease begins. Moreover, TCM's diagnostic procedures may help to detect very subtle symptoms that conventional diagnoses miss.

Serious, advanced diseases are more difficult to treat with TCM, but TCM can provide important supportive treatment. Even if TCM cannot reverse cancer, it can help to relieve pain, improve appetite, improve general functioning, and increase the sense of well-being. However, the efficacy of Chinese medicine is much more limited in surgery, emergency medicine, and trauma care—areas where Western medicine excels.

In addition, TCM is not always effective at quickly solving serious problems. Some ailments may require up to two years of regular, vigorous treatment. In our time-driven Western culture, Chinese medicine may try the patience of many people.

Furthermore, research has not definitively demonstrated the cost-effectiveness of TCM. It does appear, though, as if the costs of TCM are usually reasonable. Office visits to licensed acupuncturists generally average about $55, with the first visit typically being 50 percent higher. Office visits may be recommended at a rate of one per week, for the administration of acupuncture, moxibustion, massage, and the prescribing of herbs. If herbs alone are used, office visits might be at three- to four-week intervals. Herbal prescriptions typically cost the patient about $2 to $4 a day. If a standard course of therapy is one to three months, then the total cost of TCM treatment would be about $300 to $800. Compared to conventional medicine, these costs are modest. Some insurance companies cover TCM, and others offer discounts on the services of certain providers. Also, several clinics in the United States, especially at TCM colleges, offer discounted fees. In addition, subsidized clinics exist for treating addictions and HIV infection. Some individual practitioners also treat patients on a sliding scale.

CLINICAL RESEARCH ON TCM

Chinese medical tradition includes a long history of research, dating back thousands of years. Early masters of herbal knowledge conducted crude empirical research to determine the actions of plants. In fact, documented research on TCM herbs was begun about fifteen centuries before the first empirical research on Western drugs was begun. There is an element of either ignorance or arrogance in the frequent Western assumption that TCM is based largely on anecdotal evidence.

Furthermore, in modern China, a plethora of research is now being conducted. There are more than one hundred Chinese medical journals currently providing reports on TCM research. Even so, some of this research is considered suspect by many Western physicians, mostly because of the innate philosophical differences between the two medical traditions. TCM clinicians, for example, prefer to use complex, individualized combinations of herbal ingredients. Also, they consider it unethical to give an ineffective placebo to a patient who is suffering. When they do use placebos, they object to randomization of patients in clinical studies, because they feel that patients should have the right to choose whether they will receive the treatment or the placebo.

Within this cultural tradition, modern Chinese herbal research rarely involves a randomized, placebo-controlled study in which a life-threatening ailment is involved. Instead, Chinese double-blind studies generally compare two agents that are both presumed to be effective. TCM clinicians also tend to believe that Western research relies too heavily on laboratory test results, and not enough on the patient's relief of symptoms and the quality of life. Furthermore, because Chinese medicine does not describe health in terms of disease conditions, but rather in syndrome patterns that are unique to the individual, it is difficult to establish comparable groups of subjects for clinical trials. Similarly, treatment is individualized to the specific syndrome pattern presented in each patient, and it runs counter to the principles of TCM to provide a standardized treatment to all people.

Despite these problems, a number of Chinese herbal treatments have been adopted in the West, largely because of research conducted in China. Chinese clinical research dating back to 1972 found *Ginkgo biloba* effective in Parkinson's disease, cerebral thrombosis, and cerebrovascular spasms. This laid the groundwork for Western research published in the *Journal of the American Medical Association* in October of 1998 indicating that ginkgo was effective in alleviating Alzheimer's disease. Researchers for this study included Dr. Alan Schatzberg, chairman of the Department of Psychiatry at the Stanford University School of Medicine. This study was a double-blind, placebo-control RCT over one year. During that time, the mental functioning was stable and social functioning improved mildly in the *Gingko biloba* group while both deteriorated in the placebo group.

Acceptance of certain TCM treatments in the West appears to be growing. Following is a review of a number of medical conditions that respond to TCM therapies, and particularly to TCM herbal therapies. Conditions chosen are those that have been studied most strenuously, according to Western research concepts. However, because of this selection criterion, the studies cited are in no way representative of the full breadth and scale of Chinese herbal research. Studies do, however, illustrate that some Chinese herbal interventions can, under carefully defined conditions, be appropriate treatment for conditions that remain resistant when treated with the best Western therapies.

Asthma. Conventional drug treatment often has side effects, so asthma patients sometimes seek alternative approaches.

In a 1996 Chinese study by Shao Changrong, 100 bronchial asthma patients received Chuanxiong Antiasthma Mixture (containing cnidium, red peony, peony, *tang kuei*, salvia, vitex negundo fruit, elaeagni, magnolia flower, asarum, and licorice), and 50 patients received the drug aminophylline. The herbal preparation performed somewhat better. Therefore, this herbal formula, which can be prepared by American practitioners, offers a possible alternative.

In another Chinese clinical trial, by Li Hongfen, two *Xiaochuanling* formulas (the first containing *ma huang*, apricot seed, gypsum, scute, and coptis, and the second containing codonopsis, hoelen, atractylodes, and ophiopogon) were given to 111 patients with bronchial asthma for seven days. A control group of 30 comparable patients received the conventional drug aminophylline. Results in the herb treatment group were 28.8 percent clinically controlled and 37.8 percent markedly effective, compared to 10 and 37.8 percent, respectively, in the drug group. Thus, the herbal preparation was judged considerably more effective. A study of T-cells showed that the herbal preparations increased CD4 and decreased CD8 subsets, which was suggested as the mechanism of action for inhibiting asthma. Herbs used in this study are readily available to United States practitioners, and the treatment time is short.

Brain function. Many brain dysfunctions present difficulties for treatment by Western medicine. Recent work with ginkgo extract and huperzine for Alzheimer's disease suggests that herbal treatments may provide important assistance.

- In a study of the treatment of senile brain function, Wang Xuemei and Xie Zhufan treated 53 patients, aged sixty to eighty, with Wu Zi Yan Zong Fluid (which contains cuscuta, lycium, rubus, plantago seed, and schizandra) for six weeks. A control group of 20 patients received no treatment. In the treatment group, significant improvements were found in nervous system function, including control of the arms and legs, and improved memory, whereas no improvement was noted in the control group. Similar formulas are available in the United States.
- During an interesting study on schizophrenia by Luo Hechun, schizophrenics received *Ginkgo biloba* leaf extract for eight to thirteen weeks, and were compared with a control group of 56 comparable schizophrenics who received a placebo. Significant improvement was found with ginkgo, appearing between weeks four and twelve, with few side effects. The people treated in this study had previously received a variety of antipsychotic drugs for at least three months without showing improvement.

Cancer. A study by Tian Qiong evaluated the use of *dilong* capsule, with earthworm as its main active ingredient, in conjunction with chemotherapy, in ten people who had liver cancer. A control group of ten people received chemotherapy alone. Earthworm extract appeared to enhance the beneficial effects, and reduce the side effects, of chemotherapy. *Dilong*, available in the United States, has been evaluated pharmacologically and reported to have significant effects on immune functioning.

- For another study, by Lin Chuanrong, an herbal decoction containing fifteen herbs was given to 25 people with cancer who were suffering from pain. These people also received chemotherapy. A control group of 25 similar cases received chemotherapy alone. Pain relief was achieved in 68 percent of the people receiving herbs, but in only 40 percent of those on chemotherapy alone. Reduction of pain was partly associated with cancer remission. Eighty percent of the herb group had some degree of cancer remission, with complete remission in five cases, while only 52 percent of the people on chemotherapy alone showed some remission, with three cases of complete remission.

Cardiovascular risk factors. Lu Decheng studied the effects of *Jianyanling* capsule (rehmannia, *ho-shou-wu*, polygonatum, American ginseng, pearl, succinum, and black sesame seed) in 64 patients for three months. A control group of 64 cases received starch capsules. Statistically significant reductions of fats in the blook, or serum lipids, were found in the treatment group, which achieved significantly lower levels than the control group.

- In another study of serum lipids, Cao Tiemi treated 124 patients with *Ehuang Jiangzhi* Tablet (zedoaria, polygonatum, acorus, rhubarb, bupleurum, and crataegus) for one month, and compared the effects with a control group of 37 people who received the drug inositol nicotinate. Herbal treatment was significantly more effective in lowering cholesterol and triglycerides.
- Conducting a study of people with high blood pressure, by Shi Peiheng, researchers gave 52 people *Dasheng Jiangya* Oral Liquid (made with gynostemma, prunella, pueraria, eucommia, gastrodia, and scrophularia). A control group received the drug nifedipine. There was no significant difference in hypertension, but the group treated with herbs showed better responses in capillary bed circulation, higher HDL, and lower total cholesterol.

Digestive disorders. In a study by We Dian, people with chronic gastritis received Clearing Heat and Nourishing Stomach Decoction (containing gentiana, oldenlandia, dandelion, *tang kuei,* peony, licorice, and curcuma). A control group received the drug furazolidone. In the herb group, 57 percent were cured and 17 percent were improved. In the drug group, 36 percent were cured and 14 percent were improved.

- With a study of gastritis by You Deshi, 46 patients received an herbal decoction (bupleurum, red peony, salvia, dandelion, and dictamnus) along with the drug cimetidine. A control group of 35 patients received cimetidine alone. People receiving the herb plus cimetidine showed a cure rate of 85 percent, while people receiving only cimetidine had a cure rate of 23 percent. Six months after treatment, the relapse rate was only 9 percent in the herb-plus-drug group, but 44 percent in the cimetidine-only group.
- A 1998 study in the special November CAM issue of the *Journal of the American Medical Association* focused on irritable bowel syndrome, which affects up to 20 percent of the population with symptoms including bloating, abdominal pain, constipation, and diarrhea. For this study, 116 patients with irritable bowel syndrome were treated for sixteen weeks with herbs or a placebo. This Australian study found that the Chinese herbal formulation significantly improved irritable bowel syndrome.

Infertility. Extensive research has been done in China on the treatment of infertility. Western medicine lacks cost-effective treatments for immunologically based infertility, the type of infertility studied in the following two trials. In the first trial, male infertility was due to autoimmune attack against sperm; in the second, the female immune system attacked the husband's sperm.

- A study of immunological male infertility by Chen Xiaoping used the traditional remedy *Zhibai Dihuang Wan.* A control group received cortisone and vitamin C. In the herbal treatment group, autoimmunity measures decreased, sperm became more viable, and 80 percent of wives became pregnant within six months. In the control group, 46 percent of wives became pregnant. This traditional formula for autoimmune disorders is available in the United States.

- For a study of female immunological infertility by Chen Xiaoping, researchers used *Guyin* Decoction (ginseng, rehmannia, dioscorea, cornus, cuscuta, polygala, schizandra, and licorice) to treat 60 women with infertility attributed to antisperm immune response. Treatment time was thirty days, with the course being repeated up to three months. A control group of 25 similar cases received prednisolone and vitamin E. Immune measures decreased significantly in the herb treatment group, but not in the drug treatment group. In the herb treatment group, 32 percent became pregnant. In the group receiving drug treatment, 24 percent became pregnant. This formula is available in the United States.

Breast lumps. In the following two studies, Chinese herbal treatment was used as an alternative, or as an adjunct, to hormone therapy, which many patients in the United States wish to avoid.

- Breast lumps, which are a common concern among American women, were treated by two TCM doctors (Qiu Xiaogung and Pu Qing), who used an herbal decoction (consisting of pangolin scales, fritillaria, oyster shell, sparganium, zedoaria, melia, cyperus, corydalis, *tang kuei*, and carthamus). Two control groups received either the amino acid asparagine or the hormone methyltestosterone. In the herb group, 87.7 percent reported a reduction of lumps and a decrease in breast pain, compared with 72.7 percent in the asparagine group and 69.4 percent in the methyltestosterone group. Herbal treatment was concluded to be superior to the other two therapies. Both the herbal treatment and the amino acid treatment were found to be superior to the hormone therapy, which is of significance to women who wish to avoid hormone treatment.

Lupus. Systemic lupus erythematosus is an autoimmune disease that is typically treated in the United States with steroid therapy, but with generally poor control. Lu Youzhi treated 27 cases of lupus with an herbal decoction (rehmannia, hoelen, moutan, astragalus, codonopsis, *tang kuei*, millettia, and licorice), along with oral prednisone. A control group of 24 patients received prednisone alone. In the herb-plus-prednisone group, the effective rate was 92.6 percent, while in the prednisone-only group it was 55.6 percent. United States practitioners can readily obtain the herbs used in this study.

Arthritis. In 1989, Tao administered an extract of the TCM antiarthritis herb T-2 (*Tripterygium wilfordii* Hook F) to 70 patients with rheumatoid arthritis of at least six months' duration which had not responded to standard treatment. T-2 produced very positive results, better than the results produced by any antirheumatic drug.

One innovative TCM study involving moxibustion was reported in the 1998 special CAM issue of the *Journal of the American Medical Association*. Researchers from Italy and China tested an ancient Chinese practice, moxibustion, which has been used to reposition fetuses incorrectly oriented in the womb before birth. Moxibustion involves burning an herb near the body so that the smoke stimulates particular acupuncture points. The report said that moxibustion increased fetal movements and was effective in repositioning a significant number of fetuses who had been in a breech, feet first, presentation in the womb.

Because of the dearth of randomized, double-blind, controlled trials published in English, Chinese herbal interventions are still in a "gray area" in terms of their proven clinical success. Thousands of clinical trials have been done, but most did not meet Western standards of clinical research. However, when these clinical studies are considered in relation to the extensive pharmacological and chemical research that has confirmed the activity of constituents of Chinese herbs, these herbal treatments appear to represent reasonable therapeutic interventions.

Furthermore, these studies can only serve as illustrations of the possible efficacy of Chinese herbs, and cannot reflect the entire breadth and scope of TCM.

FUTURE EVOLUTION OF
TRADITIONAL CHINESE MEDICINE

Traditional Chinese medicine is in a unique position among CAM therapies: It is a complex and comprehensive body of practice, based on thousands of years of clinical experience, and elements of it have already been embraced by conventional physicians.

Acupuncture, an important component of TCM, is currently a licensed profession and is already being incorporated into mainstream medicine. Qi Gong, the movement discipline, has been accepted as a viable intervention in MindBody medicine and is being practiced by large numbers of people. Chinese herbal medicine, although relatively new to the United States, has become widely available.

Similar to Ayurvedic medicine, TCM is an enormously complex system, with a diagnostic and therapeutic approach that is quite foreign to the Western scientific approach. TCM offers a bewildering universe of unfamiliar concepts and materials. It appears, however, that Western-trained acupuncturists, including conventional physicians, do grasp the system and can produce positive results with it. Since herbal remedies are prescribed on the same diagnostic basis as acupuncture, and since the formulas are based on the same accumulated body of clinical experience, they can presumably prove equally efficacious when properly applied. Furthermore, in contrast with Ayurveda, TCM already has a large number of practitioners in this country. Many of the herbs used in TCM are somewhat more familiar to Westerners than those used in Ayurvedic medicine. There are also large Chinese-American communities in the United States where TCM is commonly used. For these reasons, TCM appears to enjoy a promising future in American conventional medicine.

However, TCM faces several important challenges. High priority should be given to incorporating Chinese herbal medicine into the United States training curriculum for TCM so that acupuncturists and other TCM practitioners will be able to employ these herbal remedies appropriately.

Clearly, the number of controlled clinical trials of Chinese herbs must be increased. Particular emphasis should be placed on testing herbs for conditions that often resist conventional treatment, such as cardiovascular disease, cancer, AIDS, chronic fatigue syndrome, substance abuse, chronic pain, musculoskeletal problems, and neuromuscular problems. Research should also proceed on the active constituents of Chinese herbs, leading to the development of well-researched herbal extracts and patentable pharmaceuticals. Among the NCCAM programs, Dr. Fredi Kronenberg at Columbia Medical School is undertaking extensive research focused on women's health and herbal medicine under the Center for Complementary and Alternative Medicine Research in Women's Health. For clinicians and researchers, one of the best sources of reliable, critical studies is the Institute for Traditional Medicine and Preventive Health Care in Portland, Oregon, under the direction of Dr. Subhuti Dharmananda. There are numerous monographs and reports focused on specific TCM herbals for an array of conditions ranging from solid tumors to diabetes.

As a whole system, TCM has great potential. Its diagnostic system provides a means of early detection of health problems before they become advanced illnesses. Hence, TCM can play a beneficial role in preventive medicine. Additionally, TCM has great promise as an adjunct to Western medicine, especially for serious diseases such as cancer, where acupuncture and herbal remedies may help to alleviate side effects and improve treatment. For terminal patients, TCM may provide a cost-effective and humane approach for helping people with the dying process. In addition, certain TCM therapies may help healthy people to achieve even greater heights of optimal health and longevity.

Because traditional Chinese medicine takes an individualized, holistic, nontoxic approach to health care, it is likely that as more skilled TCM practitioners become available, individuals in the United States and internationally will increasingly use Chinese medicine as a form of primary care, and as a first approach to chronic illnesses that are not life-threatening.

CHAPTER 5

ACUPUNCTURE

From Yellow Emperor to
Magnetic Resonance Imaging (MRI)

Acupuncture, which originated in China more than five thousand years ago, was only recently rediscovered by the West, and is now one of the most vital and "modern" of all areas of complementary and alternative medicine. Acupuncture is now widely used in the United States as a primary treatment for chronic pain, and is a very popular complementary therapy for substance abuse recovery, nausea, cancer, AIDS, immune disorders, stroke, and many other conditions.

A major component of traditional Chinese medicine, acupuncture was first codified as early as A.D. 25, and was described in the ancient text *The Yellow Emperor's Classic of Internal Medicine.* Use of acupuncture gradually spread to the entire Asian continent, and it was introduced to Europe by early traders and missionaries. Europeans brought the practice to America in the early 1800s, and it was also used extensively in the mid-1800s by Asian-American immigrants. In the late 1800s, it was credited by Sir William Osler, the "father of modern medicine," as the best treatment for low back pain. However, acupuncture was not accepted by many members of the modern American medical community until the 1970s, when the United States normalized relations with China. By 1998, over one million Americans annually were being treated with acupuncture, by some ten thousand licensed acupuncturists.

Despite its long history, however, no one is certain how acupuncture works. Acupuncture's healing techniques are based on principles that are very different from those of the Western scientific model. Western medicine generally deals with an illness by looking for a specific cause and trying to eliminate it. Traditional Chinese medicine takes a more holistic approach, and holds a different view of symptoms, of the causes of disease, and even of human anatomy. According to Chinese medicine, health is determined by a balanced flow of *qi* (or *chi*), the vital life energy that is said to animate all living organisms. *Qi* flows to all parts of the body through fourteen major energy pathways, or meridians, twelve of which are associated with specific organs. Thus, acupuncture anatomy is a multilayered, interconnecting network of energy channels that permit *qi* to move through the muscles and organs.

Chinese medicine views disease as the result of an excess or a deficiency of *qi* in various parts of the body. This imbalance of *qi* is influenced by many factors, including heat, cold, dampness, emotions, diet, exercise, and the spirit. Acupuncture seeks to rebalance the flow of *qi* by inserting special needles at any of 360 specific points along the energy meridians.

Most Western experts, however, while acknowledging that acupuncture is effective, believe that it works by triggering chemicals, including pain-killing endorphins and brain-altering neurotransmitters and neuropeptides, that influence the endocrine system, and thus affect mood, energy, and immunity. According to Dr. George Ulett, a psychiatrist and neurologist, the stimulation of motor points where nerves enter muscles releases neurohormones. To activate this mechanism, he observes, no ancient Chinese philosophy is necessary.

However, other modern researchers have applied scientific techniques that appear to confirm the existence of meridians. In the 1960s, microdissection procedures revealed evidence of a system of extremely fine ducts that correspond to acupuncture meridians. Also, radioactive isotope testing in 1985 suggested that the meridians exist. Other researchers have found evidence of a network of electrical currents that flow along the meridian pathways.

Debate over how acupuncture works is likely to continue for decades.

Acupuncture at correct points is generally more effective than sham or nonspecific acupuncture. However, according to Dr. Bruce Pomeranz, a professor of zoology and physiology at the University of Toronto who conducted much of the research in this area, sham acupuncture does produce improvement in some 35 to 50 percent of people with chronic pain, while true acupuncture helps 50 to 80 percent. Perhaps sham acupuncture is a very convincing placebo, or it may be that any kind of needle insertion produces a response in some people. Despite this debate, the majority of acupuncturists apply the technique in a somewhat similar way.

To perform treatments, acupuncturists begin by taking a thorough medical history. Then they perform a physical examination, noting not just obvious characteristics of health, but also subtle factors, such as the color of the skin, body language, and the tone of voice. Additionally, the tongue is carefully examined for color, coating, and surface irregularities, since it is believed to reflect the overall health of the patient.

Acupuncturists also focus on the pulse, which is considered another indicator of the patient's overall condition. In Chinese medicine, the pulse is felt at six locations and three depths on each wrist. Qualities of the pulse reveal the balance and flow of qi throughout the body. Interestingly, current Western research indicates that subtleties in the pulse do reflect the conditions of various organs.

Then the acupuncturist organizes all the information and symptoms into clusters, and identifies patterns of disharmony and disturbances in organs. Treatment is then devised to provide energy to weak areas by redirecting the flow of energy.

Sterile, hair-thin acupuncture needles are inserted at selected points. Generally about ten to twelve needles are used, but this may vary. Acupuncture is usually painless, although some points can be acutely painful, or there may be a very slight pricking sensation, followed by a feeling of heaviness, numbness, warmth, or a mild aching, which is known as "obtaining the qi."

To potentiate acupuncture's effects, heat may be applied by burning an herb above the acupuncture point. When the patient begins to feel the heat, it is removed. Another traditional treatment is cupping, in which a glass or bamboo cup is used to create suction on the skin above a painful muscle or acupuncture point. Also, in addition to needles, the acupuncturist may apply electrostimulation, ultrasound, or laser beams.

There are several styles of acupuncture, including:

Traditional Chinese medicine acupuncture, which is favored in China and taught in most U.S. acupuncture schools. It is linked with the use of herbal therapy, and acupuncture points are selected to reinforce this herbal therapy.

Medical acupuncture is the practice of acupuncture by an M.D. or osteopath, and includes elements of Western medicine. The physician may choose acupuncture points based not only on the TCM diagnosis but also on a conventional diagnosis, and may insert needles in nonacupuncture points, such as muscle "trigger points," which hold muscular tension.

Japanese meridian acupuncture emphasizes energy movement through the meridians, and uses thinner needles and gentler needling techniques, such as holding the needles on the surface of the skin.

Five Elements acupuncture, an English approach, is based on European interpretations of classical Chinese acupuncture, and has proven valuable in addressing psychogenic problems.

Ear acupuncture (or auricular acupuncture) is based on the theory that the entire body can be affected by stimulating specific points on the outer ear. It is most often used for treating pain, dyslexia, and alcohol and drug addiction.

Korean hand acupuncture applies needles only to the hand, on the theory that the palm contains a meridian microcosm of the entire body.

Scalp acupuncture, recently developed, uses points on the scalp to exert a cerebral influence on the body. This approach is also used to deal with neurological problems.

In choosing an acupuncturist, some people prefer to be treated by a Western-trained physician, who also practices conventional medicine. Insurance coverage may be easier to arrange with a licensed physician. Others seek more traditional practitioners. A typical treatment lasts about forty-five minutes and averages about $45. Initial appointments take longer and are generally more expensive. For chronic illness or physical rehabilitation, ten to twelve treatments are generally scheduled. To treat acute illness, minor injury, or a seasonal "tune-up," only one to four treatments may be needed. Visits are usually weekly, but may be more frequent early in treatment. Follow-up visits may be necessary, particularly for chronic pain.

Although acupuncture in America is most frequently used for pain, as early as 1979 the World Health Organization compiled a list of 104 conditions that acupuncture can treat, including migraine, lesions, sinusitis, common cold, tonsillitis, asthma, inflammation of the eyes, addictions, myopia, duodenal ulcer and other gastrointestinal disorders, trigeminal neuralgia, Ménière's disease, tennis elbow, paralysis, stroke, speech aphasia, sciatica, and osteoarthritis. In the United States, acupuncture is often used as a last resort for many of these conditions.

According to a review by Dr. Joseph M. Helms of the world clinical literature, the use of acupuncture throughout the world most often involves: lesions (40 percent), pain (25 percent), surgical analgesia (16 percent), neurological disorders (10 percent), substance abuse (5 percent), and psychiatric disorders (4 percent). Some conditions are beyond the scope of acupuncture treatment. It cannot relieve pain in all surgical procedures, and is not feasible for emergency medicine or trauma care.

Acupuncture presents few risks. Among the most serious common side effects are mild, transitory depression or anxiety and fatigue. Risk of infection is minimal, since needles are sterile and disposable.

Although voluminous research exists indicating the efficacy of acupuncture, much of this research does not meet Western standards. Several factors complicate acupuncture research. One is that the success of the technique is closely related to the skill of the practitioner. Another is that it is difficult to create a placebo form of acupuncture, because the patient virtually always knows when the procedure is being performed. Sometimes, researchers perform a placebo treatment by placing needles inappropriately, into "sham" acupuncture points, but it is possible that any insertion of needles will have some effect.

Nonetheless, a number of persuasive studies have been performed on many different conditions. To date, one of the best reviews of the research evidence underlying clinical acupuncture is a monograph by Stephen Birch and Dr. Richard Hammerschlag entitled *Acupuncture Efficacy: A Summary of Controlled Clinical Trials*, published in 1996 by the National Academy of Acupuncture and Oriental Medicine. For clinicians, this publication provides excellent details on a great deal of the clinical research cited in this chapter. Following is an examination of some of the best research on acupuncture, in which it was tested on some of the conditions for which it is most often used.

ACUPUNCTURE:
WHAT WORKS AND WHAT DOES NOT WORK

Pain

Chronic and acute pain is consistently the number one reason why people seek alternative medicine care. In the United States, acupuncture has found its greatest acceptance and success in the management of a wide variety of painful conditions, especially musculoskeletal pain. There seems to be an overwhelming amount of evidence for its efficacy.

Following are some of the most well-designed studies on pain.

- In a 1976 study by Dr. Jorma Laitinen of low back pain, comparing acupuncture to the conventional therapy of transcutaneous electrical nerve stimulation (TENS) for pain control, acupuncture achieved moderate to complete pain relief in 58 percent of patients, compared to 46 percent of patients undergoing TENS therapy.
- For a 1982 study by Dr. Seppo Y. T. Junnila of osteoarthritis patients, 50 percent of acupuncture patients became much improved or symptom-free, compared to 31 percent of patients taking medication. In another arthritis study, 25 percent of patients scheduled for knee surgery were able to avoid surgery after a course of acupuncture.
- With chronic neck pain, patients reported a 68 percent decrease in mean hours of pain, compared to a decrease of 0 percent in untreated patients, in a 1982 study by Dr. Richard W. Coan.
- A 1983 review by Lewith and Machin of studies showed that acupuncture provided short-term relief to 50 to 80 percent of patients with acute and chronic pain. Chronic musculoskeletal pain responded well, and so did acute musculoskeletal lesions, such as bruises, sprains, and strains.
- One 1983 study by Dr. E. Ahonen and colleagues on tension headaches indicated that acupuncture was more effective in relieving pain than treatment by physicians applying physiotherapy.

- From a 1984 study by Dr. Leng Loh of forty-eight migraine patients, 59 percent reported benefits from acupuncture, compared to 25 percent who benefited from drug therapy.
- In a 1990 study by Chen of thirty-six acupuncture patients with carpal tunnel syndrome, all but one attained excellent short-term relief of pain. In the study's long-term follow-up, twenty-four of the thirty-six patients showed 2.5 to 8.5 years of pain relief.
- Based on a 1991 study by Johansson of muscular pain of the face and head, acupuncture was as effective as conventional treatment with physiotherapy.
- Concluding a sophisticated 1994 pain study by Dr. Jurgen Hesse and Dr. Henrik Simonsen of acupuncture versus drug therapy, acupuncture was equally effective, with notably fewer side effects.
- Based on a 1987 study by well-known clinician and acupuncture practitioner Dr. Joseph M. Helms, founding President of the American Academy of Medical Acupuncture, on painful menstruation, or dysmenorrhea, 91 percent of patients showed improvement, compared to 36 percent of patients in a sham acupuncture group.

Acupuncture may not be equally helpful in controlling pain in some populations. A five-year study of 348 pain patients concluded that acupuncture was less effective for pain control in the elderly, in patients with a psychiatric history, in patients taking high doses of analgesics, and in those with long-standing pain.

Pain is a major problem for the U.S. health care system. It is estimated that 10 percent of all Americans have pain conditions that are present for over one hundred days a year. Therefore, treatments that are less expensive and relatively effective, such as acupuncture therapy, are extremely valuable.

Substance Abuse

Acupuncture, particularly when applied to the external ear, has proven valuable in managing substance abuse problems and reducing the need for prescription narcotic pain medications. In the treatment of opium and heroin addiction, acupuncture studies by Wen as early as 1973 have shown a success rate as high as 100 percent in relieving the symptoms of withdrawal.

Acupuncture has helped patients withdraw not only from opiates but also from alcohol and other addictive drugs.

Consider the following carefully conducted studies.

- In a 1985 study by Clavel of cigarette addiction, acupuncture was compared to the use of nicotine gum. Using a newly discovered acupoint (*tien mi*), as well as traditional points (primarily in the ear), acupuncturists helped 8 percent of patients to stop smoking for more than a year, while use of nicotine gum helped 12 percent to stop smoking.
- For a 1987 controlled study on hard-core alcoholics in Minnesota, funded by the NIH, a group that received acupuncture had half as many drinking episodes and admissions to detox centers as did a control group, which received sham acupuncture. "Sham" or placebo acupuncture involves placing needles in areas that are not actual acupuncture points or applying pressure at points without the actual insertion of a needle.
- During a 1993 study by Dr. Arthur Margolin and colleagues of cocaine addiction, addicts were given acupuncture treatment, or conventional pharmacotherapy (consisting of either amantidine or desipramine), or placebo therapy. Of those receiving acupuncture, 44 percent were abstinent from cocaine by the end of the eight-week trial, compared to 15 percent taking amantidine, 26 percent taking desipramine, and 13 percent on placebo therapy.
- From a 1994 study by Dr. Douglas S. Lipton of crack cocaine addicts, acupuncture was as effective as conventional drug therapy.

For the treatment of substance abuse, the best clinical evidence of the effectiveness of acupuncture is for narcotic addiction, then alcohol. Acupuncture is clearly useful as an adjuvant therapy in the treatment of substance abuse and drug dependency, and appears to be effective as a primary therapy.

Nausea

A relatively large body of evidence shows that acupuncture is effective in treating nausea and vomiting due to pregnancy, surgery, and chemotherapy. It appears as if the single most effective acupuncture point for this condition is PC-6.

Pertinent, well-designed studies include the following:

- In studies by Dr. R. G. Ghaly in 1987 and Ho in 1990 of postsurgical patients, acupuncture effectively controlled nausea for both gynecological surgeries and outpatient laparoscopy procedures.
- In a 1992 study by De Aloysio of women with morning sickness, nausea was controlled with an acupressure "Sea Band" twice as effectively as it was with a placebo.
- During a study by Dundee of chemotherapy patients with nausea, 65 percent experienced complete abolition of symptoms after undergoing acupuncture treatment.

Cancer, HIV/AIDS, and Immune Disorders

In cancer therapy, acupuncture can help control nausea and other side effects of chemotherapy and radiation. For treatment of HIV and AIDS, it has been shown to increase total white blood cells and T-cell production. In a controversial program in Miami, acupuncture is allegedly increasing life span of AIDS patients and improving quality of life, according to Dr. Harvey Grossbard. In the special CAM issue of the *Journal of the American Medical Association* in November 1998, a research team from the National Institutes of Health, the University of Minnesota, and the University of Colorado reported that acupuncture was not effective in treating nerve pain due to HIV infection. There appear to be no known effective treatments including acupuncture.

Finally, there is some preliminary evidence that acupuncture may be of general value in treating chronic fatigue syndrome, asthma, ulcerative colitis, rheumatoid arthritis, and collagen-vascular diseases.

Stroke and Nervous System Disorders

In traditional Chinese medicine, acupuncture has a long history of use for treating stroke. This form of intervention may be of value to Westerners, because the conventional approaches to stroke rehabilitation have not been definitively shown to be of value, according to some researchers. However, acupuncture's mechanism of action in stroke rehabilitation remains unclear. Several studies, however, are intriguing.

- A 1987 study by Zhang compared acupuncture to medication in rehabilitation of stroke patients with limb paralysis. The study indicated that acupuncture was an effective treatment, especially when begun as soon as possible after a stroke.
- In a well-designed 1993 Scandinavian study by Dr. Kurt Johansson, seventy-eight stroke patients with severe hemiparesis, or slight weakness or paralysis affecting only one side of the body, were treated with either acupuncture or occupational therapy. Patients in the acupuncture group showed greater improvement in balance, mobility, and in the managing of activities of daily life. Moreover, the cost of rehabilitation was almost 50 percent lower for those receiving acupuncture than for those receiving conventional treatment.
- For a 1996 Norwegian study by Dr. Susanne Sallstrom at the Sunnaas Rehabilitation Hospital, a group of stroke patients received acupuncture and was compared to a control group that did not receive acupuncture. Only the acupuncture group rated a significantly improved quality of life. Control patients improved only physical movement, and declined in quality of sleep.

According to most researchers, adding acupuncture to multidisciplinary stroke rehabilitation therapy in the subacute (acute but not chronic) stage benefits all outcome areas. Poststroke patients have untapped rehabilitation potential, which is important to utilize. Researchers suggest that acupuncture may enhance reorganization within the brain, which appears to underlie the functional reorganization that occurs after stroke.

Other Conditions

Acupuncture can be used successfully to treat many other diagnosable medical conditions, although it may need to be used in conjunction with other conventional and unconventional therapies. Following are examples of some of the conditions that respond to acupuncture.

- In a 1985 study by Drs. Luo, Jia, and Chan of clinical depression, acupuncture compared favorably to treatment with conventional medications. After five weeks of acupuncture treatment, 70 percent of depression patients were cured or markedly improved, compared to 65 percent of depression patients taking medication for the same length of time.
- Based on a 1986 study by Jobst, published in *Lancet*, of chronic obstructive pulmonary disease, three weeks of acupuncture treatment reduced breathlessness and increased perception of well-being.
- Concluding a 1992 study by Gerhard and Postneek of female infertility, acupuncture was as successful as hormone therapy for helping women to become pregnant.
- From a 1992 study by Dr. David Ehrlich and Dr. Paul Haber, which measured the effects of acupuncture on a group of healthy men, aged nineteen to twenty-nine, the men were able to extend their performance limits at aerobic exercise by 7 percent. Two control groups, which were given sham acupuncture or no acupuncture, showed no significant increase in capacity. This study indicated an intriguing movement in the direction of using acupuncture not just to overcome disease but to achieve optimal health—a welcome direction indeed.
- Among the other areas with positive results are dental craniomandibular disorder, in a series of 1992 studies by Dr. Theodore List; muscle tension headache, by Dr. Jane Carlsson in 1990; relief of severe knee osteoarthritis, by Dr. B. V. Christensen in 1992 and Dr. M. Thomas in 1991; and success in preventing recidivism with severe alcoholics, in a series of studies by Dr. Milton L. Bullock.
- A UCLA School of Medicine study by Dr. David Bresler and Dr. Richard Kroening, focused on bronchospasm in asthma patients whose illness averaged twenty-two years in duration, found that the spasms were effectively controlled by acupuncture.
- Throughout veterinary medicine, acupuncture is recognized as a valid medical procedure, used mainly for surgical analgesia and chronic pain, and to eliminate some forms of epileptic convulsions. Because animals are not susceptible to suggestion, this indicates that it is unlikely that acupuncture has purely a placebo effect.

WHAT'S IN THE WORKS

Acupuncture is certain to be even more widely used in the future, for many reasons. One reason is its cost-effectiveness. According to Dr. Joseph Helms, founder of the American Academy of Medical Acupuncture and author of *Acupuncture Energetics*, doctors who use acupuncture in at least half their cases afford their patients considerable savings in laboratory exams, hospitalizations, and prescription drugs. Acupuncture's emphasis on preventive health maintenance may also contribute to its overall cost-effectiveness, since it seeks to intervene before costly chronic diseases become manifest. Because nine to twelve million acupuncture treatments are administered each year in America, acupuncture is already reducing our national expenditure on medicine.

Another reason acupuncture is growing in acceptance is because it is being taught at many of the country's most prestigious medical schools, including UCLA, where it is taught by Dr. Helms and colleagues; the Stanford University School of Medicine, where it is taught by Dr. Yuan-Chi Lin, an associate professor of anesthesiology; and in the internationally recognized clinical and research program at the University of Maryland School of Medicine, under the direction of Dr. Brian Berman in the Department of Anesthesiology. There are now more than forty schools that teach acupuncture.

Furthermore, acupuncture is gaining acceptance by the insurance industry, in part due to its proven cost-effectiveness.

Reflecting this increasing popularity, every state now allows allopathic physicians and osteopaths to practice acupuncture, and thirty-three states and the District of Columbia currently license the practice of non-physicians. As of 1999, there were ten thousand acupuncture specialists in the United States, and three thousand are conventionally trained physicians. During the year 2000, it is estimated that over $500 million will be spent on acupuncture treatments.

Most significant of all, in November of 1997 the National Institutes of Health held its first consensus development conference on acupuncture. That expert panel concluded that acupuncture is effective against nausea and some pain, and encouraged more research on the subject. Data supporting acupuncture, noted panel chair Dr. David J. Ramsay, president of the University of Maryland, "are as strong as those for many accepted Western medical therapies." Although the consensus statement was limited specifically to pain and nausea, such a statement will help to increase acupuncture research in other conditions as well. The clinical evidence did not constitute an unqualified endorsement, but the panel indicated that acupuncture did seem to be effective in disorders such as fibromyalgia, tendonitis, postoperative pain, low back pain, drug addiction, stroke rehabilitation, carpal tunnel syndrome, osteoarthritis, headache, and asthma. In fact, the panel noted that acupuncture may possibly be safer and more effective than many accepted conventional treatments for these disorders.

At the University of Maryland School of Medicine, Dr. Brian M. Berman and his colleagues are focused on a number of NCCAM longitudinal studies on various clinical applications and basic research on the biological mechanisms through to 2005. One of the new, ongoing studies at the University of Arizona, with Dr. Fayez Ghisban and Dr. Andrew T. Weil, is examining the use of acupuncture, self-hypnosis, and osteopathic manipulation to reduce muscle tension in children with spastic cerebral palsy. Recent well-conducted research clearly indicates that acupuncture is a highly adaptable discipline, and is of therapeutic value in many kinds of pain and general medical problems. Whether it is used as a primary or a complementary therapy depends on the nature and severity of the medical problem, and on the training, orientation, and practice environment of the practitioner.

Like most medical interventions, acupuncture is most successful when used early in a medical condition, but it can be applied at almost any stage of treatment, particularly if it is combined with other therapies. Acupuncture combines well with other forms of treatment, many of which reinforce the effects of acupuncture.

Acupuncture's meridian system offers a theoretical model that may assist in diagnosing and treating disorders that Western medicine has not been able to help. Because it is a noninvasive technique, and is less expensive than traditional diagnostic and treatment procedures, acupuncture may come increasingly to be used not just as a last resort, but as a first approach, especially in conditions that Western medicine has had difficulty addressing, such as addictions and certain kinds of pain.

Studies documenting the influence of acupuncture on the body's neurotransmitters and natural pain killers have begun to explain how acupuncture might work. Innovative studies using imaging technologies such as magnetic resonance imaging (MRI) seem to verify the presence of subtle energy pathways outside of the central nervous system. However, future research should investigate how acupuncture helps to improve the well-being of the whole person. Also, this research should assess the total environment in which acupuncture is used, including the impact of factors such as thoughts and emotions, and even the impact of factors such as the season of the year. These types of factors have long been taken into consideration in Chinese medicine, but are just beginning to be explored in the West.

As more well-designed research continues to document the safety and effectiveness of acupuncture, it is likely that it will be increasingly integrated into Western health care, taking its place alongside conventional medicine, both as an adjunctive therapy and as a primary-care approach.

CHAPTER 6

WESTERN HERBAL MEDICINE

Nature's Green Pharmacy

Herbal medicine has entered the mainstream in America and abroad. It's estimated that about one-third of all adult Americans, or some sixty million people, use herbal medicinal products each year, spending over $3.2 billion. In the rest of the world, approximately 64 percent of the population relies on herbal medicines. Over 1,500 herbs are currently marketed in the United States, and are sold not only in health food stores but also in pharmacies, supermarkets, department stores, and even truck stops!

Equally indicative of herbs' importance is the fact that about one-quarter of all U.S. prescription drugs are derived from herbs. Approximately 119 plant-derived compounds are currently used as drugs, and nearly three-quarters of them were discovered by following up on folklore. Examples include quinine, from the bark of a South American tree, which is used to treat some strains of malaria; digoxin, the widely prescribed heart medication, which is derived from the foxglove plant; salacin (the source of aspirin) from willow bark; and, recently, taxol for cancer prevention from the yew tree.

In the parlance of herbal medicine, the term *herb* applies to any plant or plant part that is used to make medicinal preparations. Herbal medicine, or botanical medicine, is also known in Europe as *phytomedicine*, from the Greek *phyto*, "plant." A phytomedicine, or phytopharmaceutical, is a complex mixture derived from plant sources that is used as a medicine or drug. Parts of plants used in herbal medicine can include leaves, flowers, stems, roots, seeds, fruit, bark, or any other plant part that is used for its medicinal, flavoring, or fragrant properties.

Early in human history, herbal medicine was practiced as a magical, or religious, healing art. Out of this, systems of herbology evolved on every continent, including Europe, North and South America, and Asia.

In colonial America, botanical medicine evolved through the blending of two separate traditions. Passengers on the *Mayflower* carried with them a book on European herbology. In America, the colonists encountered not only new plants but also a population of Native Americans who were knowledgeable about them.

During the 1800s, many of the most effective American healers were those who combined European and Native American herbalism. Soon, Chinese immigrants added their own herbal tradition to the mix, especially on the West Coast.

Following the Civil War, herbology began to lose influence, partly because of improvements in conventional medicine that were achieved during the war. By the beginning of the twentieth century, chemists had become more adept at isolating the active ingredients in plants, and the use of raw, whole-plant materials began to seem crude and unscientific. In 1910, the Carnegie Foundation, at the request of the AMA, issued a study of American medicine called the Flexner Report. This report elevated pharmaceutical medicine, and was critical of schools that taught herbal medicine and other nonconventional approaches. Historically, this influential report contributed greatly to the decline of alternative medicine, including herbology.

By the end of World War II, synthetic drugs were increasingly being produced by companies that had originally sold herbs, such as Merck and ParkeDavis. Unlike herbs, these pharmaceuticals could be protected by patent, offering greater profit. Modern physicians also preferred synthetic drugs. Drugs seemed more scientific than natural products, and were supported by clinical studies. Moreover, since drugs required prescriptions from doctors, the new drugs—unlike herbs—brought the medical profession a guaranteed business.

In the 1970s, however, there was a resurgence of interest in herbal medicine, led primarily by patients who objected to the inaccessibility, high cost, and toxicity of pharmaceutical drugs. Many patients found that herbs could have actions that were similar to those of herb-derived drugs, without drug side effects. Also, many patients became aware that pharmaceutical drugs were often ineffective for the modern wave of degenerative diseases. Mild herbal medicines, however, could help prevent some of these diseases.

Interest in herbalism was also spurred by the global search for new plant products that were effective medicinally. Between 1960 and 1986, the National Cancer Institute tested more than 35,000 species of plants, and found that nearly 4 percent of them had antitumoral actions.

Renewed interest in herbs has become even stronger in Europe than in America. In Germany, 70 percent of physicians currently prescribe herbal remedies, which are paid for by government health insurance. Since 1993, the licensing examination for German physicians has included a section on herbal medicine.

One reason that Western herbalism is popular in modern America and Europe is because its principles are essentially consonant with those of conventional medicine. Unlike traditional Chinese medicine, Ayurveda, or even homeopathy, Western herbal medicine does not have its own distinct theory of disease and treatment. Also, unlike TCM or Ayurveda, Western herbalism generally uses single-plant preparations, which often have specific effects, rather than combinations of herbs or herbs that have a broad range of effects.

Unfortunately, though, we now know that purified, isolated plant products often have more side effects than whole herbs. Isolated herbal preparations, however, are at least gentler than most pharmaceuticals.

Even whole herbs that have relatively specific effects usually have a significantly wider range of effects than most drugs. For instance, pharmaceutical researchers are now scrambling to find new arthritis drugs (such as antiprostaglandins, anti-inflammatories, and antileukotrienes) that target a variety of possible receptor sites. Herbs, on the other hand, naturally address arthritic symptoms with precisely this degree of complexity. Bilberry, for example, contains nineteen phytochemicals that have a demonstrated activity against arthritis, including pain-killing compounds, general antiarthritics, antiedemics for reducing swelling, and anti-inflammatories.

Americans now use herbs mostly for a variety of minor conditions.

According to a 1997 *Prevention* magazine survey, the most common conditions for which they use herbs are colds (59 percent), followed by burns (45 percent), headaches (22 percent), allergies (21 percent), rashes (18 percent), insomnia (18 percent), PMS (17 percent), depression (7 percent), diarrhea (7 percent), and menopause (4 percent).

Among American consumers, herbs are extremely popular as adaptogens, which are products that help the body adapt to a broad range of physical and emotional stressors, and which are considered safe for longterm use. The most frequently used adaptogen is ginseng. In light of Americans' awareness of the connection between chronic stress and major killer diseases, it is not surprising that there has been a strong demand for adaptogenic herbal remedies.

Herbs are most often ingested as teas, and in capsules and tablets. They are also used in a concentrated form, as tinctures and extracts. Sometimes, herbs are added to oils and ointments and applied topically.

Current government regulations on herbs are moderate. Herb manufacturers are not required to conduct the expensive safety and efficacy studies that are necessary for new drugs. However, the FDA can remove herbal products it considers unsafe. It must justify the removal in an administrative hearing. Herb manufacturers are largely prohibited from making claims on labels that an herb can cure a disease, but they are allowed to make claims about how an herb can affect the body's function or structure.

In 1994, the FDA threatened to remove herbs from the open market, but this caused a letter-writing campaign to Congress that has been described as the most extensive since the Vietnam War. Under current regulations, consumers have been left in an informational vacuum concerning the value and safety of herbal products. Detailed information regarding therapeutic use of herbs is not permitted on product labels, and the spate of enthusiastic booklets, books, and articles touting the latest herbal crazes are not necessarily reliable.

Although herbal products are now commonly carried in drugstores, most pharmacists are not experts on herbology. Similarly, many health food store clerks may have only a smattering of knowledge, and will often be influenced by the desire to sell their products. Most naturopathic physicians will be well versed in Western herbology, but are licensed to practice in only a limited number of states.

In the absence of any organized professional body that can help unravel the complex questions about herbal remedies, consumers are often left to their own devices. Herbal medicine is not a regulated health profession in the United States, and there is no licensing body for practicing herbal medicine.

Without official standards of quality, herbal preparations may not always be pure, and may not be accurately labeled. According to a 1979 review by Dr. Ara Der Mardersosian at the Philadelphia College of Pharmacy and Science, 60 percent of fifty-four ginseng preparations contained so little ginseng that they were essentially inactive, and about 15 percent contained no ginseng at all.

In a study by Heptinstall, analyzing the herb feverfew, which is used to prevent migraine headaches, researchers found that two out of three of the feverfew products contained no active ingredient. Also, it was estimated by Awang in 1991 that more than half of the echinacea sold in the United States from 1908 through 1991 was actually *Parthenium integrifolium,* and not echinacea.

One way of dealing with the problem of variable contents in herbal remedies is to follow the European example of producing herbal preparations that are standardized, so that each unit of dosage contains a known quantity of the active constituents. This not only provides a clinically effective dosage, but is also more cost-effective.

With regard to scientifically determining the safety and efficacy of herbs, the best current research is an extensive collection of monographs published by the German government's Commission E. In late 1998, this herbal compendium was translated into English in both written and electronic text. It is considered to be the definitive text on herbal medicine and is available from the American Botanical Council in Austin, Texas, under the title of *The Complete Commission E Monographs: Therapeutic Guide to Herbal Medicines,* edited by Mark Blumenthal.

Many of these Commission E studies are referred to in the following examinations of the herbs that are among the most widely used natural medications in America today.

HERBAL MEDICATIONS: WHAT WORKS

While herbs are not the most frequently used alternative medicine, they are among the most controversial and problematic because of their increasingly widespread use, lack of quality control and standardization, as well as the potential for severe and even fatal side effects. For these reasons and particularly for this chapter, it is essential to underscore that although some common dosages, appropriate uses, cautions, and adverse side effects are noted in Part II of this book, "CAM Therapies for Specific Conditions," before using any herbal, it is imperative that an individual be aware of general cautions, such as abstaining from herbs during pregnancy; specific applications and cautions for a particular herb; and always working with a clinician experienced in the appropriate use of herbal interventions.

In Part II, recommended forms, contraindications, and adverse effects for specific herbals are noted under the specific conditions for which the herb is most commonly used. Despite the general consensus of the safety and efficacy of these guidelines, it is always advisable to use herbals with the oversight and monitoring of a clinician trained in herbal medicine. Herbs are potent and need to be used appropriately and judiciously.

Perhaps one of the most important and overlooked properties of herbs and complex herbal formulas is that they are "adaptogenic" or have the effect of normalizing body functions. If a level is too high, it is lowered, or if it is too low, it is raised. Essentially, herbs and MindBody interventions derive much of their impact from restoring the body's natural state of homeostasis or harmonic balance.

Black Cohosh (Cimicifuga racemosa). Black cohosh, a plant native to eastern North America, was used by Native Americans to treat general malaise, kidney ailments, malaria, rheumatism, sore throat, and especially menstrual irregularities. One of black cohosh's popular names is squaw root, because it was used to treat female disorders. Early settlers used it for rheumatism, and it was used in early patent medicines such as Lydia Pinkham's famed "Vegetable Compound," which women drank for menstrual distress.

Black cohosh contains triterpene glycosides, isoflavones, and aromatic acids, and affects the endocrine system, producing effects similar to those of estriol, a form of estrogen. Estriol is an antagonist of estradiol, the estrogen that is given in synthetic form to treat menopausal symptoms, and which is associated with an increased risk of ovarian, breast, and endometrial cancers. According to Murray in 1997, estriol, and perhaps also black cohosh, seems to afford some protection against these cancers.

Commission E in Germany approves black cohosh for premenstrual discomfort, dysmenorrhea, and menopausal ailments, and notes no contraindications or significant side effects (except for occasional gastric discomfort). Commission E recommends the use of black cohosh for no more than six months.

Remifemin®, a black cohosh extract manufactured in Germany, is the most widely used natural alternative to hormone replacement therapy. More than 1.5 million women in Germany have used Remifemin since 1956 for menopausal symptoms with remarkable effectiveness. Nearly 10 million monthly units of the extract were sold in Germany, Australia, and the United States in 1996.

Mark Blumenthal, executive director of the American Botanical Council, cites at least eight clinical studies that have been published on the therapeutic effects of Remifemin in treating menopausal symptoms.

- In a 1983 open study by Daiber, 36 women noted highly significant decreases in menopausal symptoms. Vorberg, in a 1984 open study, treated 50 women for twelve weeks with Remifemin for menopausal complaints, yielding significant to highly significant improvements in menopausal symptoms.
- Four studies have compared Remifemin with placebo, hormones, and/or diazepam (Valium) drugs. In a study by Warnecke in 1985, black cohosh showed a clear advantage over both of the other drugs in controlling menopausal symptoms. A 1987 study by Stoll compared Remifemin with conjugated estrogens and found that black cohosh produced better results. Researchers commented that the black cohosh extract produced such a great improvement in the vaginal lining that it should be the drug of first choice to treat menopausal symptoms.

  Studies have also explored the feasibility of switching from hormone replacement therapy to black cohosh extract.
- In a study involving 131 doctors and 629 women, in which Remifemin produced a clear improvement in menopausal symptoms in more than 80 percent of the women, researchers noted advantages of Remifemin therapy over preceding hormone treatment in 72 percent of the cases.

Although much of the research reported on black cohosh has not met the gold standard of RCTs, the benefits of the herb are well documented for treating premenstrual and menopausal conditions. Additional research with improved design will help to substantiate these findings.

Echinacea (Echinacea species). Echinacea was the best-selling herbal medicine in U.S. health food stores from 1995 to 1997.

Widely used by the Plains Indians, especially for infectious diseases and wound healing, echinacea was adopted by Eclectic physicians in the late 1800s. Once very popular, it was largely replaced by antibiotics, but is again gaining popularity.

Echinacea is primarily used to prevent and treat the common cold, flu, and upper respiratory tract infections; to enhance immune system function; and to treat systemic *Candida* infections. There is good clinical research support for its use in colds, flus, and upper respiratory infections, but research on other applications is more equivocal. Echinacea is inappropriate for HIV and AIDS, since echinacea may promote the replication of T-cells, which is where the HIV virus resides.

- A 1994 review by Melchart and associates of twenty-six controlled clinical studies examined the activity of echinacea on immunity. The authors concluded that echinacea could strengthen immunity. The most striking effects of echinacea were a reduction in susceptibility to infection and a decrease in the incidence of colds.
- Braunig in 1992 found that the dosage of echinacea was critical. One hundred and eighty subjects were divided into three groups, one receiving a placebo, one receiving 450 mg of echinacea, and one 900 mg. Improvements in the 450 mg group were only comparable to the placebo group, whereas those in the 900 mg group showed a statistically significant improvement in flu symptoms.

    When using echinacea to prevent cold and flu or to relieve their symptoms, Dr. Varro Tyler recommends taking it in small doses every few hours, with a maximum length of treatment of six to eight successive weeks.
- In a study of recurrent *Candida* vaginal yeast infections, half the women were treated with the commonly prescribed antiyeast medication econazole nitrate alone, while the other half received both econazole nitrate and echinacea. Those receiving just the drug had

a 60.5 percent recurrence rate, while those also taking echinacea had a recurrence rate of only 16.7 percent.

- At the University of California at Irvine Medical Center, See and colleagues examined cells infected with mononucleosis and found that echinacea enhanced immune function in cells in both normal subjects and those with depressed immunity.

While more well-designed clinical trials of echinacea extracts are certainly desirable, there seems to be sufficient clinical and pharmacological evidence to suggest that it is safe and effective. However, echinacea preparations on the U.S. market have proven inconsistent in quality. Relying on reputable brands and standardized extracts should help to ensure quality and proper dosage.

Feverfew (Tanacetum parthenium). A member of the daisy family, feverfew originated in the Mediterranean area and was used in Greco-Roman times, primarily for menstrual difficulties. In the seventeenth century, it was used for headaches.

Feverfew's current popularity as a remedy for preventing and treating migraine is a result of the publication of a number of clinical studies in British medical journals.

- Based on a 1983 article by Johnson and associates, 70 percent of migraineurs reported reduction in the frequency or pain of migraine.
- Reporting a small 1985 study by Johnson, feverfew reduced migraine pain and duration by about half.
- From a well-designed follow-up study of fifty-nine migraine patients by Murphy and associates, patients using feverfew showed a 24 percent reduction in the number of migraines, and a significant reduction in nausea and vomiting.
- A 1996 study in the Netherlands by De Weerdt and associates produced negative results. In this study, a dried alcohol extract of feverfew leaf was used. It was speculated that perhaps the alcohol extract did not deliver the most active constituent of feverfew, parthenolide.
- In an Israeli study by Palevitch, which used dried feverfew leaves, the herb did not perform significantly better than a placebo.

Feverfew has been proposed for adoption by the European Union as a prophylactic treatment of migraine. Despite the somewhat equivocal research findings, feverfew appears to have won acceptance for this application.

Garlic (Allium sativum). Garlic is recognized in traditional medicine worldwide as a valuable medicinal herb. In the United States and Western Europe, garlic has become one of the most popular substances for reducing cardiovascular risk factors. This medicinal application is partly based on a large number of clinical studies.

Garlic is used for reduction and stabilization of blood pressure, blood sugar, and blood lipids. It also has anticlotting, antioxidant, antimicrobial, antifungal, and antiprotozoal activity, and boosts immunity.

By 1993, at least 1,088 scientific studies dealt with garlic's medicinal effects, for both healthy people and ill people. Garlic's medicinal properties depend on its principal active constituent, allicin, which has a strong odor and is unstable under many conditions. Many people object to the bad breath caused by garlic, but deodorized garlic preparations do not have the same allicin-producing ability, and are less valuable medically. Also, cooking destroys most of garlic's medical benefits. Carefully dried garlic powder preserves the alliinase activity, but the powder should be ingested in enteric-coated tablets to protect it from inactivation by stomach acid.

Most of the clinical trials on garlic have studied its effect on lowering blood lipids, especially total cholesterol and low-density lipoproteins (LDL).

- Forty studies yielded a mean decrease of serum cholesterol of 10.6 percent. In another meta-analysis of studies by Warshafsky, researchers concluded that garlic, at a dosage of about one-half to one clove a day (or 600–900 mg) was able to reduce total serum cholesterol levels by about 9 percent.

    Other clinical studies have looked at the effect of garlic on blood pressure, as well as its antibiotic, anticancer, antioxidant, and immunomodulatory effects. Although research appears promising in these areas, the evidence is not as strong as it is for hypolipidemic activity.
- Epidemiological studies have suggested that garlic (as well as other

members of the genus *Allium,* including onions, leeks, shallots, chives, and wild garlic) can reduce the risk of certain types of cancer. Statistical studies have correlated garlic consumption with low incidence of cancer in Europe, Egypt, India, China, and in some Third World countries.

- Clinical research on garlic's anticancer properties has generally involved Kyolic®, an odorless, aged garlic extract from Japan. This preparation, however, is less effective for cardiovascular problems. In a study by Steiner, it yielded reductions in total cholesterol of about 6 to 7 percent. While these results are positive, they do not compare with the degree of blood lipid reduction that has been achieved with standardized powdered garlic preparations. Moreover, the amount of garlic given in the Kyolic study was 7.2 grams a day, a relatively large and costly dosage.

Research seems to substantiate claims for garlic's ability to reduce cardiovascular risk factors, but the precise mechanism remains unknown. Perhaps future well-designed research will confirm garlic's anticancer actions.

Ginger (Zingiber officinale). Long popular as a spice, ginger is also used as a traditional medication, especially in Chinese and Ayurvedic medicine. It is primarily used to help the gastrointestinal tract. It is approved in Germany as a nonprescription medicine, and is increasingly used in the United States for preventing nausea and motion sickness.

- Clinical investigations of ginger's antinausea properties began with a 1992 study by Mowrey and Clayson, in which a single 940 mg dose of powdered ginger root was compared with Dramamine and with a placebo in a single-blind trial. Blindfolded subjects treated with ginger lasted longer in a tilted rotating chair than either the Dramamine or the placebo group, before vomiting occurred.
- A 1994 study at sea by Schmid and associates, involving 1,741 participants in a whale-watching cruise, found none of the 203 persons taking 250 mg of ginger had seasickness. Ginger proved as effective as five other medications. Ginger has also been effective for postoperative nausea, and nausea from chemotherapy. However, in another study, the drug scopolamine was better able to prevent motion sickness.

Ginger may not be safe for morning sickness nausea, however, because some components of ginger may have mutagenic effects, which could possibly cause birth defects.

Historically, ginger has also been a popular remedy for headache, migraine, inflammation, and rheumatic conditions, but such uses are not well documented by clinical studies.

Ginkgo (Ginkgo biloba). Considered a "living fossil," *Ginkgo biloba* is the world's oldest living deciduous tree. It originated some 200 million years ago, and was almost entirely destroyed in the last Ice Age, except for a small population that survived in northern China. The trees live up to one thousand years, and are remarkably adaptable to a wide range of climates, insects, and diseases.

Ginkgo biloba extract, or GBE, is the most frequently used phytomedicine in Europe, available in Germany by prescription and over-the-counter. Commission E in Germany has approved GBE for the symptomatic treatment of dementia-related memory deficits, concentration problems, and depression; for intermittent claudication (pain on walking due to compromised blood flow to the extremities); and for vertigo and tinnitus (ringing in the ears) of senile vascular origin. Daily doses of 120 to 240 mg have been shown to elicit response.

Ginkgo leaves contain many pharmacologically active compounds, including unique flavonoids and terpenoids, with chemical properties similar to vitamin P, known as ginkolides, which are found nowhere else in nature. All the many constituents of ginkgo act together; single components do not show the same activity as the whole leaf extract. GBE's pharmacological actions include free radical destruction, reduction of lipid peroxidation, and reduction of blood platelet aggregation.

- A review of forty trials of GBE by Kleijnen and Knipschild indicated GBE's effectiveness in treating insufficient cerebral blood flow to the brain, although many of the studies were poorly designed.
- During a double-blind trial by Vesper and Hansgen in 1994, the GBE preparation kaveri was tested on ninety elderly patients with cerebral insufficiency, and improvement was found with a daily dose of the ginkgo preparation over twelve weeks.
- From a review of ten studies with people who had intermittent claudication, or temporary blood flow blockages, ginkgo appeared to be

effective. Based on some of these studies, Commission E concluded that there was enough evidence to approve the use of ginkgo for such intermittent claudication.

- Bauer in 1984 used a daily dose of ginkgo preparation for six months to treat intermittent claudication in a randomized clinical trial of patients with insufficient circulation to their extremities. Significant improvement was observed in the ginkgo group after twenty-four weeks of treatment.

  Ginkgo has been promoted for some time as a treatment for Alzheimer's disease, and recent studies indicate that it does have potential benefit in slowing progression of the disease.

- In an important 1997 study of Alzheimer's patients by LeBars and associates, published in the *Journal of the American Medical Association,* ginkgo induced modest improvement in, or a delay in the decline of, cognitive function, living skills, and social behavior.

Claims have also been made for ginkgo's ability to improve mental functioning among healthy people. Some studies have been positive. Whether the widely publicized claims for ginkgo as a "smart pill" for normal individuals will ever be proved remains a controversial but interesting question. It appears likely that ginkgo will be definitely proved capable of producing noticeable increases in intellectual performance in normal, healthy subjects.

Ginseng (Panax quinquefolius, Panax ginseng, and other species). Long valued in Asia as an adaptogen, ginseng is one of the most expensive herbs in the world and has become one of the top three herbal products in the United States. *Panax,* the genus name, comes from the Latin word *panacea,* meaning "cure-all," and indeed, the claims for ginseng, of which scientists have historically been skeptical, imply a near-miraculous ability to address a wide variety of problems. Uses of ginseng include treatment of diabetes, impotence, gastrointestinal disorders, prevention of liver toxicity, and promotion of longevity.

Thousands of pharmacological studies and hundreds of animal studies have been done on Asian ginseng root. Its active constituents are ginsenosides (or triterpenoid saponin glycosides), which may have beneficial effects on fatigue and the immune system and have antidiabetic and anti-impotence effects. Human studies are much more equivocal.

A significant number of studies have been done with a proprietary extract of *Panax ginseng* manufactured in Europe known as G115, or Ginsana®. Twenty-one placebo-controlled trials have been done on Ginsana extract, as well as six review articles, many of them following good experimental design. Ginsana is sold in the United States as a dietary supplement.

- Ginsana improved mental functioning in a study by Rosenfeld of fifty patients with psychosomatic weakness, depression, or neurological disorders. Physicians and patients, respectively, rated the success of ginseng therapy at 96 and 88 percent.
- According to a recent University of Illinois monograph, clinical studies support the use of ginseng as a mental and physical preventive and restorative agent in some cases of weakness, exhaustion, tiredness, loss of concentration, and during convalescence.
- Concluding a 1990 randomized clinical trial by Scaglione and associates, patients receiving ginseng showed improved immunity. In another study by Scaglione, research indicated that ginseng helps prevent colds and flu.
- Based on a 1995 study by Sotaniemi and associates, diabetics taking ginseng noted improvements in mood, physical performance, reduced fasting blood sugar, and overall regulation of blood sugar levels.

What Does Not Work

Not all studies of ginseng, however, have been favorable.

- In a 1997 study of thirty-one men, a standardized ginseng extract did not produce any improvement in work performance and recovery, nor a change in energy metabolism. This suggests that ginseng has not been proven to improve work performance.

One reason for the lack of definitive data about ginseng's health effects is the inherent difficulty of quantifying intangible benefits such as "vitality" and "quality of life." People who take ginseng risk paying a high price without proven benefit. Commercial preparations of ginseng can cost up to $20 an ounce and vary tremendously in quality. Adverse reactions to ginseng are rare, although hypertension and tachycardia have been reported.

Another problem with ginseng is product quality. Studies in the late 1990s found that ginseng products were of widely variable quality, and that many contained little or no ginseng. Nevertheless, ginseng products enjoy great popularity, both in the United States and abroad, and research will undoubtedly continue to evaluate this highly prized and puzzling plant.

Hawthorn (Crataegus species). Hawthorn has long been used as a longevity remedy in China, and has now found favor in Europe and the United States. Hawthorn is presently the plant medicine of choice in Europe for regulating heart functions. It has a long history of use, and a high level of safety, with clinical evidence to support its cardiovascular benefits, especially its cardiotonic activity.

Many German studies document its effectiveness in treating heart disease.

- From a 1993 RCT by Leuchtgens of 30 patients with stage II heart conditions, patients receiving hawthorn showed significant improvement in exercise tolerance, and also mild reduction in blood pressure.
- During an intervention by Weikl of 136 patients with stage II cardiac insufficiency, patients receiving hawthorn showed a statistically significant improvement in blood pressure and heart rate output, with improvement in quality of life.
- Based on an eight-week German study by Schmidt, which used high daily doses of hawthorn (900 mg), the symptoms of heart failure decreased by a mean of 66 percent by the end of treatment, with stage I cardiac insufficiency patients becoming largely symptom-free.
- Hawthorn has also been shown by Hanack and Bruckel to help combat anginal pain, which results from insufficient blood flow to the heart muscle.

With growing public awareness of the benefits of hawthorn in treating heart disease, healthy individuals are also beginning to use the herb as a heart tonic, for prevention, and for minor heart problems. Caution is advised in self-medication of heart problems, since any heart symptoms should receive professional medical attention. Until cardiologists become more familiar with the benefits of this safe botanical remedy, however, it is likely that hawthorn will usually be self-prescribed.

Milk Thistle (Silybum marianum). A bristly plant native to the Mediterranean, milk thistle has a long history of medicinal use in Europe. It was used in Greco-Roman times for a variety of ailments, particularly liver problems.

Milk thistle must be prepared in standardized, concentrated form to protect the liver. Preparations of milk thistle are generally standardized to a concentration of 70 to 80 percent of several substances known collectively as silymarin. This concentration of silymarin is required to avoid destruction by gastric fluids.

Germany's Commission E recommends daily doses equivalent to 200 to 400 mg of silymarin, and approves the use of silymarin to treat toxic liver damage, and as supportive treatment in chronic inflammatory liver disease and hepatic cirrhosis. Some 120 clinical studies have been done.

Milk thistle changes the structure of the outer membrane of liver cells, preventing toxins from entering the cells. It also stimulates the formation of new liver cells.

Milk thistle extract has been shown in clinical studies to be effective for hepatitis, alcoholic cirrhosis, and liver damage from exposure to harmful chemicals. It has also been successfully employed to prevent or treat poisoning by the death cap mushroom.

- A review of European clinical studies dating from 1971 to 1988, by Hikino and Kiso, concludes that silymarin is effective not only for toxic and metabolic liver damage, but also for acute and chronic hepatitis.

Treatment of liver damage due to alcohol is one of the most effective uses of silymarin.

- During a study by Fintelmann and Albert of 66 patients, most of whom had alcohol-induced toxic liver disease, 31 patients received the standardized milk thistle preparation legalon, and showed significant improvement in liver enzyme levels.

Some forms of hepatitis have responded to treatment with silymarin.

- In a 1971 study by Poser, 67 subjects were treated for toxic metabolic liver damage, chronic hepatitis, and bile duct inflammation. After three months of treatment with silymarin, chronic hepatitis was significantly improved, with bile duct inflammation particularly responsive to the treatment.
- Silymarin was evaluated in the treatment of liver cirrhosis in an RCT by Ferenci and associates. Eighty-seven of 170 patients received silymarin and 83 received placebo. Survival rate for the silymarin group was 58 ± 9 percent, whereas in the placebo group it was 39 ± 9 percent.

Milk thistle has become a popular dietary supplement in the United States. Milk thistle extracts are being used by many people to promote proper liver function and to aid detoxification. Future research may explore the use of milk thistle extract as an adjunct to cancer chemotherapy.

Saw Palmetto (Serenoa repens). Saw palmetto berry is the most widely used botanical preparation for prostate problems. Saw palmetto is native to the West Indies and the southeastern United States. Native Americans used saw palmetto berries to treat genitourinary problems. In the early part of this century, saw palmetto berry tea was commonly recommended by medical professionals for benign prostatic hypertrophy (BPH).

Although a number of controlled clinical studies have verified the use of saw palmetto preparations as a safe and effective treatment for relieving the symptoms associated with BPH, results overall have been somewhat variable. Claims that the herb reduces prostate enlargement, or helps prevent the onset of prostate cancer, are not well documented.

- A twenty-eight-day study of 110 BPH patients by Champault and associates found that saw palmetto was able to reduce painful urination, nighttime urination, and residual urine in the bladder, with significant improvement in flow rate.
- In a trial in Belgium, 505 patients with mild to moderate BPH symptoms were treated with an oral saw palmetto preparation. At the end of three months, the 305 patients who were available for evaluation

showed a significant decrease in prostate symptom scores.

- A critical review by Lowe and Ku, however, argued that no clear mechanism of action has been proposed for BPH, that there is conflicting evidence in some areas, and that some trials were of poor quality.
- Saw palmetto extract has been compared with finasteride (Proscar®), a commonly used synthetic pharmaceutical for the treatment of BPH. In a six-month RCT of 1,098 men, prostate symptom scores showed equivalent decreases with both treatments, but saw palmetto use resulted in fewer complaints of impotence and reduced libido.
- Most recently, in the special CAM issue of the *Journal of the American Medical Association* in November of 1998, researchers at the Minneapolis Veteran Affairs Medical Center reported another positive study on the effectiveness of saw palmetto. This study also found that saw palmetto was as effective as the drug Proscar in relieving symptoms and increasing urine flow with fewer side effects than the commonly prescribed drug.

Biochemical and anatomical evidence is lacking to support claims that saw palmetto actually reduces enlarged prostate size. While some research suggests it may help to prevent prostate cancer, more research in this area is needed. In the United States, the FDA currently prohibits the sale of over-the-counter products for treating BPH, arguing that none have been proven efficacious, and that their use may cause delays in seeking medical attention. Under proper medical supervision, lipophilic saw palmetto extract, sold as a dietary supplement, may afford a low-cost and nontoxic alternative to conventional pharmaceutical treatment.

St. John's Wort (Hypericum perforatum). St. John's wort (SJW) is one of the powerhouses of contemporary herbal medicine. It has become very popular in the United States in a short period of time, and is used primarily to combat depression.

Ancient herbalists, including the Greeks and Romans, used SJW for wound healing, as a diuretic, and for treatment of neuralgic pain. It was brought by early European colonists to the United States, where it was valued for its astringent, sedative, and diuretic properties. It was also used in the nineteenth century for depression.

St. John's wort is currently of keen interest to AIDS researchers, who are looking into the possible antiviral activity of one of its primary active compounds, hypericum.

In Germany, sixty-six million daily doses of SJW were taken in 1994 for the treatment of depression. German doctors now prescribe SJW far more frequently than Prozac, at ratios variously reported as twenty to one, six to one, or four to one (depending on the specific product cited).

Germany's Commission E recommends an average daily dosage of 2 to 4 grams of dried herb, containing 0.2 to 1.0 mg of hypericin, the constituent considered responsible for some of the herb's activity. However, there may be as many as ten active constituents.

- In 1992, Reh and Laux compared SJW to placebo in a study of 50 depressed patients. Given daily for eight weeks, it produced a significantly greater improvement than the placebo in the patient's mood and ability to carry out daily activities, with no side effects.
- In a study by Harrer and Sommer, SJW produced notable improvement in depression after only two weeks.
- During a 1994 study by Woelk and associates of 3,250 patients with depression, depression was resolved or improved in about 30 percent of cases.
- Based on a 1996 meta-analysis of twenty-three studies, reported in the *British Medical Journal,* SJW was compared with conventional tricyclic antidepressants. In the trials, 63.9 percent of patients responded favorably to SJW preparations, compared to 58.5 percent of those receiving tricyclics.

What's in the Works

St. John's wort is currently being evaluated in comparison with Prozac, but studies are incomplete. SJW's mechanism of action may be an inhibition of the reuptake of neurotransmitters, including serotonin, which is the mechanism for Prozac. Half the people who take drugs like Prozac experience side effects, some of them serious. There is hope that SJW will prove as effective as Prozac, without similar side effects.

At the present time, the Office of Alternative Medicine is conducting a major, multiyear randomized clinical trial at several university sites to determine the efficacy of SJW with depression. This study is being coordinated by a research team at the Duke University School of Medicine. For this study, the extracts of SJW were carefully standardized. Such a combination of standardization, RCT, and multiple sites is precisely the kind of definitive research needed for CAM therapies and therapeutics.

St. John's wort has been known to produce reactions to sunlight in livestock that feed on the plant. This photosensitivity has never been demonstrated in humans, but it is wise to be cautious, and to refrain from using the herb if one is taking a drug that produces photosensitivity, such as tetracycline. Fair-skinned people, or those with a history of photosensitivity, might want to reduce sun exposure when they are using this herb.

Standardized hypericin dosage is 400 mg of the extract, at 0.3 percent hypericin. Typically, it takes a few weeks before the antidepressant effects of the herb will be noticed.

Valerian (Valeriana officinalis). For more than one thousand years, valerian has been used for its calmative properties. More than any other herb, valerian has a solid reputation as a safe and effective mild sedative and sleep aid.

A common misconception about valerian is that it is the source of the benzodiazepine drug Valium.

Despite its long use, the active constituents of valerian remain unknown. It is commonly believed that the plant's activity results from the synergistic action of several ingredients.

- Participating in a German study by Schmidt-Voigt, 11,168 individuals received valerian tablets for ten days. Among subjects who had difficulty falling asleep, 72 percent reported cessation of the problem, and 22 percent reported improvement. Among those who had difficulty staying asleep through the night, 72 percent reported resolution of the problem, and 20 percent reported improvement. Results occurred in an average of less than two days.
- In a study by Seifert of 1,689 children and adults with sleep disorders, 75 percent reported a significant reduction of sleep disturbances.
- For a multicenter RCT by Vorbach and associates, 121 patients diagnosed with insomnia received either powdered valerian root or placebo. Doctors rated the effectiveness of the herb at 61 percent.

In this study, most of the statistically significant results did not appear until after twenty-eight days.

In Germany, it is common for valerian to be combined with hops, lemon balm, or passionflower. These combinations have been tested against both placebo and benzodiazepine drugs, with favorable results.

Research thus far confirms the claims for valerian as a mild sedative and sleep aid. Valerian is very safe, and unlike barbiturates and other conventional drugs for treating insomnia, it does not interact synergistically with alcohol.

WHAT DOES NOT WORK

A number of reports have appeared in the popular press recently about alleged poisonings by herbal products. Many plants do contain potent toxins, but these plants are not commonly used in herbal medicine. Only a few of the more than one thousand medicinal plants that are commonly available present any serious risk of adverse reactions.

According to a 1988 story in *U.S. News & World Report,* of 1.2 million reports of poison exposure in the United States, only 7 percent involved plants. Of the twelve most frequently reported plants in poisoning incidents, only one, pokeweed (*Phytolacca decandra*), is used medicinally. Most of the plants involved in poisonings were ornamentals, not commercial herbal products.

Nonetheless, a long history of folk use does not necessarily guarantee that a plant is safe. There is always a danger of mislabeling or contamination, and some plants do contain potentially harmful constituents. Some herbs currently available in the United States do present serious concerns. Here we will look at the most common of them.

Comfrey (Symphytum officinale). Comfrey has a long history of medicinal use. It's used to help heal wounds, to help mend broken bones, and to improve respiratory and digestive symptoms. Many American herb enthusiasts consider comfrey a miracle plant, and refuse to believe that it may present toxic risks. However, comfrey contains pyrrolizidine alkaloids, which have been associated with death and illness among livestock that graze on them. They are particularly toxic to the liver, causing a blockage of the hepatic veins, which can lead to fatal reactions.

Comfrey roots contain a higher concentration of pyrrolizidine alkaloids than do the leaves, but both can lead to cirrhosis, liver cancer, and damage to the lungs and other organs. Therefore, comfrey cannot be recommended for internal use. Comfrey products for internal use may still be available in some stores, but have supposedly been removed from the market.

Comfrey is safe to use externally, but should not be applied to broken skin. However, Dr. Andrew Weil reports using comfrey leaves to treat the ulcerated bites of the brown recluse spider, which are notoriously resistant to healing.

Other common plants besides comfrey also contain pyrrolizidine alkaloids, including coltsfoot, liferoot, and borage. Borage seed oil is now being sold for its gammalinoleic acid (GLA) content, but borage oils containing more than 0.5 to 1 mcg per gram of pyrrolizidine alkaloids are not considered safe.

Ephedra (Ephedra species). Ephedra is also known as *ma huang* in Chinese medicine, and in the United States as Mormon tea (actually a different species with little or no ephedrine or pseudoephedrine). This twiggy herb has proven valuable in treating colds, asthma, and cough, and in combination with caffeine, it has also been shown to produce greater weight loss than can be achieved with caloric restriction alone.

Active constituents of ephedra are the alkaloids ephedrine and pseudoephedrine. These potent substances increase blood pressure and heart rate, and pose dangers for people with heart disease, high blood pressure, thyroid problems, or enlarged prostate, and for pregnant and lactating women.

Some 1.5 million pills and tablets containing ephedrine and pseudoephedrine are reportedly taken every day in the United States in cold, hay fever, sinus remedies, and diet aids.

In recent years ephedrine developed a reputation as a recreational drug, and began to be packaged in products with such names as Herbal Ecstacy (*sic*), which supposedly produced safe and pleasurable stimulation. Abuse of these products, as well as some of the more conventional preparations, has resulted in hundreds of reports of adverse reactions, and the FDA has reportedly received notice of fifteen deaths. Most of these cases involved excessive doses.

In response to reports of toxic reactions, the FDA is currently considering banning any products that contain more than 8 mg of ephedrine. This is probably an excessively low limit, since many of the OTC cold and hay fever remedies contain upwards of 30 mg. Some states have suspended the OTC status of ephedrine- and pseudoephedrine-containing drugs, making them available only by prescription. Herb industry spokespeople consider the attempts to control ephedra somewhat overzealous. They point out that whereas some eight hundred adverse reactions per year may have been reported for ephedra, users of acetaminophen, a common aspirin substitute, experience as many as fifty thousand toxic reactions a year. However, this statement is somewhat misleading given the much greater prevalence of the use of acetaminophen than ephedra at the present time.

A major study is presently being conducted at Harvard and Vanderbilt Universities in which seventy-five people will take 90 mg a day of ephedrine alkaloids along with caffeine to determine whether they lose weight, and also to monitor for harmful effects.

Ephedra is probably safe, especially as a whole plant, in modest doses for people who do not have the medical conditions that contraindicate its use.

Chaparral (Larrea tridentata and other species). Chaparral, or creosote bush, is a desert shrub that was a traditional Native American remedy for rheumatism and other illnesses. Chaparral would in itself be a misnomer, as *chaparral* refers literally to dwarf evergreen oak, and broadly to the brushy areas where they and other desert shrubs grow. In California, the creosite bush is one of many common desert shrubs. Its primary active constituent, NDGA, is a powerful antioxidant that has been valued commercially for its preservative properties. More recently, chaparral has been investigated for possible anticancer activity, but that research is inconclusive.

In the 1990s, isolated reports began to appear about liver disease from chaparral. Thirteen cases showed evidence of liver toxicity, with symptoms appearing three to fifty-two weeks after ingestion, usually resolving one to seventeen weeks after intake of the herb stopped. Four individuals progressed to cirrhosis, and two required liver transplants. While chaparral may indeed cause liver damage, its toxic impact is not well established. In some of the reported cases, the people were also taking drugs with established negative effects on the liver, and others had a history of liver disease.

For a time, the American Herbal Products Association requested its members to voluntarily stop selling chaparral. Then, after a medical review of cases of liver dysfunction, they merely suggested that chaparral products be labeled with the appropriate cautions, and with a phone number for reporting adverse effects.

Senna (Cassia species) and other herbal laxatives. Many products labeled as "dieter's teas" contain plant-based laxatives such as senna, aloe, and buckthorn, which can cause uncomfortable and dangerous symptoms when consumed in excessive amounts. Product labels often do not include information about the teas having laxative effects.

Short-term adverse effects of herbal laxative use can include stomach cramps, nausea, vomiting, and diarrhea. With chronic use, laxative dependency can develop, causing sluggish bowel and even loss of colon function, accompanied by severe pain and constipation, which in some cases can require surgical removal of the colon. Severe laxative abuse reactions include fainting, dehydration, and electrolyte disorders, which can lead to death. Four deaths have been reported to the FDA involving women with histories of these medical problems, and the herbal teas may have been a contributing factor in their deaths.

Garcinia cambogia. One additional negative finding was reported in the November 1998 CAM issue of the *Journal of the American Medical Association.* According to a report from the obesity research center at Columbia University College of Physicians and Surgeons, overweight patients who took a TCM herbal remedy, *Garcinia cambogia,* which is found in many commercial weight-loss products, were no more successful at shedding pounds than were those who took a placebo.

Finally, there are four additional negative findings with regard to herbs in the September 17, 1998, issue of the *New England Journal of Medicine.* Doctors from Alberta Children's Hospital in Canada report two cases in which parents opted to treat their children's cancer with shark cartilage or the herb astragalus instead of standard medicines. In both cases, the cancers progressed, and one child died. From a second report, a research team from Robert Wood Johnson Medical School in New Jersey tested a mixture of eight herbs, sold as PC-SPES, on men with prostate cancer. They found that the herb blend has potent hormonal effects. In a third article, the FDA described an episode in which the herb plantain was contaminated with a naturally occurring form of digitalis, a heart stimulant that can cause cardiac arrest. Citing a case report, a group of doctors from Arizona reported the case of a man found driving erratically after taking a supplement promoted as a way to increase growth hormones. Findings such as these and others underscore the need for consumer caution, further research, and the absolute necessity of herbal manufacturers to provide a safe, standardized product with full disclosure to the consumer of the contents, appropriate use, and cautions regarding any and all herbal supplements.

Consumers should be cautious in the use of teas whose labels imply that they promote weight loss, and should examine the list of ingredients carefully for laxatives.

What's in the Works: The Future of Herbal Medicine

In the immediate future, Americans can expect to hear more about a virtual inundation of herbs in the consumer and medical marketplace. For the most part, consumers are driving the demand for more herbal products. However, large drug companies and pharmacy chains are also keenly interested in herbal sales, recognizing the potential for profit. In all likelihood, these companies will sponsor more high-quality studies on herbs. This will make these herbs easier for the consumer to evaluate.

Among the NCCAM research centers, the University of California at Davis under the direction of Dr. M. Eric Gershwin and Dr. Judith S. Stern is focusing on evaluating the clinical applications and underlying biochemical mechanisms for ginseng. Another NCCAM research team at the University of Michigan under Dr. Keith Aaronson and Dr. Susie Zich, a naturopathic physician, is investigating the effect of hawthorn on patients with congestive heart failure (CHF). This series of studies, concluding in 2002, will compare the effectiveness of hawthorn with and without other forms of medication such as digoxin. Researchers at the University of Arizona will be evaluating two new treatments involving herbs and osteopathic manipulation for children with recurrent ear infections.

No matter what, consumers should be cautious. Because the herb industry is essentially unregulated, the practice of botanical medicine is not formalized, and since herbal medicine is not taught in medical and pharmaceutical schools, consumers have essentially been left to their own devices in determining how they will use botanical products.

To ensure the safe and effective use of botanical medicines, consumers should observe the following precautions:

- Herbal preparations should not be used to self-treat serious medical conditions, or persistent symptoms.
- Herbs should not be used for children without medical supervision, by women during pregnancy, or by women who are nursing.
- All people should tell their doctors about any herbal remedies they are taking, because herbs can interact with conventional drugs.
- People should never take more than the recommended dosage of an herbal preparation. They should stop ingestion immediately if they notice an adverse reaction, and should report it to the FDA Med-Watch line at (800) 332-1088.
- Individuals should purchase herbal preparations from reliable, trustworthy sources.
- People using herbs should choose products that give the Latin botanical name and the quantity of herb contained, thus allowing them to calculate the amount of active constituents in each dose.
- It is preferable for people to use preparations that are standardized, according to their active constituents. Many herbal preparations on the market contain insufficient active constituents.
- When people take laboratory or drug tests, they should advise the person administering the test of any herbal preparations they are taking. These herbs can trigger false findings in tests for drug abuse, and can invalidate routine lab tests.

Despite these reasonable cautions, however, herbal medicine is virtually certain to remain a growing area of personal self-care, as well as medical care. Herbal medicine has been used effectively for thousands of years throughout the world. With the help of modern scientific studies, it can become even more effective in the future. Perhaps even more important, the global recognition of nature's green pharmacy will inspire more individuals and nations to protect this extraordinary resource that predates human evolution by hundreds of millions of years.

CHAPTER 7

NATUROPATHIC MEDICINE

"Do No Harm"

Naturopathic medicine includes the diagnosis, treatment, and prevention of disease, as well as the promotion of health. Naturopathy is not a single-modality treatment, but draws upon an array of natural healing interventions and diagnostic techniques. It particularly emphasizes the adage "do no harm," by stressing the use of interventions that are largely free of side effects rather than pharmaceutical medicines and surgery.

Naturopathy is one of the oldest forms of medicine known to humankind, tracing its roots to the healing techniques of ancient China, India, and Greece, and to Native American cultures. It weaves these healing traditions together with modern scientific principles and technology.

Modern American naturopathy grew out of the natural healing movements of the eighteenth and nineteenth centuries, when the popular European practice of "taking the cure" at natural mineral springs and spas spread to the United States. Naturopathy was introduced as a formal American health care profession at the turn of this century by Dr. Benedict Lust, who came from Germany to the United States in 1896 to teach hydrotherapy, which he had used to help cure himself of tuberculosis. After completing his medical training, he founded the first school of naturopathic medicine in New York City, and taught herbal medicine, nutrition, physiotherapy, psychology, homeopathy, and manipulation techniques. During the same period, Dr. James Foster established a similar school in Idaho, and Lust and Foster together named the new profession "naturopathy." Because it drew upon a variety of techniques, it was also referred to as Eclectic medicine.

Naturopathy gained rapidly in popularity; by the 1920s there were more than twenty naturopathic colleges, and the profession was licensed in most states. However, with the consolidation of power by conventional medicine, and with the increasing reliance of allopaths on pharmaceutical drugs, naturopathic medicine entered into a decline. It virtually disappeared until the 1970s, when a revival of popular interest in alternative medicine gave rise to a new generation of highly trained naturopathic practitioners. Today, among the foremost naturopathic physicians are Dr. Michael T. Murray and Dr. Joseph Pizzorno, founding president of Bastyr University, authors of the definitive book *Encyclopedia of Natural Medicine*, which is the defining text of conventional naturopathy.

Modern naturopathy is founded on six basic principles:

1. *Nature has the power to heal.* It is the physician's role to support the self-healing process by removing obstacles to health.
2. *Treat the whole person.* Disease rarely has a single cause, so every aspect of the patient must be brought into harmonious balance.
3. *First, do no harm.* A physician should utilize methods and substances that are as nontoxic and noninvasive as possible.
4. *Identify and treat the cause.* Rather than suppress symptoms, the physician should treat the underlying causes of disease.
5. *Prevention is as important as cure.* A physician should help create health, as well as cure disease.
6. *Doctors should be teachers.* "Doctor" originally meant "teacher." Part of the physician's task is to educate the patient and encourage self-responsibility.

Naturopathic physicians help mobilize their patients' own natural healing powers. Because symptoms represent the body's attempt to heal itself, the naturopath does not try to suppress them. For example, fever and inflammation are not only symptoms but also healing mechanisms. Inflammation is an increase in healing blood flow to an area, and fever is part of the body's way of killing harmful organisms. However, taking aspirin or an antihistamine combats these efforts by the body to heal itself. In actuality, several scientific studies have verified that antihistamines actually may prolong the course of a cold. Instead of using the symptom-suppression approach, a naturopath might encourage a patient to drink extra liquid to help flush out the membranes, and to take nutrients and herbs that stimulate the body's immune system. Naturopaths believe that if a certain healing response is repeatedly suppressed, the body's ability to produce that response may become weakened. Therefore, they believe that symptom-suppression drugs may temporarily relieve discomfort, but can undermine the body's self-healing mechanisms. When the body loses its ability to produce healing responses, chronic disease can become established.

Treatment Methods of Naturopathy

Naturopathy draws upon a variety of modalities, combined to fit the needs of the individual patient. None of these modalities is unique to naturopathic medicine.

Any one of the following modalities can become an area of specialization for a naturopath. Naturopathic colleges offer advanced training in a number of them, leading to specialized degrees. Practitioners may also specialize in a specific problem area, such as pediatrics, family medicine, or allergies.

- *Clinical nutrition.* Therapeutic use of nutrition and diet is the cornerstone of naturopathic medicine. Naturopaths may make dietary recommendations and suggest nutritional supplements, including herbs, vitamins, and minerals. They may order laboratory tests to determine a patient's nutritional status and to monitor changes in his or her condition.
- *Physical medicine.* Naturopaths often use hydrotherapy; exercise; massage; naturopathic manipulation techniques, which are somewhat similar to chiropractic; immobilization, by using braces and

splints; ultrasound, diathermy, or heat therapy; electrical stimulation; and light therapy.

- *Homeopathy.* Homeopathy, discussed in detail in another chapter, is a frequent area of specialization among naturopathic practitioners, and is a healing system that stimulates the body's own natural force.

- *Botanical medicine.* Naturopathic physicians are trained herbalists who believe that using whole plants is generally more effective and less harmful than using either isolated chemical substances derived from plants or drugs that are synthesized from plants. Medicinal herbs, when properly used (either alone or in combination), address the underlying problem that caused the patient's symptoms, and are used in a way that minimizes undesirable side effects.

- *Natural childbirth.* Studies of naturopathic obstetrical care have demonstrated that naturopaths achieve much lower complication rates during and after childbirth than conventional care.

- *Traditional Chinese medicine.* A common area of specialization among naturopaths is traditional Chinese medicine, which includes the use of Chinese herbs and acupuncture. (TCM is described in Chapter Four.)

- *Ayurveda.* Originating in ancient India, Ayurvedic medicine is the world's oldest organized system of natural medicine (discussed in Chapter Ten). Bastyr University, a naturopathic college in Seattle, now offers a specialization in Ayurveda, leading to the degree N.D. (Ayurveda).

- *Counseling and psychotherapy.* Naturopaths are trained in counseling, psychotherapy, behavioral medicine, hypnosis, stress management, and biofeedback, and use these techniques, in part, to motivate patients to comply with lifestyle changes.

- *Minor surgery.* Naturopaths are trained to perform a variety of minor surgical techniques (which are done in the office under local anesthesia), such as superficial wound repair, removal of foreign masses, sclerosing therapy for spider and varicose veins, minor hemorrhoid surgery, circumcision, and the setting of fractures.

An initial appointment with a naturopathic physician takes about an hour, though patients may fill out a questionnaire ahead of time. The naturopath takes a complete medical history and evaluates the patient's lifestyle. Diagnostic procedures may include a physical examination, conventional blood and urine tests, and tests that are not used in conventional medicine, such as the urine indican test (to determine the degree of intestinal putrefaction, a cause of toxemia), or the Heidelberg test (to measure stomach acidity). Using all of this information, the naturopath arrives at a functional and constitutional assessment, as well as a conventional disease diagnosis.

Treatment is individualized, generally using a combination of therapies. A significant amount of time is spent on lifestyle counseling, and recommendations are made on diet, exercise, and stress management. Follow-up visits typically average about half an hour. Naturopaths monitor the progress of their patients through their own observations, the patient's reports, and laboratory tests.

Naturopathic practitioners can prescribe certain classes of drugs in some states, but they do not generally have prescribing privileges. In the state of Washington, naturopaths are allowed to prescribe antibiotics, thyroid medication, progesterone, and selected other drugs.

Naturopaths treat a variety of disorders, but the most common complaints they treat are allergies, fatigue, colds, headaches, digestive prob-

Treatments Used by Naturopaths for Selected Disease Conditions

Condition	Diet	Nutr. Suppl.	Botanic Med.	Homeopathy	Physical Med.	Couns./ Psy.
Osteoarthritis		X	X		X	
Asthma	X	X	X	X	X	X
Atherosclerosis	X	X	X			
Back pain		X			X	X
BPH		X	X			
Depression	X	X	X		X	
Diabetes mellitus	X	X	X		X	X
Eczema	X	X	X			X
HIV	X	X	X	X	X	X
IBS	X			X		X
Migraine	X	X	X	X	X	X
Middle ear inf.	X			X		
PMS	X	X	X		X	
URI		X	X	X		
Vaginitis	X		X			

lems, middle ear infections, menstrual problems, chronic pain, upper respiratory infections, sinusitis, and hormonal imbalances (including menopausal problems). They also often work with allopaths in treating thyroid problems, irritable bowel syndrome, cancer, heart disease, and high blood pressure. Naturopaths also offer natural obstetric care, and their prenatal and postnatal care employs noninvasive, drugless treatment.

A naturopath's treatment may reflect his or her specialty, such as traditional Chinese medicine or homeopathy. In addition, some naturopaths try to cure illnesses by aggressively stimulating general health; this is called the "vitalistic" approach. Most naturopaths, however, seek to remedy the specific biochemical factors that are causing an illness, using particular herbal medicines and other interventions that are especially tailored to the illness.

Because naturopathy focuses relatively more on the whole person than the treatment of isolated disease entities, practitioners tend to employ highly developed counseling and communication techniques. At Bastyr University, students study counseling almost as much as nutrition. Patients generally benefit greatly from these communication skills.

Naturopathy is particularly strong in the areas of preventive medicine, treatment of acute illness, and in chronic and degenerative diseases that may not have responded to other forms of treatment.

However, naturopathic practice does have its limitations. Naturopaths acknowledge that conventional medicine excels in the treatment of acute trauma, childbirth emergencies, treating broken bones, performing corrective surgery, and treating acute, life-threatening illnesses. Nevertheless, naturopaths can provide excellent supportive treatment for all these conditions.

Naturopathic methods have also been used successfully in the treatment of cancer. Thousands of patients have reported astonishing recoveries from cancer using naturopathic methods, such as fasting, therapeutic diet, hydrotherapy, herbal formulas, and other health-building techniques that stimulate immunity. However, naturopaths are often reluctant to publicize such successes because in many states only allopaths are allowed to treat cancer. Even so, naturopaths may work collaboratively with oncologists, especially to ameliorate side effects from cancer treatment.

Collaborating with conventional doctors is, in fact, one of the most valuable services that naturopaths provide. Their solid grounding in biomedical sciences prepares naturopaths to recognize dangerous conditions that require conventional medical intervention. Also, naturopaths often help patients to recognize the potential dangers of some of the popular forms of self-treatment, such as the use of powerful herbs.

Naturopaths are certainly sufficiently trained to work alongside conventional doctors. Naturopaths and allopathic physicians receive similar training in anatomy, cell biology, physiology, pathology, neurosciences, clinical and physical diagnosis, histology, genetics, biochemistry, pharmacology, laboratory diagnosis, pharmacognosy, biostatistics, and epidemiology. Two of the most prominent naturopathic schools, the National College of Naturopathic Medicine and Bastyr University, require more hours of training in these subjects than many allopathic medical schools. In addition, naturopathic students also receive training in botanical medicine, homeopathy, traditional Chinese medicine, hydrotherapy, and naturopathic manipulative therapies, none of which is taught by conventional medical schools. Naturopathic schools also require significantly more training than medical schools in nutrition and in psychological counseling.

WHAT WORKS AND WHAT MAY WORK

A growing body of evidence documents the effectiveness of the various therapies used in naturopathy. However, there are almost no studies of the efficacy of naturopathic medicine as a whole. Only very recently have research techniques been developed for comparing to conventional medicine the efficacy of various whole practices, such as naturopathy, traditional Chinese medicine, or homeopathy.

Many problems have thwarted research on naturopathy as a whole system. One problem is that naturopathic treatment may resolve a wide range of problems in a patient and prevent their return, but these multiple gains are not reflected by most randomized clinical trials, which generally examine only one disorder at a time. Also, funding agencies typically make their decisions on the basis of biomedical theories that naturopathy may directly challenge. Furthermore, most research tends to focus on the efficacy of single, specific substances, rather than multimodal programs or lifestyle changes.

However, some research projects that examine natural, multimodal approaches have been performed recently. Here are two examples.

- During a series of studies by Dr. T. Hudson in 1991 and 1993, forty-three women with abnormal Pap smears engaged in a naturopathic program consisting of botanical and nutritional supplements, topical cleansings, and herbal and nutritional suppositories. After the program, thirty-eight of the forty-three women no longer had abnormal Pap smears.
- From a pilot study at Bastyr University, HIV patients showed improved immune function after engaging in a comprehensive program of herbal and nutritional therapies.

Another current source for naturopathic intervention is research done by mainstream medical researchers. This research tends to focus on single modalities rather than whole programs. An extensive review of this research was completed in 1998 by Dr. Carlo Calabrese of Bastyr University. For fifteen different conditions which are frequently treated by naturopaths, research studies done by conventional practitioners indicated that many of the modalities used by naturopaths were effective. Virtually all of the studies cited by Dr. Calabrese consisted of randomized clinical trials. On page 182 is a table showing these fifteen conditions, along with the treatments that had been found to be effective for them. It's important to remember that combinations of these therapies are likely to be more effective than any single therapy.

Reviews of the clinical literature in naturopathy for this chapter, including the excellent review by Dr. Calabrese, selected only those studies where natural treatments were found effective in addressing the disease conditions included in his table. Negative findings were not included in the clinical literature cited. Partially, this is due to the fact that negative findings are found less frequently in conventional research publications. This shortcoming is compounded in virtually every CAM area, including naturopathy, since research funding is much more limited than in conventional research. Increased attention and research into naturopathy will result in an increase in both positive and negative outcomes and serve to further the scientific basis for the effective practice of clinical naturopathy. Moreover, as with virtually all clinical trials of alternative treatments, many of the studies are seriously flawed in terms of methodology, or included too small a sample size to be conclusive.

Following is a more detailed examination of the research reviewed by Dr. Calabrese. This research clearly indicates that many of the modalities used by naturopaths are effective.

Osteoarthritis

- *Nutritional supplements.* In 1979, Dr. Innocenzo Caruso compared the nutrient SAMe with use of the nonsteroidal anti-inflammatory drug naproxen, and found that SAMe was equally effective, and better tolerated. Also, glucosamine sulfate was found to be as effective as ibuprofen, with fewer adverse reactions.
- *Botanicals.* During a 1991 study, the herb capsaicin reduced pain in a study of seventy arthritis patients by Dr. C. L. Deal. Other studies confirmed the value of cartilage extracts, as well as combinations of herbs and minerals.
- *Physical medicine.* Dr. David H. Trock and colleagues at Danbury Hospital in Connecticut found in 1993 pulsed electromagnetic field stimulation to be significantly more effective than sham treatment. Since electromagnetic fields are not detectable by participants, the sham or placebo treatment uses the same instrument but it is turned off.

Asthma

- *Diet.* A study by Dr. Kim A. Ogle in 1980 yielded a 91 percent improvement of both allergic rhinitis and bronchial asthma with an elimination diet by selectively removing specific parts of the diet. Restricting tryptophan, an essential amino acid, from the diet was found in a 1983 study at the Kardinska Institute to help improve asthma symptoms.
- *Nutritional supplements.* In a 1975 RCT by Dr. Platon J. Collip, pyridoxine reduced asthma attacks. A 1982 Nigerian study of asthmatics by Anah showed that supplementation with 1,000 mg per day of ascorbic acid for fourteen weeks produced less frequent and less severe attacks.

Also, in a very early 1931 English study, treatment with hydro-chloric acid before meals, and exclusion of food allergens, produced improvement in asthma patients. In a 1979 study by Dr. Saroj Gupta, the herb *Tylophora indica* produced improvement in 135 patients with bronchial asthma.

- *Homeopathy.* At the University of Glasgow in 1994, Dr. David Reilly elicited improvement in 77 percent of patients with allergic asthma, using homeopathic remedies.
- *Physical medicine.* In a 1992 study by Dr. Michel Girodo of the University of Ottawa, patients were taught a method of deep diaphragmatic breathing that produced a significant reduction in symptom intensity and use of medications in 67 asthmatic adults.
- *Counseling and psychotherapy.* Twenty-four asthma patients were randomized in a 1993 research project by Henry and colleagues to receive either autogenic training or supportive group therapy. Autogenic training is a relaxation technique developed in Germany in the 1930s. It consists of practices that an individual patient uses to focus and enhance sensations of heaviness and warmth in the body to induce deep relaxation. Today, autogenic training is used extensively in Canada and Europe for treating a wide array of chronic conditions. Those in the autogenics group showed a significant improvement in respiratory function.

Atherosclerosis

- *Diet.* A 1995 study of 605 heart attack patients by Dr. Michel de Lorgeril in France documented the value of a Mediterranean-type diet, rich in alpha-linolenic acid, bread, root vegetables, green vegetables, fish, and fruit; and low in meat, butter, and cream. After twenty-seven months, there were 73 percent fewer heart attacks, and 70 percent fewer deaths in the group on the experimental diet.
- *Nutritional supplements.* A study of 8,341 men with damage to the heart muscle due to prior heart attacks demonstrated the long-term benefits of niacin. In a fifteen-year follow-up study by Dr. P. L. Canner and colleagues of the Maryland Medical Research Institute in 1996, niacin supplementation was associated with an 11 percent reduction in mortality in the 8,341 men who'd had heart attacks.

Also, in a 1985 study by Cherchi and colleagues at the University of Cagliari in Italy, supplementation with the amino acid L-carnitine was found to increase exercise tolerance in 44 patients with angina.

* *Botanicals.* In a 1990 study by Atani of 50 patients with ischemic heart disease, subjects received eight weeks of either the Ayurvedic herbal combination Abana or placebo. Abana reduced the frequency and severity of angina, and improved ventricular function. A 1989 study by Weng of 46 patients with angina found that the herb *Crataegus pinnatifida,* which traditionally has a positive effect on the heart's action, improved symptoms in 84.8 percent of patients.

Back Pain

* *Nutritional supplements.* An innovative 1990 study by Dr. G. Bruggermann of Heidelberg, Germany, indicated that vitamins increased the efficacy of conventional drug therapy for back pain.
* *Physical medicine.* A physiotherapy program, plus exercise, was more effective than education alone in a 1995 study by Dr. H. Frost, of Oxford, for low back pain. Also, in a study of 741 patients with low back pain, chiropractic manipulation was compared with hospital management by Dr. T. W. Meade in England. Those who received chiropractic treatment showed greater improvement in pain scores than those under hospital care.
* *Counseling and psychotherapy.* Cognitive therapy, relaxation training, and cognitive therapy plus relaxation training all decreased back pain in a 1993 study by Dr. Judith A. Turner of the University of Washington. Improvement was sustained at six- and twelve-month follow-ups. In another 1989 study by Dr. Steven J. Linton of Sweden, behavioral pain control training produced significant decreases in pain intensity and pain-related absenteeism as well as improvements in other measures of quality of life in 66 women with back pain.

Benign Prostatic Hypertrophy

* *Botanicals.* Saw palmetto was compared with placebo in a 1984 study by Dr. G. Champault, and produced improvement in urinary symp-

toms and flow rate. In other studies, the herb *Pygeum africanum*, and also a pollen extract, decreased prostate size.

- *Nutritional supplements.* Forty-five patients with enlarged prostates received a combination of the amino acids glutamic acid, alanine, and glycine, and 40 received only placebo. Those receiving amino acids showed a reduction in urinary problems, and a nonsignificant decrease in prostate size.

Depression

- *Diet.* During a 1988 study by Dr. Kelly Kreitsch of Texas A&M University, 23 depressed subjects were placed on a diet free of caffeine and sucrose for one or two weeks, then challenged, in a blinded fashion, with caffeine and sucrose. When challenged, 50 percent responded with significant and sustained deterioration of their moods.
- *Nutritional supplements.* For a study by Tempeste and colleagues in Rome, 24 depressed elderly patients showed significant improvement on one gram of the amino acid L-acetylcarnitine taken daily for one month, as compared with a placebo. A 1978 study by Dr. Bernardo Heller of the University of Buenos Aires found that 100 mg of the amino acid d-phenylalanine produced a higher proportion of recovery or improvement than 100 mg of the antidepressant drug imipramine.
- *Botanicals.* Most significant, a 1996 meta-analysis by the internationally recognized German physician Dr. Klaus Linde of Munich of 23 randomized trials of St. John's wort indicated that the botanical was as effective as standard antidepressants, with fewer adverse effects.
- *Physical medicine.* Treatment of winter depression using light stimulation resulted in less depression, according to a study by Dr. David H. Avery of the University of Washington School of Medicine.

Diabetes Mellitus

- *Botanicals.* Capsaicin cream produced a significant reduction in the pain of peripheral neuropathy, or problems with the nervous system, in a 1992 study of 277 diabetes patients. Also, fenugreek seed powder produced significant improvements in fasting blood sugar, glucose tolerance, and glucose excretion, compared to a placebo, in a study by Sharma in 1990.

- *Counseling and psychotherapy.* Research by Dr. George Moran, of London, indicated that diabetic children receiving psychotherapy showed better diabetic control, with improvement maintained at one year.
- *Nutritional supplements.* In a study of 162 patients with type I and II diabetes mellitus, treatment with 200 mcg of chromium reduced patients' needs for insulin.

Eczema

- *Diet.* According to Atherton in 1978, 14 of 20 afflicted children who completed a twelve-week diet excluding eggs and cow's milk responded favorably. In Fergusson's 1994 study in which a group of children was followed from birth, 1,265 children who received a diverse solid-food diet during their first four months had a higher risk of developing eczema than those who did not.
- *Botanicals and specific foods.* In a 1992 study of 40 adults with longstanding refractory dermatitis, or treatment-resistant skin problems, treatment with ten traditional Chinese herbs resulted in improvement in symptoms. Also, a 1981 study by Antoun of seed extracts (*Lupinus termis*) verified that their effectiveness in treating chronic eczema was comparable to cortisone therapy.
- *Counseling and psychotherapy.* A 1995 research project by Dr. Anke Ehlers of Oxford showed that autogenic training and cognitive-behavioral treatment resulted in improved skin condition and less use of topical steroids.

HIV Disease

- *Diet.* A 1996 Harvard study by Dr. Christine A. Wanke showed that a diet based on medium-chain triglycerides reduced chronic diarrhea and malabsorption, compared with a long-chain-triglyceride-based diet.

- *Nutritional supplements.* In a 1993 study by Dr. Gregg O. Coodley of Oregon Health Sciences University, beta-carotene produced an improvement in immune system function. A 1995 study of 118 children born to HIV-infected mothers indicated that children who were given vitamin A died less often.
- *Homeopathic remedies.* In a 1993 study by Dr. D. P. Rastogi in India, 129 asymptomatic HIV carriers were treated with individualized constitutional homeopathic remedies, and 12 became HIV-negative after three to sixteen months. A 1994 study by Wolffers of homeopathic treatment of HIV and AIDS patients in the Netherlands showed an improvement in CD4+ cells in 23 of 34 cases.
- *Physical medicine.* In a very small 1993 pilot study by Dr. Michael T. Carpendale in San Francisco, five AIDS or ARC patients with intractable diarrhea improved markedly after daily colonic insufflations, or blowing of gases, of medical ozone. In a larger 1996 study of massage therapy by Dr. Frank Scafidi of the University of Miami School of Medicine, newborns with HIV showed improved behavioral measures and greater weight gain.
- *Combination therapy.* From San Francisco, Dr. Jon D. Kaiser has used a program of diet, exercise, vitamins, herbs, and stress management that has shown promising results in halting the progression of AIDS among HIV-infected individuals. Based on his clinical experience, Dr. Kaiser considers HIV a potentially dormant virus that can remain in the system for years without causing symptoms if an inhospitable environment for the virus is maintained in the body. Over a five-year period, which included limited use of drugs, 89 percent of 134 HIV-positive patients improved or remained stable on the program.

Irritable Bowel Syndrome

- *Diet.* A 1982 study by Dr. V. Alun-Jones at the University of Cambridge, England, showed that patients who had been symptom-free on an allergy-free diet reexperienced symptoms when food allergens were reintroduced.
- *Homeopathy.* Using asafoetida, Dr. V. W. Rahlfs of Stuttgart elicited improvements in 100 patients.

- *Counseling and psychotherapy.* At the University Hospital of Wales in 1991, Dr. G. Shaw and his colleagues found significant improvement of symptoms in a group taught stress management skills, compared with a group receiving the medicine Colpermin. Also, a 1984 study supported use of hypnotism in treating IBS.

Migraine Headache

- *Nutritional supplements.* According to Dr. T. McCarren, studies have shown the efficacy of treating migraine with fish oil fatty acids and with the amino acid tryptophan. A 1991 study by Dr. Fabio Faccinetti of the University of Pavia in Italy indicated improvement when subjects were given daily magnesium supplementation.
- *Botanicals.* In 1988, Dr. J. Murphy noted reduced symptoms in patients receiving herbal treatment.
- *Homeopathy.* Based on a 1991 study by Drs. Brigo and Serpelloni, 80 percent of patients treated over four months improved with homeopathy, compared with 13 percent on placebo. However, two follow-up and better designed studies by Gaus in 1992 and Whitmarsh in 1997 were both totally negative. Homeopathy does not appear to be effective in migraines.
- *Physical medicine.* Successful therapies include transcutaneous electrical nerve stimulation (TENS) and cryotherapy, which is treatment with cold applications. TENS therapy consists of applying electronics to an injured area and passing a low-intensity electrical current through the involved injury. An uncontrolled trial in 1989 by Dr. Lawrence D. Robbins of the University of Illinois showed that 64.5 percent of patients found a cold wrap mildly effective and 9 percent judged it completely effective.

Middle Ear Infections

- *Diet.* A large 1993 retrospective study by Dr. Burris Duncan of the University of Arizona of 1,220 infants showed that there were significantly fewer occurrences of a type of middle ear infection, otitis media, in infants who were exclusively breast-fed for at least four months. Food allergy has also been implicated in otitis media, as demonstrated by Dr. David S. Hurst in a 1990 study of 20 patients. In another study, Dr. T. M. Nsouli of Georgetown University elicited significant improvement in 86 percent of children with recurrent otitis media, using an allergy-exclusion diet.

• *Homeopathy.* As reported by Dr. K. H. Friese, the average duration of treatment in a homeopathic group was four days, compared with ten days with conventional care. Although this was not an RCT, relapses within one year occurred in 29.3 percent of the homeopathic group, and 43.5 percent of the conventionally treated group.

Premenstrual Syndrome

• *Diet.* Dr. D. Yvonne Jones of the National Cancer Institute found that women on a low-fat diet (20 percent of calories) had significantly fewer physical PMS symptoms than women on a high-fat diet (40 percent of calories).

• *Nutritional supplements.* Alpha-tocopherol supplementation for three menstrual cycles produced significant reduction of symptoms, according to Dr. Robert S. London of the Johns Hopkins University School of Medicine. Daily calcium carbonate supplementation also reduced symptoms, according to Dr. Susan Thys-Jacobs of the New York Medical College.

• *Botanicals.* For a large 1985 study by Dr. J. K. Pye, 92 patients were given three grams daily of evening primrose oil for three to six months, and experienced a significant decrease in cyclical breast pain. In a 1993 study by Tamborini, 165 women with congestive premenstrual difficulties who were treated with *Ginkgo biloba* had significantly reduced symptoms, particularly in breast complaints.

• *Physical medicine.* In a 1994 study by Dr. Julie A. Aganoff of the University of Queensland in Australia, 97 PMS sufferers found that regular exercise improved their concentration, disposition, and pain.

Upper Respiratory Infection

- *Nutritional supplements.* A 1992 study by Dr. Ranji Kumar Chandra found that 96 elderly subjects who were given a multivitamin in modest dosage had significantly less frequent infection-related illness than a placebo group. In a 1994 study of the use of zinc gluconate lozenges, Dr. George A. Eby reported that after seven days of treatment, 86 percent of 37 patients who took zinc lozenges were symptom-free, compared with 46 percent of 28 placebo patients.
- *Botanicals.* During a 1994 study by Mumcuoglu of patients with influenza B, those treated with an herbal extract of *Sambucus nigra* and *Rubus idaeus* became symptom-free significantly more quickly than a placebo group.
- *Homeopathy.* In a 1989 study by Dr. J. P. Ferley of Grenoble University Hospital in France, 17.1 percent of influenza patients taking Oscillococcinum recovered within forty-eight hours, compared to 10.3 percent of a placebo group.

Vaginitis

- *Diet.* Patients who consumed eight ounces daily of yogurt containing *Lactobacillus acidophilus* had a threefold decrease in infections and candidal colonization, compared with those on a yogurt-free diet, as reported by Dr. Eileen Hilton in 1992 in *Annals of Internal Medicine.* Acidophilus capsules are widely available in health food stores and commonly used to restore the intestinal flora after diarrhea or use of antibiotics.
- *Botanicals and specific foods.* Women with certain vaginal infections, including trichomonal vaginitis, an acute bacterial infection, who received *Malaleuca alternifolia oil* achieved results equivalent to those of standard treatment in 50 of 96 cases, according to Dr. Eduardo F. Pena in 1962. In a 1993 study by Dr. Alexander Neri of Tel Aviv, 84 women with bacterial vaginal infection during pregnancy received yogurt, acetic acid, or no treatment. Yogurt was found superior to the other forms of treatment.

What's in the Works

At Bastyr University, Dr. Leanna Standish served as the research director of the previously funded OAM research center. Although Bastyr is not currently a funded NCCAM center, Dr. Standish and Dr. Carlo Calabrese are currently examining naturopathic treatments in people infected with HIV. She has found that herbal and nutritional therapies have produced improvement in some measures of immune functioning and slower progression of AIDS, as compared to controls who received only conventional therapy.

Naturopathic colleges have also conducted studies in a number of other areas, such as the antitumor activity of maitake mushrooms; the absorption of zinc in various forms; the effects of garlic oil on blood clotting, blood lipids, and blood pressure; treatment of intestinal yeast infection with acidophilus, and with homeopathy; colon hydrotherapy; and herbal treatment of sinus inflammation.

Research currently under way or recently completed at naturopathic colleges includes a study of outcomes of alternative cancer therapy among patients attending three Mexican cancer clinics; allergenic properties of primitive wheat strains; the effects of homeopathic treatment of osteoarthritis of the knee; the use of shark cartilage in treating Kaposi's sarcoma; techniques for clinical assessment of food sensitivities; effects of aloe vera on migraine; and a clinical trial of odorless garlic in treating yeast infections.

At the Colorado Health Sciences Center in Denver, Dr. Kedarn Prasad was funded by OAM to study the use of high doses of multiple antioxidant vitamins in cancer treatment, to determine whether they can enhance the effectiveness of chemotherapy and radiation therapy. From the University of Minnesota School of Public Health, Dr. Lawrence Kushi, with funding from OAM and the Kushi Foundation, a leading center for macrobiotic education, is developing data collection procedures to be used in clinical trials of macrobiotic diets in the treatment of cancer.

The Future of Naturopathy

Naturopathy is increasingly being integrated into conventional medicine. One reason for this is its cost-effectiveness. Naturopathic office visits cost about half as much as visits to a conventional practitioner. Naturopaths often have lower office overhead than conventional doctors since they place less emphasis on high-technology equipment. Their malpractice insurance costs are also much lower, because they are rarely involved in litigation. In Germany, the government requires conventional doctors and pharmacists to study naturopathic methods, since the approach has proven so cost-effective.

Naturopathic medicine also offers inexpensive natural alternatives to common medical procedures that are expensive, risky, and often overused, such as hysterectomy, prostate surgery, and tonsillectomy.

During recent years, naturopathic medicine has gained increasing respect not only from American health care consumers but also from government bodies and from the conventional medical community. It has become common for medical organizations, which in the past opposed naturopathic medicine, to endorse naturopathic techniques. Because of their broad training in complementary and alternative practices, as well as in basic biomedical sciences, licensed naturopaths are considered by many authorities to be the best prepared of all CAM practitioners for integration into the mainstream.

Insurance coverage for naturopathic treatment varies by state and by carrier. Many insurance companies now cover naturopathic medicine, and in Connecticut, state law requires 100 percent coverage of naturopathic treatment. In fact, HMOs and insurance carriers may do well to use naturopaths as gatekeeper physicians, allowing patients to opt for more natural and cost-effective approaches to their overall health care. Ultimately, our health care system will probably recognize the benefits of this approach.

Another important factor, besides simple proof of the efficacy of these treatments, is the skill of the naturopathic practitioner in making the correct choice of interventions in each individual case. It is not enough to know that a certain treatment modality was proven successful in a clinical trial in dealing with a certain health condition. It is just as important that the naturopath select appropriate treatments and combinations of interventions for the individual patient. Many treatment options require professional supervision to ensure that they are working and that no untoward effects are being produced. Naturopaths adjust and change treatment modalities depending upon the patient's response, as in all clinical practice.

While this brief review provides considerable positive evidence for the effectiveness of common naturopathic interventions in the illnesses listed, it does not constitute conclusive proof of the efficacy of naturopathy in its entire scope of practice.

In the future, it is likely that naturopathy will act as a complementary treatment for a wide variety of patients, including cancer patients and postsurgical patients. Natural therapies will probably help to speed recovery, and reduce undesirable side effects, when used alongside allopathic techniques. Groundbreaking work is already being conducted to evaluate combination therapies for some of today's most troublesome diseases, including AIDS. Naturopathy might provide alternative protocols for treating certain forms of cancer, and has already proven fruitful in the treatment of heart disease.

Economic incentives may ultimately fuel greater interest in naturopathy. Naturopathy appears to be a cost-effective alternative to conventional approaches. Furthermore, many of the most common naturopathic interventions are well supported by studies. Therefore, naturopathic medicine will in all probability enjoy a bright future.

CHAPTER 8

HOMEOPATHY

Like Cures Like

Homeopathy is a two-hundred-year-old system of medicine based on the principle of "like cures like." It uses extremely dilute preparations of natural substances to stimulate the body's self-healing mechanisms.

At the end of the eighteenth century, Dr. Samuel Hahnemann first formulated the principles of homeopathy. A well-known German physician, Hahnemann was disillusioned by the harmful medical practices of his day, and set out to find a gentler approach.

In the 1790s, Hahnemann undertook an experiment with Peruvian bark, the source of quinine, which is now used to treat malaria. Twice a day he gave himself a dose of quinine bark, and soon developed symptoms of malaria. When he stopped taking the bark, the symptoms went away. He theorized that the same substance, taken in smaller doses by someone suffering from malaria, might stimulate the body to fight the disease. Thus he developed the Principle of Similars, or "like cures like."

He then successfully experimented with other substances. He called his new system homeopathy, from the Greek words *homeo* (similar) and *pathos* (suffering or illness). Emphasis in homeopathy remains in the principle of "like cures like," and the belief that the body's own healing and regenerative capacity can be elicited to restore health.

For the remainder of his life, Hahnemann conducted experiments in which he gave common herbal and medicinal substances to healthy people to see what symptoms they produced. He also began testing his theory on sick people. Hahnemann's subjects sometimes experienced dramatic and uncomfortable symptoms, so he tried giving smaller and smaller doses, to find the smallest amount of a substance that still produced its characteristic effects. For sick people, Hahnemann found that highly diluted remedies were not only less harmful, but also more effective.

Hahnemann's gentle new approach to medicine quickly spread in Europe, and reached the United States in the 1820s. One of the main reasons for the popularity of homeopathy was its success in treating the devastating epidemics of the time. Death rates for some of these diseases were markedly lower among patients treated in homeopathic hospitals. According to contemporary homeopath Dana Ullman, author of *Everybody's Guide to Homeopathic Medicine* and other books, during an 1849 cholera epidemic in Cincinnati, only 3 percent of the patients treated homeopathically died, compared with 40 to 70 percent among those treated with conventional medicine.

Homeopathy's fortunes began to decline with the growth and political advances of organized allopathic medicine, and by 1930 homeopathy had all but disappeared in America. In Europe, however, homeopathy remained relatively popular. Since the 1970s there has been a revival of interest in homeopathy in the United States.

Homeopathy's underlying theoretical principles appear to contravene the principles of modern scientific medicine. It is largely for this reason that homeopathy is often attacked by the medical establishment. However, proponents of homeopathy sometimes point out that the principle of "like cures like" was the basis for the development of vaccines and allergy desensitization treatments. This analogy, though, is not really accurate, since the substances used in immunization and desensitization are identical or similar to the disease-causing agents, whereas homeopathic remedies are usually substances different from those that cause disease.

Hahnemann believed that homeopathic remedies operate by influencing what he called the "vital force," the organizing, animating principle that maintains health in a living system. There is no concept parallel to vital force in Western medicine, but it is somewhat similar to *qi* in Chinese medicine, or *prana* in Ayurveda. A properly selected homeopathic remedy is believed to provoke the vital force, so that the body's own healing power can produce the cure. Homeopaths believe that modern pharmacological medicine may actually interfere with the body's efforts to heal by artificially suppressing symptoms and weakening the vital force.

Today, the leading theoretician and clinical practitioner of homeopathy is George Vithoulkas, author of *The Science of Homeopathy*, who teaches homeopathy curriculum in Athens, Greece. Training at the Vithoulkas school is limited to conventional physicians and osteopaths only, resulting in clinicians who are well versed in both conventional and homeopathic medicine.

Homeopaths have some two thousand remedies, prepared from plants, herbs, animal products, minerals, and chemicals. Remedies are prepared through a process of repeated dilution.

Classical homeopathy is considered a complete medical system, capable of addressing a wide array of health problems. It can treat acute and chronic illnesses, especially in the earlier stages, before there is tissue damage. Migraines, allergies, autoimmune disorders, arthritis, and chronic viral and bacterial infections have all been reportedly treated successfully. Many laypeople also consider homeopathy an excellent method for self-treating minor illnesses, such as flu and colds, and for stimulating general health. In the case of flu, a properly prescribed remedy, such as the popular Oscillococcinum, can provide relief within a few hours to a day or two. Homeopaths do caution that there is no one remedy for the annual varieties of flu, and that self-diagnosis and care are often ineffective. Chronic conditions generally require a longer time, perhaps from a few months to two years.

Homeopathic practitioners may use laboratory testing to help establish an allopathic diagnosis or to determine how severe an illness is. This can help to define expectations about the course of treatment. Clarification of the appropriate use of diagnostic laboratory procedures is reviewed in an excellent 1996 book, *Healing with Homeopathy*, by Dr. Wayne B. Jonas and Dr. Jennifer Jacobs. Laboratory testing is not a major part of homeopathic practice, since prescribing is based on a patient's detailed symptoms rather than on laboratory tests per se. Homeopaths use lab tests much less frequently than do allopaths. According to a survey by Jacobs in 1996 for the American Institute of Homeopathy, diagnostic testing was used among homeopaths less than half as much as by allopaths, 30 percent of the time as compared with 68.5 percent.

For clinicians practicing homeopathy, the two books widely recognized as among the most definitive modern texts are those published by homeopath and conventional physician Dr. Roger Morrison of the Hahnemann Medical Clinic. These books are the *Desktop Guide to Keynotes and Confirmatory Symptoms,* from 1993, followed by *Desktop Companion to Physical Pathology,* published in 1998 as a companion volume.

Homeopathy has always been considered particularly helpful for children. It is reported to resolve, gently and effectively, such problems as recurrent ear infections, colic, croup, diarrhea, bladder infections, teething pain, hyperactivity, emotional problems, and even learning disabilities. Children apparently respond very quickly, because their symptoms are often relatively simple and uncomplicated. Many parents prefer homeopathy, since pharmaceutical drugs can have unpredictable and long-lasting, even toxic effects on children. Homeopathy is also a valued approach for treating health problems in pregnant women and nursing mothers, since they must avoid many pharmaceutical drugs that could be passed on to the infant.

Homeopaths warn patients about the possibility of canceling out the beneficial effects of a remedy with certain substances. These substances, called antidotes, vary with the individual but are thought to include coffee, camphor, mint, some prescription and recreational drugs, strong-tasting or -smelling substances, electric blankets, and dental anesthetics and drilling. Although coffee does appear to antidote or nullify the effects of homeopathic remedies in some cases, Dana Ullman has noted in *The Consumer's Guide to Homeopathy* that homeopathy is used widely and effectively in Europe despite the fact that Europeans have tended to drink strong, espresso coffee more frequently than in the United States until quite recently. Although various substances can antidote remedies, they do so quite rarely. Homeopathic physicians often advise patients to avoid these potential antidotes "just in case," especially during and immediately after treatment. Homeopaths disagree as to how great a danger there is of antidoting a remedy. Many believe that a properly selected remedy is less vulnerable to antidoting. Susceptibility to antidoting also varies from individual to individual.

Problems that homeopathy cannot address include broken bones and surgical emergencies, although homeopathy can help to speed the healing process. Genetic illnesses and diseases cannot be cured by homeopathy, and serious infections may require immediate antibiotic treatment, although homeopaths often report treating such infections successfully. Homeopathy cannot replace the insulin required by diabetics, but in some cases may help reduce certain diabetic complications. One of the greatest risks of homeopathy, in the eyes of critics, is that it may discourage a patient from seeking medical treatment.

Surely, the most controversial aspect of homeopathy is the claimed curative power of highly diluted homeopathic remedies. However, homeopaths are not particularly dismayed at the inability of science to demonstrate the postulated principle by which the remedies work. They point out that for many commonly prescribed allopathic drugs, including aspirin and some antibiotics, the mechanism of action remains equally unknown.

In 1990, Dr. Emilio Del Giudice, an Italian physicist, theorized that water molecules form structures that can store minute electromagnetic signals. This theory is bolstered by the findings of German biophysicist Dr. Wolfgang Ludwig, who has conducted preliminary research showing that homeopathic substances give off electromagnetic signals, indicating specific dominant frequencies in each homeopathic substance, according to physicist Dr. Beverly Rubik of Temple University in 1991. Using nuclear magnetic resonance (NMR) imaging, a 1968 study demonstrated subatomic activity in twenty-three different homeopathic remedies, while such activity was not found in placebos. Similar NMR findings have been confirmed by Dr. J. L. Demangeat and colleagues in a series of 1992 studies.

Most recently, two research papers by physicist Dr. Shui-Yin Lo and his colleagues at the California Institute of Technology indicated that there are novel, stable structures which occur in water molecules at room temperature and under normal atmospheric pressure. These stable molecular forms occur in water containing "very dilute solutions" through a mechanism apparently similar to the formation of ice crystals at low temperatures. While such basic research is preliminary, it does suggest that a proposed mechanism of dilute remedies as residing in the "molecular memory" of the water molecule may ultimately have a basis in modern physics.

Most recently, several studies conducted in both immunology and chemical engineering at UCLA have replicated Dr. Lo's findings. These results are so new that they have only been reported at conferences and have not yet been published and subjected to peer review.

HOMEOPATHY: WHAT WORKS

A team of Dutch medical professors, led by the noted Dutch physician Dr. Jos Kleijnen, none of them homeopaths, conducted a meta-analysis of controlled clinical trials of various forms of homeopathy dating from 1996 to 1990, and published their results in the *British Medical Journal* in 1991. Of the 107 controlled trials studied, 81 showed that homeopathic medicines had some clinical benefits, 24 showed they were ineffective, and 2 were inconclusive. Most of the studies were flawed in some way, but of 22 high-caliber studies identified by the researchers, 15 showed that homeopathic medicines were effective. This suggests that the better-designed and -conducted studies were more likely to find homeopathic medicines effective. Actually, the Dutch professors expressed surprise at the positive results of their study, which included:

- 4 of 9 trials showing benefits in treating vascular disease;
- 13 of 19 showing benefits in treating respiratory infections;
- 5 of 5 successful in treating hay fever;
- 5 of 7 showing faster return of bowel function following abdominal surgery;
- 4 of 6 successful in treating rheumatological disorders;
- 18 of 20 beneficial in treating pain or trauma;
- 8 of 10 helpful in mental or psychological problems;
- 13 of 15 successful in a variety of other conditions.

Since that time, a recent Cochrane review of the literature through 1995 by Dr. Wayne B. Jonas, immediate past Director of the NIH NCCAM, examined nearly 90 well-designed, randomized clinical trials, and the combined results from all these studies also tended to support homeopathy compared to placebo.

More recently, *The Lancet* published a state-of-the-art meta-analysis in 1997 of homeopathic clinical trials by Dr. Klaus Linde and Dr. Wayne Jonas. Working from the published literature, as well as reports from conferences and personal communications, the authors found a total of 186 clinical trials, 89 of which were randomized, double-blind, placebo-controlled, and had adequate statistical data for analysis. Based on this analysis of these 89 placebo-controlled studies, Dr. Linde and his colleagues concluded that "Results of our meta-analysis are not compatible with the hypothesis that the clinical effects of homeopathy are completely due to placebo. However, we found insufficient evidence from these studies that homeopathy is clearly efficacious for any single clinical condition. Further research on homeopathy is warranted, provided it is rigorous and systematic." Such a well-articulated research position characterizes the research and clinical practice of homeopaths, who increasingly rely upon scientific research for support.

Following are a number of conditions that appear to respond to homeopathic treatment, according to studies.

Seasonal Allergic Rhinitis or Hay Fever

- A series of studies by Dr. M. Weisenauer investigated a single remedy, Galphimia glauca, for seasonal allergic rhinitis, or hay fever. A total of nearly six hundred people were involved in the trials, which showed a statistically significant improvement in symptoms among people using homeopathy.
- Two other studies of nasal allergies were conducted by noted clinician Dr. David Reilly and associates of Scotland in 1985. Their pilot study, involving thirty-nine patients, found statistically significant results in favor of the homeopathic remedy. In a similar, larger study by Reilly in 1996, patients using homeopathy showed a statistically significant decrease in symptoms.
- From the Harvard Medical School, a 1995 study by Dr. Mark Abelson indicated that Similisan produced a statistically significant reduction in redness and itching among allergy patients.

Postoperative Ileus

- A series of experiments carried out by researchers in France investigated the use of homeopathy for postoperative ileus, or bowel inactivity following surgery. Three of five of these studies showed a shorter time following surgery until the passage of the first stool among patients using homeopathy.

Childhood Diarrhea

- Three RCTs were conducted, two in Nicaragua and one in Nepal, evaluating the effect of homeopathy on the duration of acute diarrhea in children, which is the leading cause of disease and death in children worldwide. Two had positive results; the third has not yet been published.
- Several other high-quality studies with positive, statistically significant results have been published in peer-reviewed mainstream journals in Europe on homeopathic treatment of childhood diarrhea.

Rheumatoid Arthritis

- In a 1980 study by Dr. R. G. Gibson on rheumatoid arthritis, at the end of three months patients receiving homeopathic treatment showed a statistically significant improvement in pain, stiffness, and grip strength as compared to placebo.
- Studies by Dr. Thomas Kohler in 1991 and Dr. M. Weisenauer also in 1991, conducted in Germany, each involving 176 patients, found statistically significant improvement in patients receiving homeopathic remedies, compared to placebo.

Fibromyalgia

- During 1989, Dr. Peter Fisher and colleagues reported in the *British Medical Journal* that 25 percent more of the homeopathically treated fibromyalgia patients experienced pain relief than those receiving placebo, and almost twice as many had improved sleep. Individuals were given Rhus toxidendron.

Influenza

- In the largest clinical trial to date of a homeopathic medicine, Dr. J. P. Ferley and associates in 1989 studied the use of a homeopathic preparation sold under the trade name Oscillococcinum, made from a highly dilute extract of duck heart and kidney, which is thought to be a reservoir of wild influenza virus. Oscillococcinum is the best-selling flu remedy in France, and is also popular in the United States. It was given to 237 patients with influenza symptoms, while 241 other flu patients received placebo. After forty-eight hours, 17.1 percent of the treatment group had recovered, compared to 10.3 percent of the placebo group. Patients under age thirty were found to respond better than those over thirty. However, the remedy was not found to be effective in patients with severe flu.

Allergic Asthma

- At the University of Glasgow, Dr. David Reilly treated allergic patients with homeopathy in 1994 and achieved an improvement rate of 82 percent, compared to 38 percent of placebo patients.

Sprains

- During two well-designed German studies, a homeopathic complex injury ointment, Traumeel, was compared with placebo in treating sprained ankles. A statistically significant improvement in joint motion was found in the homeopathically treated patients, as compared with the placebo group, in each of the two studies.
- A study of Traumeel in the treatment of eighty patients with hemarthrosis, joint swelling of the ankle, also reported significant results, according to Dr. Jennifer Jacobs in 1997.

WHAT DOES NOT WORK

Plantar Warts

- In a 1992 study by Dr. Michel Labrecque of the homeopathic treatment of plantar warts, 174 patients were treated with three homeopathic medicines—Thuja 30C, Antimonium crudum 7C, and Nitric acid 7C—or with placebo. After six weeks, there was no noticeable difference in the disappearance of warts between the treatment and placebo groups. This suggests only that this particular treatment regimen was unsuccessful.

Osteoarthritis

- According to a 1983 study often cited by critics of homeopathy, thirty-six patients with osteoarthritis were treated in a double-blind crossover design by Dr. Michael Shipley. One-third of the patients were given the homeopathic medicine Rhus tox in the 6C potency, one-third received a conventional nonsteroidal anti-inflammatory, and one-third were given placebo. Patients who were given the conventional drug showed some relief of symptoms, but there was no change among those receiving either the homeopathic remedy or the placebo. However, there were design flaws in the study, and according to Ullman in 1996, Rhus tox is a commonly prescribed remedy for rheumatoid arthritis, but is less commonly prescribed for osteoarthritis.

Preventive Use of Homeopathy

Homeopathy has not been proven effective for preventing illness. Several studies used various homeopathic combination remedies to prevent upper respiratory infections, and failed to show a difference between homeopathic medicine and placebo.

- In a study of Oscillococcinum, which has been shown to be effective in the treatment of influenza, it was given weekly to 1,573

patients during the flu season and compared to placebo. Among
treated patients, the rate of influenza was 21.6 percent, compared
to 23.5 percent in those receiving placebo.

- A study using the remedy Euphrasia 30C to prevent conjunctivitis
was similarly unsuccessful.

WHAT MAY WORK

Most research in homeopathy falls into a "gray zone," with inconclusive
results. Following are research areas that indicated equivocal results.

Recurrent Upper Respiratory Infections

- A 1994 study by Dr. E. S. M. de Lange de Klerk falls into this gray
area. Children with recurrent respiratory tract infections who
received homeopathic remedies had 15 percent better daily symptom scores than those receiving placebo. The treatment group
reduced its use of antibiotics by 55 percent, compared with 38 percent in the placebo group.

Migraine Headache

- During 1991, Dr. Brigo conducted an RCT of sixty patients with
migraines and reported a significant reduction in the frequency and
duration of migraine attacks in the patients receiving homeopathic
remedies. However, subsequent attempts to replicate the results
using International Headache Society guidelines have not been successful.
- Two well-controlled studies on the homeopathic treatment of
migraines did not show that homeopathy was any more effective
than placebo. One 1997 study, using the remedy Cephalgia, was
particularly well designed, and appears to indicate that homeopathy
is probably not effective with migraine headaches.

Mustard Gas

- In London and Glasgow during World War II, homeopathy was used to prevent or treat skin lesions induced experimentally by mustard gas, according to Paterson in 1943. Statistically significant results were obtained in two experiments, but three other homeopathic remedies did not produce any noticeable benefits.

Gastrointestinal Disorders

- Ritter in 1966 used Nux vomica 4X to treat patients with gastritis. Forty-three of seventy-four patients receiving homeopathy responded to treatment, compared to twenty-seven of seventy-three receiving placebo. However, other studies of the use of homeopathy in treating gastritis and irritable bowel syndrome showed no difference between homeopathic medication and placebo.
- A large study using Asafoetida 3X to treat irritable bowel syndrome found a statistically significant improvement in symptoms in those receiving active medication. While not of high quality, these studies do suggest areas for further, more rigorous research.

Women's Health

- In 1987, Dr. Pierre Dorfman of the Unité de Rechercher en Immunologie in Montpelier, France, found a decrease in complications during labor and delivery in patients pretreated with a homeopathic combination remedy.
- Based on a study on "honeymoon cystitis" by Dr. P. A. Ustianowski in 1974, improvement was reported by more women receiving the homeopathic remedy than receiving placebo, but the study was of poor methodological quality.

Otitis Media or Ear Infections

• For the treatment of middle ear infections, or otitis media, in children, a 1996 study by Dr. K. H. Friese comparing individualized homeopathic treatment with conventional antibiotic therapy found a decrease in the degree of pain as well as fewer relapses within one year among children receiving homeopathy.

Respiratory Illness

• A 1997 study by Dr. Jennifer Jacobs examining the use of potentized common cockroach, *Blatta orientalis*, for treating childhood asthma showed no difference in the group receiving homeopathy, compared with placebo. For homeopaths, "potentized" solutions are increasingly diluted in the somewhat paradoxical state that less is actually more potent.

Pain and Healing

Several studies have examined the popular remedy Arnica montana in various applications, with variable results, as summarized in Jacobs's 1997 survey of the literature. Arnica is used extensively in homeopathic practice for pain and wound healing.

• When Arnica was used alone for wounds in the lower pelvis area, no significant difference was found between homeopathy and placebo.
• Combined with Hypericum 15C, Arnica 7C was found to significantly improve dental pain, compared to placebo.
• Arnica 5C, when used in the treatment of hematoma, or blood-filled tumor, from blood transfusions, was found in two studies by Amadeo in 1987 to produce statistically significant results compared to placebo.
• A study using Arnica 200 to treat pain following tooth extraction showed no significant difference from placebo.

Based on the above research, there is credible evidence that homeopathy is effective in the following situations:

- Using a single remedy, Galphimia glauca, in low potency, and iso- pathic mixed grass pollens in the 30C potency, for allergic rhinitis or hay fever.
- Homeopathic combination ophthalmic solution Similisan for aller- gic conjunctivitis or allergy-inflamed eyes.
- Individualized classical homeopathic treatment using the 30C potency for childhood diarrhea. Within homeopathy the "C" dosages contain the most molecules of the substance and are the lowest potency.
- Classical individualized treatment and a homeopathic complex for rheumatoid arthritis.
- Single remedy Rhus toxicodendron in the 6C potency for fibromyal- gia, painful benign tumors in the connective tissues of the muscles and joints, in patients whose symptoms match the remedy.
- A high-potency isopathic preparation, Oscillococcinum, for influenza.
- Isopathic preparations of allergens for allergic asthma.
- Homeopathic complex ointment Traumeel for ankle injuries.
- Homeopathic Rhus tox for fibrositis or inflammation of the white body tissues of the muscle sheaths causing considerable pain and stiffness.

Studies with negative findings illustrate the difficulty of proving that homeopathy is not effective for a particular condition. For each negative study it can be argued that the treatment regimen was wrong, that there was not a large enough sample size, or that the study design was flawed. Therefore, we can only conclude that a specific remedy is ineffective for a specific indication. Frustrating as this may be for critics of homeopa- thy, it is not possible to make meaningful generalizations that disprove homeopathy when such a wide variety of homeopathic practices are being used.

WHAT'S IN THE WORKS

Starting in 1999, a very significant study will be completed under the overall coordination of noted homeopath and conventional physician Dr. David S. Riley of Santa Fe, New Mexico. This is an observational outcomes study, called the International Integrative Primary Care Outcomes Study. This study incorporates the research principles from continuous quality improvement and classical methodological techniques for examining various complex phenomena. Such a study will not be able to separate the effectiveness of the homeopathic care relationship from the effectiveness of the remedy itself. This choice is intentional, because it allows a scientific study to respect the integrity of a different philosophy of care, which is based upon the belief that the two are inseparable, and should not necessarily be split during research.

One objective of the study is to evaluate the effectiveness of homeopathy for six specific clinical conditions commonly seen in the primary care setting: upper and lower respiratory complaints, including allergies; ear complaints; abdominal pain/cramps; injury/bruising; and teething. This study is an international, multicenter, prospective, observational effectiveness study, containing one pilot test before the main outcome study begins.

Such a large, comprehensive study is badly needed because, from the viewpoint of conventional scientific medicine, homeopathy remains an unproven treatment modality, however popular it may have become. Scientific skepticism about homeopathy largely focuses on the fact that its mechanisms of action are unknown. If homeopathy is truly effective, as its proponents claim, it is necessary to rethink our conventional understanding of some of the basic laws of nature. Even if well-designed studies show that homeopathy has benefits, the question remains whether any therapy should be accepted whose mechanisms we do not understand.

FUTURE DIRECTIONS

A great deal of clinical evidence now exists, some of it of very good quality, suggesting that conventional scientists can no longer ignore the issue of homeopathy's efficacy. Future research, involving both homeopathic practitioners and objective investigators, should address the methodological errors in homeopathic research, the failure to replicate significant experimental work, the publication bias, the tendency to report only studies with favorable outcomes, and the lack of understanding of the mechanism of action.

While homeopathy is currently recovering from a profound decline in the United States, it has remained in widespread use throughout Europe, Latin America, and India. In the United Kingdom, there are five homeopathic hospitals, and approximately 40 percent of British physicians refer patients to homeopathy. Homeopathic treatment by physicians in Great Britain is reimbursable under the National Health Service. Members of the royal family have been using homeopathy for four generations, and Prince Charles has reportedly used Arnica to treat bruises incurred in falls during polo matches. France has eight schools of medicine offering advanced degrees in homeopathic medicine, and some 40 percent of French physicians use homeopathy. Virtually all French pharmacies, as well as German, carry homeopathic medicines along with conventional medicines. Today the homeopathic preparation Oscillococcinum is the country's most popular cold and flu remedy.

In Germany, medical schools have been required since 1993 to offer courses in homeopathy, and all medical doctors must take one course in the subject. Twenty percent of German physicians use homeopathy. Germany's National Health System reimburses for homeopathic treatment by physicians, and German insurance companies offer reduced rates to people who have taken a homeopathic first-aid course. Homeopathy is also widespread in India, according to Kishore in 1983; it is practiced under the national health service, with more than one hundred homeopathic medical colleges and more than one hundred thousand homeopathic physicians.

With the upsurge of interest in natural healing in the past two decades in the United States, homeopathy has enjoyed a revival of popularity, and is now being practiced not only by physicians but also by other health professionals. According to Eisenberg's 1993 report in the *New England Journal of Medicine,* 2.5 million Americans used homeopathic medicines in 1990, and 800,000 patients received treatment from homeopaths in that year. From the repeated *Journal of the American Medical Association* survey by Eisenberg in 1997, this use of homeopathy has nearly doubled since 1990, and homeopathy is one of the most rapidly increasing areas of CAM use.

An estimated three thousand physicians and other health care practitioners currently use homeopathy in the United States, and the number is increasing every year. Only a few hundred American physicians practice homeopathy full-time, many having turned to homeopathy after becoming disillusioned with the limitations of conventional medicine. In naturopathic medical schools, homeopathy is one of the most popular specializations.

In keeping with the growing recognition of homeopathy as a viable alternative therapy, the NCCAM in 1993 approved two grants for research on homeopathy. One of these studies is currently being conducted at the University of California at Los Angeles.

Recently, a petition was circulated before the FDA to require that all OTC homeopathic remedies be required to meet the same safety and efficacy standards as nonhomeopathic remedies to be effective, according to Winston, in 1995. However, this was not acted upon by the FDA. Additionally, a series of lawsuits has been filed in California against drug chains, claiming that inserts and packaging for homeopathic preparations constitute false advertising. However, these have either been settled or dismissed, as of 1998.

Historically, with the long heritage of homeopathy, its apparent efficacy in an array of chronic and acute conditions, and growing current consumer and scientific interest, there is every indication that homeopathy will endure and thrive as one of alternative medicine's most promising healing approaches.

CHAPTER 9

CHIROPRACTIC

Thigh Bone Connected to the Knee Bone

BACKGROUND

Chiropractic is a hundred-year-old health profession that was developed in the United States as an alternative to the often harsh medical practices of the late nineteenth century. Central to chiropractic is the belief that the body has an inherent ability to heal itself if nerve impulses are allowed to travel freely between the brain and the rest of the body. Manipulation of the spine is chiropractic's primary means of ensuring proper function of the nervous system. Chiropractors now make up the third-largest group of health care providers in the United States, after physicians and dentists.

Chiropractic was founded in 1895 when Daniel David Palmer, a successful, self-taught healer in Davenport, Iowa, received a visit from the janitor of his office building, who had been deaf for seventeen years following a straining injury. Palmer, who had a background in spinal therapeutics, physiology, anatomy, magnetic healing, and laying on of hands, examined his patient and found a prominent, painful, misaligned vertebra in the upper spine, in the area the man had injured just before he'd lost his hearing. Palmer administered a sharp thrust to the bone, and the janitor's hearing was restored. Palmer believed that by adjusting the misaligned vertebra, he had relieved pressure on a nerve that affected hearing.

Palmer christened his new approach *chiropractic*, meaning "done by hand," from the Greek words *cheir* for hand, and *praxis* for practice. In 1897 he set up a school to teach his system.

From its beginnings, chiropractic had a stormy relationship with orthodox medicine. In the 1960s, the American Medical Association declared that its members could not ethically consult with any members of the "cult of chiropractic." However, after legal actions against the AMA and other medical organizations in the 1970s and 1980s, the profession began to gain increasing acceptance among conventional physicians. Currently, chiropractic is widely accepted as a legitimate therapy for musculoskeletal pain, and particularly back pain.

Early chiropractors believed that misalignments of the spinal vertebrae, or "subluxations," were responsible for virtually all diseases because they interfered with the body's natural functions, including immunity. This theory was hotly disputed by conventional physicians. Currently, most chiropractors believe that subluxations are only one factor in disease. Even this theory, however, is not accepted by most conventional practitioners.

Yet a great many chiropractors no longer seek to address general disease issues, but focus instead upon merely relieving joint dysfunction. Most clinicians now believe that this is a valid application for chiropractic. Actually, the primary intervention used by chiropractors is the manipulation of joints through "adjustments" of misaligned vertebrae and other joints. A typical chiropractic adjustment is a high-velocity, low-amplitude thrust which lasts about one-tenth of a second. Practitioners apply a small, highly controlled force to stretch a joint just beyond its usual range of motion. Procedures are painless when done properly, and are usually accompanied by an audible snapping or popping sound, resulting from the release of tiny gas bubbles that have built up in the joint fluid because of immobility. Properly done, the adjustment immediately produces an improvement in joint function with increased range of movement, relief of pain, and relaxation in the area.

Spinal manipulation is not limited to the chiropractic profession. Osteopaths, allopathic doctors, and physical therapists also use it. However, according to a 1994 RAND Corporation report by chiropractor Dr. Paul D. Shekelle, chiropractors perform 94 percent of all manipulative procedures.

Chiropractors also perform low-velocity, variable-amplitude maneuvers called "mobilizations." In addition, they perform soft tissue manipulation, trigger point manipulation, and direct deep tissue massage. Chiropractors employ exercise and rehabilitation procedures, and physical therapy modalities. Many of them offer advice on nutrition, hygiene, and health promotion. Many also use other modalities, such as acupuncture or homeopathy.

Chiropractors often use a variety of external physiotherapy treatments to help relax muscles before they make manual adjustments. These treatments also support the body's healing. Among them are:

- *Heat therapy* (for pain relief and to promote healing)
- *Cold therapy* (to decrease swelling and relieve pain)
- *Immobilizing therapies* (such as splints, casts, wraps, and traction to protect and heal damaged tissues)
- *Hydrotherapy* (to soothe muscles and increase circulation)
- *Electrotherapy* (to provide deep tissue massage and improve circulation)
- *Ultrasound* (to reduce swelling, eliminate fluids, and soothe muscle spasms)

In addition to standard adjustments and physiotherapy, chiropractors sometimes also use other manipulation techniques and therapies, including:

- *Cranial manipulation,* which focuses on the bones of the skull and on the spinal fluid. Various forms include Sacro-occipital Technique, which emphasizes the relationship between the cranial bones and the bones of the lower back; and Craniopathy, in which delicate force is applied to the spine, skull, and pelvis.
- *Activator technique,* which employs a small instrument that gently moves vertebrae.
- *Network chiropractic,* a system developed in 1979 by Dr. Donald

Epstein, which uses light, subtle touch, and a combination of manipulation techniques.

Currently, only about 15 percent of chiropractors practice only one form of adjustment therapy. The rest use a wide variety of techniques and approaches.

One of the most common approaches used by chiropractors is the use of nutritional therapy. Seventy-four percent of some 2,400 chiropractors surveyed by a leading chiropractic newspaper in 1988 reported that they used nutritional supplements in their practice. Many supplement companies sell their products exclusively through chiropractic offices, and some critics argue that these supplements are overpriced and may not be helpful.

Another approach used by many chiropractors is applied kinesiology (AK), a system for diagnosing and treating illness based on the belief that every organ dysfunction is accompanied by a specific muscle weakness. Applied kinesiology technique is based on the theory that complementary muscles can indicate the strength or weakness of corresponding organ systems. Skilled practitioners say they can use AK to test the health of organ systems, and to determine whether a supplement is effective, and at what dosage. In a 1994 national survey, 37 percent of chiropractors said that they used AK.

Many critics argue that such unorthodox approaches as AK go beyond the appropriate scope of chiropractic practice, and that chiropractors would do better to confine their activities to the use of manipulative techniques.

An initial visit with a chiropractor often includes a discussion of the patient's history and current problem; a standard physical examination; an observation of how the patient walks, bends, and sits; and palpation of the spine, to determine whether there are any muscle imbalances or subluxations. Many chiropractors also take X rays.

Chiropractic treatment usually involves a series of visits. In an uncomplicated low back condition, significant improvement should be noted within twelve visits. If a disc is bulging or protruding, it may take longer.

Cost varies by region and location. An initial chiropractic visit generally takes forty-five to sixty minutes and may cost from $50 to $150 or more, though some practitioners give a free initial consultation. Subsequent treatments may range from $20 to $50 for a ten- to twenty-five-minute visit. However, ancillary charges can add to the cost; supplements might cost an additional $10 to $200 or more per visit. Approximately 75 percent of insurance companies, including Medicare, pay for chiropractic care, and workers' compensation plans in all states cover chiropractic treatment. Supplements are not covered.

Chiropractic's greatest strength is in the treatment of neuromusculoskeletal conditions, which account for more than 90 percent of cases. Back pain is second only to the common cold as a reason for visits to doctors' offices, and second only to childbirth as a reason for hospitalization. Based on a review of literature by Dr. William C. Meeker of the Palmer College of Chiropractic in 1997, an estimated 40 percent of chiropractic patients seek care for low back pain. Other conditions for which patients commonly seek chiropractic care include upper back, neck, and head pain, and extremity, joint, and muscle problems. A much smaller proportion of patients seek chiropractic care for nonmusculoskeletal conditions, often of a chronic or visceral nature. According to chiropractic theory, chiropractic manipulation has a general health-enhancing effect, and there do exist clinical anecdotes and case reports that support this view. According to chiropractor Dr. Chester Wilk of Chicago, chiropractic has helped respiratory problems, gastrointestinal disorders, sinusitis, bronchial asthma, heart trouble, high blood pressure, and the common cold.

Children have become a focus of chiropractic outreach, a trend which is alarming to critics of the profession and to many chiropractors. Approximately 10 percent of chiropractic patients, or as many as two million, are seventeen or younger, according to a survey cited in *Consumer Reports* in 1994. However, according to Dr. Meeker in 1997, patients younger than eighteen do not comprise such a large percentage of chiropractic practices.

Chiropractic clinicians and researchers almost always acknowledge their limitations, as do all responsible practitioners. Chiropractors do not prescribe medications, perform major surgery, or treat fractures. They cannot provide emergency care or provide stand-alone therapy for life-threatening illnesses. While all chiropractors are trained in obstetrics and gynecology and can deliver babies, most states limit their ability to do so.

There are very few published reports of serious complications arising from spinal manipulation, but such complications may be underreported. In 1993, a survey of literature reported in the journal *Neurosurgery* found 138 cases of complications in English-language journals. All the reports of complications came from conventional physicians who had been called in to treat the problems.

Documented risks of chiropractic manipulation include increased pain, ruptured disks, and paralysis. Manipulation of the neck tends to produce the most serious injuries, including stroke and other neurological problems. Nevertheless, the *Neurosurgery* article found only 112 published case reports of complications due to neck manipulation, over a period of some sixty-five years.

Chiropractors have among the lowest malpractice insurance premiums of all physicians, because the percentage of chiropractic physicians who have been sued for malpractice is lower than the percentages of virtually all other medical and legal professionals, according to Brady in 1994 and the *Medical Liability Monitor* in 1996. Low malpractice incidence has made chiropractic increasingly prominent in the management of workers' compensation and work-related injuries.

WHAT WORKS

Historically, chiropractic has not had an adequate basis in scientific and academic research; it has not attained adequate research funding from government or the public sector. However, there are more than fifty RCTs in the chiropractic research literature, and the scientific basis for chiropractic is growing steadily. Following are the primary areas in which chiropractic care appears to be efficacious.

Low Back Pain

According to the prominent chiropractor Dr. Paul Shekelle, a formal meta-analysis of the literature in 1992 revealed that spinal manipulation was of short-term benefit for patients with uncomplicated, acute low back pain. However, Dr. Shekelle noted that there was insufficient evidence about patients with nerve root pain and chronic back pain.

A 1991 blinded systematic literature review by Koes of thirty-five randomized clinical trials concluded that although the results of chiropractic were promising, the efficacy of manipulation had not yet been convincingly demonstrated.

Both of the meta-analyses did indicate that spinal manipulation appeared to be at least as effective for low back pain as most standard medical treatments.

There are at least thirty-six RCTs comparing manipulation to other treatments for low back pain (LBP). Based on Meeker's 1998 analysis, twenty-four of the thirty-six trials favored manipulation, while twelve did not. However, in no case was the comparison treatment found to be more effective than manipulation. These LBP trials can be broken down into acute and chronic categories.

- Twelve studies evaluated patients with acute LBP and compared manipulation with exercise, diathermy, infrared, electrical stimulation, movement education, massage, and drugs. Six of the studies favored manipulation, three found no statistically significant differences, and three trials found statistically significant differences only in subgroups of the study samples.
- Eight trials focused on chronic or subacute low back pain. Five of the eight studies reported better results with manipulation, and two reported no additional benefit from manipulation. One did not draw a statistical conclusion.
- Twelve interventions included a mixture of acute, subacute, and chronic LBP patients. Eight favored manipulation, one reported a favorable result only in a subgroup, and the others did not find a statistically significant difference in favor of manipulation.
- One of the most noteworthy of the literature reviews was by Dr. Paul Shekelle, and was published in the *Annals of Internal Medicine* in 1992. Shekelle evaluated twenty-five controlled clinical trials and concluded that with manipulation, there was a 17 percent greater likelihood of recovery from uncomplicated, acute low back pain within three weeks than without it.
- Based on a single, long-term, 1995 study by Meade and colleagues, reported in the *British Medical Journal*, chiropractic was compared to hospital outpatient management for low back pain in 741 patients. After three years, the chiropractic group had improved 29 percent more than the hospital group.
- From a paper by Assendelft, published in a 1995 issue of the *Journal of the American Medical Association*, a group of Dutch epidemiologists from Vrije University in Amsterdam looked at fifty-one

reviews of literature. Thirty-four of the reviews concluded that the evidence favored spinal manipulation for low back pain, while seventeen were neutral. The reviews were coded for quality and scholarship, and nine of the ten highest-rated reviews were in favor of manipulation.

A landmark event in support of spinal manipulation came in 1994, when the federal Agency for Health Care Policy and Research (AHCPR) issued practice guidelines for treating acute low back pain. After reviewing more than four thousand studies focused on low back pain, the expert panel concluded that spinal manipulation appears to provide temporary relief.

In summary, there is sufficient published evidence to support the efficacy of spinal manipulation for low back pain, especially during the first three months of the condition. While some studies have reported favorable long-term results, the long-term data are insufficient to draw reliable conclusions.

Neck Pain

Manipulation of the cervical spine for neck pain has also been evaluated in randomized clinical trials.

- A landmark government-sponsored study by chiropractor Dr. David Cassidy on "whiplash associated disorders" appeared in *Spine* in 1995. It concluded that there was a dearth of high-quality research on the topic, but did single out spinal manipulation and mobilization as having at least weak cumulative evidence of efficacy.
- A review conducted in 1996 at the RAND Corporation "think tank" by Hurwitz and associates examined sixty-seven studies. Fourteen were randomized trials, which varied widely in quality. None indicated that the comparison treatment was more effective than manipulation.
- Hurwitz's 1996 review at RAND included nine trials for acute, subacute, and chronic neck pain. Most of these studies favored manipulation, but not all of them were statistically significant.

In summary, randomized clinical trials, along with meta-analysis of research, support the efficacy of spinal manipulation for acute and chronic neck pain, even though the findings have not always been statistically significant.

Headache

For the 1996 RAND study on cervical spinal manipulation, Hurwitz and associates reviewed five randomized trials that assessed the effectiveness of spinal manipulation for headache. One trial focused on migraine, and the rest focused on muscle tension headache.

- In the one randomized trial on migraine headache, by Parker in 1978, chiropractic patients had significantly less pain intensity than those who received manipulation and mobilization by a physical therapist or conventional physician.
- During the highest-quality study on muscle tension headache, by Boline in 1995, chiropractic was compared with low-dose amitriptyline over six weeks. Both approaches achieved initial favorable results. However, four weeks after the end of treatment, patients who had received manipulation maintained their improvement, while the patients on amitriptyline did not. Statistically significant differences were found in headache intensity and frequency, medication use, and functional status. Significant differences in favor of manipulation were also found in the three other tension headache studies.
- Cervical spine manipulation for headache was compared with low-level laser treatment and deep friction massage in a 1995 study by Nilsson. Patients receiving manipulation showed greater improvement in all variables, but not at statistically significant levels.

Although the effectiveness of chiropractic interventions for headache is promising, it is not clearly effective, based on the findings to date. Relief of common headache would be significant if it resulted in long-term relief and avoided the intestinal bleeding complications from too frequent use of aspirin and other pain medications.

WHAT MAY WORK AND
WHAT DOES NOT WORK

There is great debate about whether or not spinal manipulation can produce significant effects for conditions other than musculoskeletal complaints.

Spinal manipulation is clearly not recommended in the presence of such problems as fractures, rheumatoid arthritis, severe osteoporosis, bleeding disorders, or infection or inflammation of the spine. Manipulation of the neck can be relatively risky, especially if the patient is taking oral contraceptives or blood-thinning medications, or has high blood pressure or other risk factors for stroke.

Although available evidence suggests that the risk of a serious complication following spinal manipulation is very low, many complications attributable to spinal manipulation might never be reported. Estimates of complication rates based on case reports will inevitably underestimate the true incidence. Risks of cervical manipulation appear to be higher and would be more devastating. It would be important for future research to identify subsets of patients at risk of complications from cervical manipulation and determine whether there are specific manipulative techniques that should be avoided or modified.

A small body of published clinical evidence now suggests that spinal manipulation might be helpful for fibromyalgia, high blood pressure, asthma, menstrual pain, infantile colic, otitis media, childhood enuresis (bedwetting), dizziness and vertigo, chronic pelvic pain, and other conditions. Following are pertinent studies.

- Two studies of hypertension yielded conflicting findings. In one study, by Morgan in 1985, manipulation was found to have no effect on high blood pressure. However, Yates, in 1988, noted a reduction in blood pressure in a group receiving active treatment, compared to placebo and no-treatment groups.
- In a study by Brennan in 1991 at the National College of Chiropractic, researchers found evidence in chiropractic patients of enhanced immunity, including significant increases in blood levels of substance P, an immune-stimulating chemical.
- A 1992 comparison by Kokjohn of chiropractic manipulation and

sham manipulation in the treatment of severe menstrual pain found no difference between the two treatment groups.

- From a study cited in a 1994 *Consumer Reports*, 316 babies with infant colic were treated with spinal manipulation, and almost all got better within two weeks. However, the study had several design flaws.
- Reporting in a 1994 study by Reed of 46 children with enuresis or bedwetting, the researchers found that children who received manipulation had fewer wet nights than those who received sham manipulation, but the findings were not statistically significant.
- Following a study of patients with chronic asthma, by Nielsen in 1995, no significant difference was found between the group receiving manipulation and that receiving sham manipulation, although both reported a 36 percent improvement in symptoms.
- Based on a 1996 study reported by William Collinge comparing chiropractic treatment with medical treatment of otitis media, a common middle ear infection in children, preliminary findings suggest that chiropractic adjustment had a significantly beneficial effect. It is speculated that chiropractic may improve the nerve supply to the inner ear, or may enhance immune function.
- A review of literature by Brontfort, presented at the 1996 International Conference on Spinal Manipulation, concluded that manipulation seemed probably not to be efficacious in the treatment of hypertension and chronic asthma of moderate severity, but that the evidence was inconclusive.
- In a 1997 Canadian study by chiropractor Dr. Kelli L. Blunt, chiropractic improved patients' cervical and lumbar ranges of motion, straight leg rise, and pain.

Most recently, in October of 1998, Dr. Daniel C. Cherkin and his colleagues at the University of Washington provided new data in a study published in the *New England Journal of Medicine*. They assigned 321 people with low back pain that had lasted for at least a week to nine visits with a chiropractor, a similar number of sessions with a physical therapist, or no special treatment other than an educational booklet on back pain. While the results did not contradict the AHCPR recommendations about chiropractic, they didn't show that spinal manipulation was any better than performing back exercises. Both the chiropractic and physical therapy groups recovered at the same rate, which was slightly faster than that of the control group. There was no difference among the three groups in terms of missed work, reduced activity, or recurrent episodes of low back pain during the subsequent year.

Again in October 1998, the special CAM issue of the *Journal of the American Medical Association* reported that spinal manipulation by a chiropractor failed to alleviate tension headache in a Danish study. Finally, in 1998 a second *New England Journal of Medicine* reported study included chiropractors from the Canadian Memorial Chiropractic College. For this study, eighty children with asthma were randomized into chiropractic treatment versus a simulated or placebo treatment. From this study, the researchers concluded that in children with mild or moderate asthma, the addition of chiropractic spinal manipulation to usual medical care provided no benefit.

Writing an editorial in the *New England Journal of Medicine* that contained these studies, noted researcher Dr. Paul G. Shekelle at the West Los Angeles Veterans Affairs Medical Center concluded that nearly twenty years after a similar editorial by Dr. Arnold Relman, there appears to be little evidence to support the value of spinal manipulation for non-musculoskeletal conditions. His conclusion is tempered by his acknowledgment that it is no longer an issue of whether or not chiropractic should be included in mainstream, conventional care, but rather what are the most appropriate conditions for treatments and role of the chiropractor within the evolving health care system.

WHAT'S IN THE WORKS

Presently, the future of chiropractic, which appeared to be in doubt as recently as a decade ago, now seems assured. Chiropractic is being increasingly accepted as the primary intervention for back pain, one of the world's most common medical complaints. Furthermore, chiropractors now function as the most frequent providers of many CAM interventions, such as nutritional therapy and lifestyle modification.

One reason for chiropractic's increasingly acceptable status is cost-effectiveness. A number of retrospective actuarial studies have attempted to compare the cost of medical care and chiropractic care, usually for low back pain. A study by Canadian health economist Pran

Manga, funded by the Ontario Ministry of Health in 1993, concluded that the evidence is overwhelmingly in favor of much greater use of chiropractic care.

Other studies confirm this view, including the following:

- In a 1991 review of workers' compensation claims in Utah, Jarvis and associates compared the costs of medical and chiropractic claims for patients with the same diagnosis and found that the costs of patients who received medical treatment were ten times more.
- A 1996 study by Mosely concluded that chiropractic care reduced the use of expensive technology, maintained a high level of patient satisfaction, and did so at a lower cost than conventional medical care.

Another key reason for chiropractic's sunny future is its ability to evoke satisfaction among patients. A 1989 study by noted researcher Dr. Daniel C. Cherkin, of the Group Health Cooperative of Puget Sound, found that the satisfaction level of patients receiving chiropractic care for low back pain was three times higher than that of patients receiving allopathic care. Other studies, reported by Collinge in 1996, have found that patients being treated for low back pain by a variety of practitioners, including chiropractors, were least satisfied with conventional medical practitioners.

Because of these two important factors, as well as chiropractic's general efficacy, chiropractic is gradually gaining acceptance by many members of the conventional medical community. More and more chiropractors have hospital staff privileges, are recruited by health maintenance organizations, work at multispecialty back centers, are appointed to medical examination boards of workers' compensation, and are commissioned as health care providers in the armed forces.

Much work needs to be done, however, in proving the efficacy of chiropractic through well-designed RCTs. Research should be undertaken to determine the relative efficacy of chiropractic as a stand-alone therapy, or as a therapy that works best when used in conjunction with other CAM therapies, such as acupuncture and MindBody medicine interventions. It would also be helpful to make more direct comparisons between chiropractic and conventional conservative approaches, such as encouraging return to normal activity, or using nonsteroidal anti-inflammatory drugs, such as ibuprofen. Also, since many orthopedists and rheumatologists now collaborate with chiropractors, researchers should compare this collaborative treatment with stand-alone orthopedic and rheumatologic treatment.

Some of this future research will be facilitated by recent government grants. In 1998, the NCCAM at the National Institutes of Health initiated funding of chiropractic research efforts. This new OAM center is directed by well-respected chiropractor Dr. William C. Meeker, dean of the Palmer College of Chiropractic. It was the first time that NIH formally recognized chiropractic as a significant research topic. Funding is for research with the Consortial Center for Chiropractic Research, a network of chiropractors that will attempt to bring chiropractic research to the level of the "gold standard" of high-quality RCTs.

Chiropractic research has acquired further acceptance by gaining recognition from the American Public Health Association, which voted in 1995 to establish a full-fledged chiropractic health section. In addition, chiropractic research is now being presented at several important medical conferences, such as the North American Spine Society.

There is sufficient evidence from clinical research to conclude that spinal manipulation is effective for some forms of common low back and neck pain, and is probably effective for at least some headache patients, but additional research is required in the latter area. Beyond these research efforts, which focused on randomized trials, the chiropractic profession has been taking significant steps to develop a research infrastructure, including creating the previously noted Consortium for Chiropractic Research, defining and prioritizing research topics, linking with nonchiropractic research centers, designing and executing pilot studies, and establishing peer-reviewed and indexed journals. Among other future directions would be to compare different types of spinal manipulation with conventional physical treatments that are already in common use, such as McKenzie physical therapy and massage.

Additionally, clinical research should be undertaken to determine the relative efficacy of chiropractic as a stand-alone and/or combined intervention for specific conditions in conjunction with other CAM therapies, such as acupuncture and MindBody medicine interventions. Direct comparisons of chiropractic with other conventional conservative approaches, such as encouraging return to normal activity and nonsteroidal anti-inflammatory drugs (NSAIDs), would be helpful. Since many orthopedists and rheumatologists report that their patients use chiropractic simultaneously with their treatments, it would be a significant opportunity to compare outcomes of such conventional treatments with or without chiropractic, to determine which singular or combination of interventions are efficacious for specific comparable diagnoses.

Addressing the integration of conventional rheumatology and chiropractic is a 1999 pilot study conducted under the NCCAM alternative medicine program at Stanford in collaboration with the Palmer Center for Chiropractic Research. Thirty-six rheumatologists identified by rheumatologist Dr. Gerson Bernhard were each sent 50 surveys. These 1,800 surveys were to be given to patients being provided care by these rheumatologists. Overall, 47.2 percent of the patients reported having used some form of CAM. Among the most frequently used therapies were dietary supplements (16.4 percent), chiropractic (15.5 percent), acupuncture (10.9 percent), yoga (10.1 percent), special diets (7.0 percent), meditation (5.0 percent), and herbs (4.1 percent). Seventy-one percent of those using CAM reported that these therapies were of help to them. Among those patients reporting use of chiropractic, 70 percent stated that they had seen the chiropractor prior to their seeing a rheumatologist, while 30 percent reported using chiropractic after having seen the rheumatologist. Findings such as these can help bridge the gap between conventional rheumatology and chiropractic in order to coordinate care for the ultimate greatest benefit to the patient.

Chiropractic is increasingly being integrated with other medical traditions, as evidenced by the growing number of chiropractors who include nutritional counseling, homeopathy, and other natural therapies in their practices. Some chiropractors do not employ manipulation at all, using their broad mandate as licensed health professionals to concentrate on other complementary health modalities. Most significant, a working integration and collaboration by chiropractic physicians with other health care providers will provide improved care for the millions of individuals suffering daily from a broad array of back and musculoskeletal traumas and pain. That is a laudable goal for any and all of the healing professions.

Osteopathy

Chiropractic is sometimes confused with osteopathy, which is a recognized primary care medical profession with a holistic perspective. Osteopathy combines allopathic techniques with the use of manipulation, physical therapy, and postural education. At the present time, doctors of osteopathy, or D.O.s, have essentially the same scope of practice as conventional allopathic physicians. Osteopaths are licensed to perform all aspects of medicine, including surgery, emergency medicine, and prescribing. They are also proficient in a variety of manual treatments, aimed at making changes in the musculoskeletal system to increase the body's own healing potential.

Osteopathic medicine was founded by Dr. Andrew Taylor Still, a registered physician who served as a surgeon in the Union Army during the Civil War. Still was disenchanted with the medicine of his day, having lost his wife and three children in an epidemic of spinal meningitis. Searching for a better method of treating illness and promoting health, he formulated a theory emphasizing the integration of the body's communication and regulatory mechanisms. He believed that this approach enhanced the inherent healing powers of the body.

From the late 1800s, Still's holistic approach went head to head with the allopathy of the era, which focused on surgical and pharmacological treatment of illness. Osteopathic and allopathic schools and hospitals evolved separately, and until the 1940s, osteopaths were denounced by the AMA as cultists.

Today there are over fifty thousand D.O.s in this country, as compared to over six hundred thousand M.D.s. Osteopaths can be members of the American Medical Association, but they also maintain their own organization, the American Osteopathic Association (AOA). Osteopaths practice all the same specialties as allopaths.

Some osteopaths use manipulation as the central focus of their practice, but most use allopathic techniques liberally, and align themselves professionally and politically with allopathy. Osteopathic physicians are trained in very much the same way as conventional doctors, except that D.O.s have additional training in osteopathic and holistic interventions.

Osteopathy's greatest strength is its versatility; it can use all the methods of allopathy as well as its own manipulative techniques.

Osteopathic treatment costs approximately the same as allopathy, and insurance coverage is the same. Fees may be slightly lower in rural areas, where osteopaths have a disproportionately large concentration of practice.

CHAPTER 10

AYURVEDIC MEDICINE AND YOGA

From Buddha to the Millennium

Ayurveda is India's traditional system of natural medicine. It was first described around 3500 B.C. in the ancient Hindu texts known as the Vedas, and means "science of life," from the Sanskrit *ayur,* or life, and *veda,* or science. An integral part of classical Ayurvedic medicine is the practice of yoga, or "union." In considering this discipline, both Ayurveda and yoga are included, out of respect to this centuries-old tradition.

Ayurveda has been continuously practiced for approximately 5,500 years in India and Asia, and is claimed to be the oldest system of natural healing on earth, the original source of many other medical traditions, and the traditional medicine of Buddha.

With the introduction of Western medicine into India, Ayurveda lost its eminence, but has since made a comeback and is now practiced side by side with Western medicine. It has also aroused increasing interest in

Western countries, including the United States. In 1978, the World Health Organization recognized Ayurveda as one of the forms of traditional medicine that could especially help developing nations.

Ayurveda is preeminently a comprehensive approach to healthy living. Its primary goal is preservation and promotion of health, with an emphasis on enhancing immunity. A secondary goal is the treatment of mental and physical illnesses, and the restoration of spiritual peace.

Taking a holistic approach to the individual, Ayurveda believes that all aspects of life contribute to health, including nutrition, hygiene, sleep, weather, and lifestyle, as well as physical, mental, and sexual activities. Emotional factors are also taken into consideration. Anger, fear, anxiety, and unhealthy relationships are believed to contribute to illness. A healthy emotional state is considered the very foundation of physical health.

Because the wider social environment is considered an important contributor to health and disease, Ayurveda is concerned with maintaining a healthful physical, social, and spiritual environment, and uses collective meditation to try to influence society.

Of the major approaches to health, Ayurvedic medicine is one of the least well understood and least researched. This critical review was possible only with the assistance of Dr. Shri K. Mishra, a prominent researcher of Ayurveda, professor of neurology and dean of the school of medicine at the University of Southern California School of Medicine.

According to Dr. Mishra, in Vedic philosophy, each living organism is a microcosm that reflects the macrocosm of the entire cosmos. In Vedic philosophy, all of creation is made up of five "elements": earth, ether, air, fire, and water. These five basic elements represent principles of action and interaction that guide and shape everything that exists, and they form the basis for understanding health and illness.

From the five elements come three essential, overriding qualities that are present in all things. The relative balance of these three qualities in each person determines that person's unique psychophysiological constitution and functional body type. The three qualities, or *doshas*, are *vata*, *pitta*, and *kapha*. *Vata* represents air, and is personified by people who are active, changeable, and energetic. *Pitta* represents fire, or transformative energy, and is personified by people who are aggressive, explosive, and efficient. *Kapha* is the densest of the three qualities, or humors, and is personified by people who tend to be slow-moving, conservative, stable, and sometimes overweight. Each *dosha* is thought to predominate in particular sites; for instance, *vata* is concentrated more in the intestines, skin, ears, and thighs.

When these three *doshas* are balanced within a person, it is conducive to health and longevity. In Ayurvedic medicine, individuals use various interventions, such as diet and exercise, to restore and maintain balance of the three doshas.

The table below describes the *doshas.*

Doshas can be increased or decreased by a variety of factors, including food, sleep, lifestyle, and other physical and mental activities. *Vata* is disturbed by eating raw vegetables, by excessive travel, sleeplessness,

Characteristics of the Three *Doshas*

DOSHA	Vata	Pitta	Kapha
Elements	Ether + Air	Fire + Water	Earth + Water
Build	Tall and slender	Medium, stable weight	Heavy, strong tendency to overweight
Physiological function	Motion, activity	Metabolism	Physical structure
Activity and habits	Movement, activity, restless, wasteful	Moderate, efficient, organized	Accumulation
Sleep and digestion	Erratic	Regular	Slow digestion, strong appetite, easy, deep sleep
Emotional/ mental	Anxious, unpredictable, alert, restless	Fiery, angry, aggressive, biting, explosive	Slow, tranquil, stubborn, procrastinating, stable, grounded
Organs	Large intestine, pelvic cavity, skin, ears, thighs	Small intestine, stomach, sweat glands, blood, skin, eyes	Chest, lungs, spinal fluid
Cyclic	Evening, summer, old age	Midday, autumn and late spring, adulthood	Morning, winter and early spring, youth

exercise, drink, or sexual activity, and is manifested primarily in people with a predominantly *vata* constitution. *Pitta* is disturbed by consuming too much hot food, tea, coffee, or alcohol, and by excess exposure to heat and sun. *Kapha* is deranged by eating excess sweets, or fatty or cold foods (including dairy products), by too much sleep during the daytime, and by an inactive lifestyle.

Doshas are also subject to natural cycles of change, on a daily and seasonal basis, and during the stages of life. *Kapha* is emphasized in the morning, in winter and early spring, and during youth. *Pitta* increases at noon, in the autumn and late spring, and in adulthood. *Vata* predominates in the evening, in summer, and in old age.

Abnormalities in the levels of the *doshas* lead to abnormalities in the tissues, the excretory system, the digestive system, and enzymatic systems. As bodily humors become agitated, they begin to accumulate in their respective sites in the body—*vata* in the colon, *pitta* in the small intestines, and *kapha* in the stomach. With continued aggravation, the accumulated *dosha* overflows from its original site and spreads throughout the body, creating lesions in one or more susceptible target tissues, and interfering with metabolism.

In Ayurvedic medicine, it is important that a disease be recognized early in its course, and that its root cause be correctly identified. Otherwise, it may disseminate to other tissues and produce secondary effects on other *doshas*, which can lead to serious consequences, including possibly death.

Most people have problems associated with their predominate *dosha*. *Vata* people are most likely to have *vata* conditions, such as nervous system problems, arthritis, sciatica, lower back pain, or intestinal gas. *Pitta* people are more likely to have liver and gallbladder problems, gastritis, hyperacidity, peptic ulcer, inflammatory disease, and skin problems. *Kapha* people are more likely to have tonsillitis, bronchitis, sinusitis, and lung congestion.

Because the principal focus of Ayurveda is not on disease but on restoring balance, diagnosis is different in Ayurveda. Practitioners try to determine the individual's constitution, and then to rebalance the *doshas*. Rather than using instruments or laboratory tests to make a diagnosis, the Ayurvedic physician relies on observation, and on questioning of the patient. Clinicians obtain a detailed family, social, personal, and past history, and gain information about environmental and nutritional factors.

Physical examination includes an evaluation of three superficial and three deep pulses on a person's right and left wrists. The three pulses are believed to correspond to the three *doshas*. The physician also examines the surface of the tongue for discoloration, irregularities, coating, and sensitivity, believing that these characteristics reveal information about the balance of the *doshas* and the condition of internal organs. In addition, the physician examines urine samples for color and odor.

Following diagnosis, a treatment program is designed, and is likely to include the following procedures:

* *Poorvakarma.* This is a three- to seven-day preparatory program that involves toxin-removing massage, sweating, and use of herbs.
* *Pancha karma.* This is an intensive, one- to two-week detoxification regimen that includes induced vomiting, purgation with laxatives, herbal enema therapy, herbal cleansing of the nasal cavity, and cleansing of the blood through a form of bloodletting, such as donating blood to a blood bank. Detoxification is also achieved by purification of the diet and lifestyle.
* *Shaman.* Also called "palliation," this intervention focuses on the spiritual dimensions of healing. It can include fasting, sunbathing, yoga, and use of herbs.
* *Rasayana.* Also known as "rejuvenation," this phase of the treatment comes after detoxification, and employs yoga, breathing exercises, and herbs to restore vitality.
* *Satvajaya.* This phase focuses on psychotherapy, and helps reduce stress, employing measures such as the chanting of mantras to change vibratory patterns in the mind.

Of considerable importance in this comprehensive healing regime is the use of herbal medicines. Herbs are added to the diet for preventive and rejuvenative purposes, and also for treating specific disorders.

Ayurvedic herbal preparations generally have no equivalent in Western medicine. Unlike allopathic medicine, Ayurveda uses combined herbal preparations, often including whole plant products, rather than isolated chemicals from plants. Herbal preparations may contain ten to twenty different herbs. The goal of using medicinal compounds is to rebalance the *doshas,* so herbs are classified according to their action upon the *doshas,* such as *vata*-stimulating or *vata*-reducing. Herbs are also divided into some fifty groups, based on their therapeutic actions, such as vitalizing agents, heart tonics, or pain relievers. Many of the substances used in Ayurvedic herbal preparations have been studied with modern laboratory techniques. *Amala,* for example, is a rich source of vitamin C, and a potent antioxidant. *Bacopa,* which is used as a brain tonic, is also a powerful antioxidant, and has been shown in studies to increase intelligence and mental clarity.

Ayurvedic preparations manufactured by herbal companies in India are currently being imported into the United States, but there is a lack of quality control in the manufacture of these products, resulting in questionable standards of purity and sanitation. Many herbal compounds from India are contaminated with biological materials, as well as with heavy metals, such as arsenic, mercury, or lead. However, some common Ayurvedic preparations are now being produced by American companies, and these are much safer. Some Ayurvedic herbs themselves also have potentially harmful side effects, and should not be used without an understanding of the full range of their biological activity, and the advice of a physician.

Typically, Ayurvedic treatment consists of an initial forty-five- to ninety-minute consultation, and one or two shorter follow-up consultations several weeks or even months apart. Costs vary greatly. An initial consultation may range from $100 to $200, with follow-up visits being proportionately less. Usually there are few follow-up visits, so Ayurvedic treatment is relatively inexpensive. Herbal remedies may cost from $50 to $100 a month. Insurance coverage is generally limited to licensed health professionals who are covered because of their other qualifications.

Ayurvedic education in the West is limited, in both the availability and extent of training. Ayurveda has the smallest number of practitioners of any medical tradition in the United States, although its popularity is growing. Only a few hundred physicians in the United States have received some degree of training in Ayurvedic medicine. However, Ayurveda is also practiced in the United States by health educators and health consultants who do not have specialized degrees. In addition, a number of graduates of Indian Ayurvedic medical schools have come to this country to practice or teach.

A major stimulus for an expansion of Ayurveda in the United States has been the development by followers of Maharishi Mahesh Yoga of an

Ayurvedic approach called Maharishi Ayur-Ved, which incorporates Transcendental Meditation (TM) as part of its array of practices. However, Maharishi Ayur-Ved does not necessarily follow classical Ayurveda, and the scientific papers describing it may be oriented toward commercialism of its products. Today, the College of Maharishi Ayur-Ved, which offers degree and nondegree courses in their form of Ayurveda, has a well-structured academic curriculum that begins at the undergraduate level and culminates in a doctoral degree in clinical Ayurveda.

In addition to Maharishi Ayur-Ved's highly organized approach to Ayurveda, there are many independent Ayurvedic teachers and practitioners who have established practices, institutions, and training programs in this country. A prime mover in the popularization of Ayurveda in the United States is prominent author Dr. Deepak Chopra, an endocrinologist who was formerly chief of staff at New England Memorial Hospital in Stoneham, Massachusetts. Among the other leading figures in Ayurveda in the United States are Dr. Vasant Lad, a former Indian medical school professor who founded the Ayurvedic Institute in Albuquerque, New Mexico, and Dr. David Frawley of the American Institute of Vedic Studies in Santa Fe, New Mexico.

One of the earliest articles to explicate Maharishi Ayur-Ved was published by Dr. Hari M. Sharma, Dr. Brihaspati Dev Triguna, and Dr. Deepak Chopra in the *Journal of the American Medical Association* in 1991. This important article was eclipsed by a controversy when *JAMA* editors accused the authors of failing to disclose a potential conflict of interest through affiliations with the marketers of products noted in the article. More recently, the controversy continued with a *Newsweek* cover story entitled "Spirituality for Sale," with Dr. Chopra's photograph on the cover. There tends to be a fusion and confusion of Ayurvedic medicine with a particular approach to this complex area. There are many significant insights in Dr. Chopra's books, and it is surely premature at best to judge, much less dismiss, the significance of Ayurvedic approaches to health care based on accusations and conjecture.

What Works and What May Work

While the primary emphasis in Ayurveda is on disease prevention and promoting longevity, treatment of illness is an important secondary aim.

Proponents consider Ayurveda particularly helpful in dealing with chronic, metabolic, and stress-related conditions. Ayurveda is considered to be potentially more effective when it addresses illness early in the disease process, before extensive tissue and organ damage has occurred.

Ayurveda is also used to alleviate the side effects of toxic allopathic therapies, such as cancer chemotherapy. In addition, it helps patients recover from surgery and encourages healing in a wide range of conditions.

As a stand-alone therapy, Ayurveda generally does not address such problems as traumatic injuries, acute pain, and advanced disease. Surgery is not commonly done by Ayurvedic practitioners today, although it was historically part of Ayurvedic practice.

Following are general conditions that are treated with Ayurveda, often quite effectively.

- *Neurological.* Some forty neurological disorders are classified in Ayurveda as *vata* disorders. Herbs commonly used for neurological disease include *Brahmi*, which is said to enhance memory, reduce insomnia, and act as a mild sedative, and *Centella asiatica*, or *Gotu kola*, valued as a memory enhancer. In the treatment of dementia, Ayurveda uses a number of herbal compounds as memory enhancers, including *Withania somnifera (Ashwaganda)*, *Brahmi*, and *Centella asiatica.*
- *Cardiovascular.* A number of herbal compounds have been used to prevent atherosclerosis, and to address other risk factors, such as obesity, elevated cholesterol, high blood pressure, and diabetes. Among the most promising is *guggul*, an extract from the mukul myrrh tree, since it is widely used in India for the reduction of cholesterol.
- *Musculoskeletal.* Ayurvedic herbs are used both internally and externally to treat arthritis and muscle disorders. Herbal compounds and massage also help relieve chronic pain.
- *Respiratory.* Ailments are treated with yogic breathing and Ayurvedic preparations, including the herbs *Sida cordifolia* and *Tylophora asthmatica*, which are used to treat asthma.
- *Gastrointestinal.* Ayurvedic preparations have been used to treat upper and lower gastrointestinal disease, and are considered especially useful in liver disease. Irritable bowel disorder, as well as pep-

tic, gastric, and duodenal ulcers, are treated with Ayurvedic herbs. Ginger is recognized as a digestive aid in Ayurveda.

- *Cancer.* Ayurveda places a great deal of emphasis on preventing cancer with diet, lifestyle changes, exercise, and the use of various Ayurvedic compounds, most notably the extract of *Semicarpus anacardium* nut and the flowers of *Calotropis procera,* as reported by Smit in 1995.
- *Metabolic and endocrine.* Diabetes is treated in Ayurvedic medicine with herbal remedies, including guar gum and fennel, which have been shown to lower blood sugar when used as adjuncts to primary drug treatment, according to Sadhukhan in 1994. Ayurvedic herbal preparations are also used to treat obesity, and as antifertility treatments.
- *Mental disorders and psychosomatic illness. Brahmi* is highly valued as an anti-anxiety compound, and *Rauwolfia serpentina* is an Ayurvedic herb that is the source of the antihypertensive and tranquilizing drug reserpine. Substance abuse is treated with herbs, detoxification, diet, and yoga, and so are stress-related conditions, such as tension headache, colitis, and insomnia.

In the past, research on Ayurveda was sparse and often poorly designed. Since Ayurveda has been practiced in India for thousands of years, the efficacy of the system is accepted there without question. However, during the last several decades, a great deal of effort has been made to study the scientific basis of Ayurveda. Much of the more recent research in India has applied Western biomedical research methods. More than forty research institutions in India have conducted clinical trials. In the United States, many of the well-designed studies on Ayurveda have been carried out by adherents of Maharishi Ayur-Ved, who have conducted both basic and clinical research on herbal products. However, USC's Dr. Mishra points out that much of this research is controversial, since it may be biased by a business agenda.

Another factor complicating research is that, as with any comprehensive system of medicine, it is difficult to demonstrate the efficacy of Ayurveda as a whole through RCTs of specific substances. As with all clinical practices, Ayurvedic treatment is individualized for each patient, and consists of extremely complex combinations of interventions.

A few attempts have been made in the United States in recent years to evaluate the efficacy of overall Ayurvedic treatment, or of complex Ayurvedic programs such as *pancha karma*. In reporting these studies, only last names are given in this chapter, since first names are traditionally omitted in Indian scientific journals and articles.

- A 1989 pilot study carried out in the Netherlands by Dr. G. W. H. M. Janssen evaluated the effectiveness of multiple Maharishi Ayur-Ved interventions among a group of 126 adults who had ten different chronic diseases, including rheumatoid arthritis, sinusitis, bronchitis, asthma, eczema, psoriasis, diabetes, hypertension, constipation, and headache. Each participant received an individualized nutritional program, herbal preparations, and daily lifestyle guidelines. Seventy-nine percent of the participants showed improvement, 14 percent showed no change, and 7 percent became worse. There were highly significant improvements, or strong trends toward improvement, in all ten of the medical conditions being studied, with complete cures for ten patients. The study suggests that Ayurveda as a whole system does have benefit.

- During a 1993 study by Dr. Sharma and associates, the researchers evaluated the effects of *pancha karma* on risk factors for heart disease in thirty-one adults. Patients who participated in a multimodal program were found to have an 80 percent increase in dilation capacity of their circulatory system three months after the treatment, indicating improved function. Total cholesterol was reduced in all the participants, with a reduced measure of free radical damage and significantly reduced anxiety.

- Among the most recent demonstration projects is one funded by NCCAM and carried out by Dr. David Simon at the Sharp Institute for Human Potential and MindBody Medicine in San Diego. This study compared the effects of an Ayurvedic health promotion program with the effects of a Western program among ninety healthy individuals. Participants were randomized to one of three groups: a group that received no treatment; one that received Ayurvedic treatment in the form of meditation, Ayurvedic diet, and yoga; and a group that received a Western program of Jacobsen progressive relaxation training, a low-fat, low-salt diet, and aerobic exercise. Eighty-eight subjects completed the one-year trial.

    In both treatment groups, health-related quality of life was found to be improved, with the Ayurvedic group showing greater improvement than the Western group in health perceptions, and in decreased use of Western prescription medications. Among subjects in the Ayurvedic program, those who were highly adherent to the prescribed therapy showed a decrease in depression. Also, adherence to Ayurvedic meditation was found to be higher than to the Western progressive muscle relaxation technique, which suggests that meditation may be more attractive. Estimated health care costs over the year of the study were more than double for the untreated group, compared with the two treatment groups. Researchers concluded that the health promotion programs, especially the Ayurvedic interventions, were effective.

More studies have been done on specific herbal substances than on the system as a whole. Following is an examination of that research.

- A 1988 Indian study by Dr. S. K. Verma and colleagues evaluated forty patients with high blood lipids, who were treated with *guggul* (the crude gum of *Boswellia serrata*). In the *guggul*-treated group, serum cholesterol decreased by 7.8 percent, 15.78 percent, and 21.75 percent at the end of the fourth, eighth, and sixteenth weeks, respectively. Triglyceride levels decreased by 6.7 percent, 17.1 percent, and 27.1 percent, with "good" HDL cholesterol showing a gradual increase up to about 35.8 percent by the end of the sixteen weeks. There was also a significant decrease in low-density lipoprotein (LDL) levels. Researchers concluded that *guggul* was safe and highly effective in lowering the various lipid fractions that are known to contribute to coronary heart disease.

- In the United States, some of the most significant research on Ayurvedic compounds has been done by advocates of Maharishi Ayur-Ved. A number of studies have evaluated two versions of a traditional metabolic tonic, *Maharishi Amrit Kalash*, known as MAK-4 and MAK-5. Each of these preparations contains a large number of ingredients, and has shown great versatility in basic and clinical research. A series of test tube studies, funded by the National Cancer Institute, investigated the anticancer properties of MAK-4 and MAK-5. Preliminary studies by Dr. J. T. Arnold and associates in 1991 showed that these substances were able to significantly inhibit cancer cells grown in both human tumor and rat cells. Another study, by Dr. M. L. Prasad and colleagues of the All India Institute of Medical Sciences in New Delhi, found that various forms of MAK-4 and MAK-5 were able to inhibit growth of mouse and human melanoma cells. In a study by Engineer and associates in 1992, MAK-4 and MAK-5 were able to reduce mortality and reduce toxic side effects in mice treated with Adriamycin, a human chemotherapy drug.

- One innovative 1990 study by Dr. Paul Gelderloos and associates utilized a double-blind study to evaluate the effect of MAK-5 on alertness. As compared with the placebo group, members of the MAK group, all age thirty-five or over, showed significant improvement in their ability to identify a symbol in a cluttered visual array after three and six weeks of treatment. Researchers concluded that MAK may help improve alertness and attentional capacity, and perhaps reverse some of the harmful effects of aging on cognitive functioning.

- Using a double-blind, placebo controlled trial, Dr. J. L. Glaser of the Maharishi International University in 1991 studied the effects of MAK-5 in forty-six patients with hay fever. Significant reductions in allergy symptoms were produced by MAK-5.

- Focusing on arthritis treatment, Dr. K. K. Kulkarni and associates in 1991 tested an Ayurvedic formulation consisting of *Withania somnifera, Boswellia serrata, Cucurma longa,* and a zinc complex. The Ayurvedic formulation produced a significant reduction in the severity of pain and in the disability score, although neither group showed significant changes on X ray.

- An article by Srivastava in *Medical Hypotheses* in 1992 reported on fifty-six patients with rheumatoid arthritis, osteoarthritis, or muscle pain who were treated with powdered ginger. More than three-quarters of the arthritis patients achieved relief from pain and swelling, and all of the patients with muscular discomfort had pain relief. None of the patients reported adverse effects.

- A combination of turmeric and neem (*Azadirachta indica*) was found by Dr. Victor Charles of the Medical and Cancer Research and Treatment Centre of Nagercoil, India, in a 1992 study of 814 subjects, to be useful in treating scabies, with a 97 percent rate of cure within three to fifteen days of treatment. Such herbal preparations commonly have many fewer undesirable side effects than the pharmacological compounds that are used to treat parasites.

- During a 1994 study in India by Drs. Dwivedi and Agourwal, a bark preparation of *Terminalia Arjuna* was evaluated in fifteen patients with stable and unstable angina. Among patients with stable angina there was a 50 percent reduction in anginal episodes, but among patients with unstable angina there was a statistically insignificant reduction in frequency of angina, and these patients also needed to use other medications.

- In an Indian study by Dogra and associates in 1994, thirty patients were evaluated to determine the effect of MAK-4 and MAK-5 on angina. Eighty percent of patients showed a significant improvement after six months of treatment, with a reduction in the mean frequency of angina from 8.87 to 3.3 episodes per month. Five out of eleven patients with high blood pressure also reported a drop in systolic blood pressure. There was a statistically insignificant rise in HDL. Ten patients showed improved exercise tolerance. No side effects or drug interactions were observed.

- Another study of *Terminalia,* by Dr. Arjuna Bharani and associates in 1995, evaluated its effectiveness in congestive heart failure in a double-blind placebo-controlled clinical study of twelve patients with refractory congestive heart failure. Patients receiving *Terminalia* showed short-term regression of signs of heart failure, and improvement in symptoms such as shortness of breath and fatigue, as compared to placebo. In a two-year extension of the trial, patients continued to show improvements in heart failure, as well as quality of life, for about two to three months. Two patients died during the second phase of the study, but the deaths were apparently not related to the use of *Terminalia* or placebo therapy.

- In a 1995 RCT, Drs. Paranjpe and Kulkarni evaluated Ayurvedic formulations used to treat acne vulgaris. Eighty-two patients were randomized into five groups. Four of the groups received different Ayurvedic formulations orally for six weeks, while one group received placebo. One of the formulations, *Sunder Bati,* produced a significant reduction in acne lesions as compared both to placebo and to the other Ayurvedic formulations, which failed to produce any significant improvement.

- For a study of more than 260 patients by Dr. Etzel in 1996, a special extract of *guggul* (the crude gum of *Boswellia serrata*), known as H-15, was used in the treatment of rheumatoid arthritis. Patients who received H-15 were found to have reduced swelling and pain, compared with those who received placebo. Patients also reported reduction of morning stiffness and were able to cut back on their intake of NSAIDs during the treatment period. Symptoms of rheumatoid arthritis were reduced in 50 to 60 percent of the patients. Unfortunately, this form of *guggul* is not currently approved for use, since its classification has been changed from a known traditional medicine to an unknown, or new, chemical entity that will require special testing prior to approval.

- At the Southern Illinois University School of Medicine, Dr. Bala Manyam evaluated the potential of a powdered preparation of the Ayurvedic herb *Mucuna pruriens* in the treatment of Parkinson's disease. During the twelve-week 1997 study, patients showed significant improvement. Some reported mild side effects. Researchers concluded that the herbal preparation, known as HP-2000, was an effective, low-cost treatment for patients with Parkinson's disease.

- Conducting a 1998 study of 280 people with acne vulgaris at the University of Poona in India, Dr. V. Shanbhag evaluated the traditional Ayurvedic formula *shanka bhasma*. Patients were assigned to groups based on their *dosha* constitution. At the end of the four-week study, the *vata* and *pitta* patients showed significant improvement, but the *kapha* patients did not. This study indicates that individualized treatment based on the *doshas* may be a meaningful approach.

Guggul, also identified as *Commiphora mukul,* has been used traditionally in Ayurvedic medicine for the last one thousand years for a variety of inflammatory problems, including rheumatoid arthritis, osteoarthritis, and cervical spondylitis. *Guggul* also lowers cholesterol and triglyceride levels and helps maintain a healthy HDL/LDL, "good" to "bad" cholesterol, ratio. This improved ratio protects against cardiovascular disease and atherosclerosis, and is also beneficial to the liver.

A number of animal studies have investigated the anti-inflammatory potential of *guggul* as well as turmeric, which does not show the same side effects and toxicity that are common in the usual anti-inflammatory medications, such as corticosteroids or nonsteroidal anti-inflammatory drugs (NSAIDs). There is also preliminary clinical evidence that the traditional Ayurvedic remedy, phyllanthus, may be an effective treatment for hepatitis. Such traditional herbals require further research but offer great promise to be incorporated into a more integrative medicine encompassing both conventional and alternative therapies of proven value.

WHAT DOES NOT WORK

Given the relative dearth of quality, randomized clinical trials for Ayurvedic medicine as a whole, it is not surprising that an exhaustive literature search did not identify any published negative studies. This is not to say that such negative outcomes are lacking. With future rigorous research, the effectiveness, limitations, and caveats regarding Ayurvedic medicine will empower both clinicians and patients to exercise truly informed choices.

YOGA

Yoga is an ancient system of practices originating in India, aimed at integrating mind, body, and spirit to enhance health and well-being. Yoga, which involves mental and physical practices, literally means "union," from the Sanskrit word *yukti*. Its principles were first set down systematically by Patanjali in the second century B.C. in the *Yoga Sutras*. According to a recent Roper Poll, more than 6 million Americans practice yoga, with 1.69 million practicing it regularly.

There are many different forms of yoga. In its original form, it was part of a larger philosophical and spiritual system, but yoga has proven beneficial to millions of practitioners who have not been grounded in the original traditions and meanings of yoga.

Hatha yoga is the most widely known form of yoga in the West, and the most closely allied with Ayurvedic medicine. It includes three practices that have been found highly beneficial for health. They are:

Asanas. Yoga *asanas* are a variety of physical postures and exercises. They help to align the spine and head, improve blood flow, induce a state of relaxation, energize glands and organs, and enhance well-being. There are more than eighty-five postures.

Some *asanas* have been applied in the treatment of specific medical conditions. In Ayurvedic practice, specific *asanas* have traditionally been prescribed to rebalance the *doshas* by stimulating the organs associated with the prevailing *dosha*. For example, as Dr. Vasant Lad explains, *vata* is seated in the pelvic cavity, and so *asanas* that help stretch the pelvic muscles are good for *vata* individuals. These include the forward and backward bends, spinal twist, and shoulder stand.

Pranayama. *Pranayama* is the control of breath, from the Sanskrit *prana*, or life energy, and *ayam*, or control. *Prana* is the life force, and is roughly equivalent to such concepts as *qi* or *chi* in traditional Chinese medicine, or "vital force" in homeopathy. Yoga teaches that interruption of the flow of *prana* by such factors as stress, toxins, or improper diet can have a harmful effect on physical, mental, and spiritual health. *Pranayama* breathing exercises are intended to remove such blockages. *Pranayama* exercises often emphasize slow, deep abdominal breathing.

Meditation. *Dhyana,* or meditation, is a third aspect of classical yoga. Meditative practices have been demonstrated to induce a relaxed state in the autonomic nervous system, which has a beneficial effect on other systems, including the immune system. For more information, see Chapter Two on MindBody medicine.

Yoga has proven beneficial in treating a variety of medical conditions, including heart disease, high blood pressure, breathing problems, asthma, musculoskeletal problems, stress-related illnesses, and mood disorders. Yoga is also helpful in the management of pain, for improving respiratory endurance and efficiency of breathing, for muscle strength, and for motor control. It helps prevent musculoskeletal problems and is beneficial for people with arthritis and those recovering from bone fractures.

Thousands of studies on yoga have been done in India, and more recently in the United States. Unfortunately, much of the research done outside America was poorly designed. Yoga first came to the widespread attention of researchers in the United States when the Menninger Foundation in Topeka, Kansas, conducted biofeedback studies on Indian yogis who were found capable of controlling supposedly automatic physiological functions, such as heart rate or thyroid function. Although medical researchers in the West have been looking into yoga for only a few decades, the work that has been completed is certainly very promising. Yoga programs have shown the potential for helping to reduce heart disease by influencing such risk factors as blood pressure, anxiety, and unhealthy reaction to stress.

Yoga is an essential component of the cardiovascular program developed by Ornish and colleagues to manage and reverse heart disease. This program includes at least one hour of yoga a day. Researchers found that those who benefited most from the program were those who did yoga at least two hours a day.

Following are some selected studies conducted on yoga.

- From a classic study by London cardiologist Dr. Chandra Patel in 1973 of yoga and biofeedback as a combined relaxation therapy, five of twenty patients with high blood pressure were able to stop using their antihypertensive drugs, while seven others were able to reduce their dosage by 33 to 60 percent.

- According to an Indian study by Telles and associates in 1993, forty male physical education teachers who were already very fit practiced yoga daily for three months, and showed a significant reduction in blood pressure, heart rate, respiratory rate, and body weight, with decreased autonomic or involuntary arousal.

- A 1994 RCT of osteoarthritis patients, by Dr. Garfinkel and associates of the University of Pennsylvania School of Medicine, found that after eight weeks of yoga training, pain, tenderness, and range of motion were improved.

- In a 1994 controlled study of healthy female volunteers by Dr. F. J. Schell at the University of Würzburg in Germany, one group of women practiced yoga, and a control group sat and read. There was significant improvement among the yoga group in psychological parameters, such as a higher score in life satisfaction, with a decline in excitability, aggressiveness, and psychosomatic complaints. Heart rate fell during the reading activity in the control group, but rose at follow-up. Among the yoga practitioners, heart rate remained low.

- At the Harvard Medical School, a NCCAM-funded study was carried out by Dr. Howard Shaffer in 1997 focused on sixty-one drug-addicted methadone clinic patients engaged in either group psychotherapy or yoga. Both programs resulted in significant reductions in drug use and criminal activities. This study indicated that yoga might provide a viable alternative for methadone patients who are resistant to group therapy, or who are unable to receive it.

WHAT'S IN THE WORKS

Medical research on yoga is in its early stages in the West, and further well-designed, controlled studies need to be done to extend the promising findings. While yoga has thus far proven to have potential in treating some diseases, research also needs to be done on whether it can help to prevent the onset of illness, or slow its progression.

Due to the fact that yoga lacks the risks of high-impact aerobic activities, research should be conducted to determine if yoga might be beneficial for people who are reluctant to engage in routine exercise, such as patients with heart disease and arthritis. Yoga may be particularly beneficial for older adults or individuals with disabilities.

Beyond their physical and mental benefits, the practices of *asanas*, *pranayama*, and meditation have traditionally been believed to contribute to an integration of mind, body, and spirit. This has not always been a recognized goal of yoga practice in the West. It would be interesting to know whether regular practitioners of yoga report spiritual benefits, as well as physical and mental benefits.

Ayurveda has achieved sufficient stature in the United States to have attracted the interest of the NCCAM, which has funded some preliminary research on Ayurvedic approaches to health maintenance and disease. However, Ayurvedic medicine faces significant challenges in its attempt to become integrated into conventional health care. Ayurvedic medicine is embedded in thousands of years of cultural tradition that may not translate readily into a modern Western context. Ayurvedic philosophy and principles of medical practice are extremely complex, and may try the patience of Western practitioners who use Ayurveda either as a primary or adjunctive therapy.

Furthermore, Ayurvedic medicine depends on a diagnostic system based on constitutional types, or *doshas*, which may not be equally applicable in the West, or may be colored by Western cultural values. Ayurvedic practitioners often point to the hurried pace of the Western lifestyle as contributing to stress-related *vata* disorders, and thereby seem to attach a negative value to the quick, active *vata* type. Similarly, slow-moving or overweight *kapha* types in the West may resist Ayurvedic treatment directed at restoring their inborn *dosha* balance, since some *kapha* characteristics described earlier in this chapter are not fashionable or valued traits in the West.

In the future, Ayurveda can appropriately be used alongside Western medicine. Ayurveda can be especially valuable for its preventive and health-maintaining benefits. It can help to strengthen the constitution, to increase resistance to illness, and to support recuperation following treatment with drugs or surgery.

Presently, the aspect of Ayurvedic medicine that will probably be most investigated in the West is its potential for conversion into new pharmaceuticals. Many Ayurvedic herbs are currently being analyzed for the treatment and prevention of cancer, heart disease, congestive heart failures, diabetes, arthritis, cholesterol reduction, psychological and emotional problems, and other diseases prevalent in the West. Most likely, these herbs will come to be used outside the context of the whole practice of Ayurveda, often in the form of isolated active chemicals, and will be prescribed allopathically to address specific symptoms.

Caution should be exercised in purchasing Ayurvedic herbs manufactured in India, since the toxicity of many of these compounds has been well documented. As with all CAM therapies, people using Ayurveda should inform their physicians.

Some practices associated with Ayurveda have already been well investigated, and have been shown to have benefit in maintaining health. Meditation, especially in the form of Transcendental Meditation and the generic relaxation response, has been adopted as a powerful intervention against stress. Yoga has been demonstrated to be a beneficial form of exercise, with positive impact on body, mind, and spirit. Yogic breathing exercises, while less well studied in the West, also seem to offer promise as a way of influencing mental states and assisting in the treatment of respiratory and other diseases.

Purification practices included in the *pancha karma* procedures may strike Westerners as obsessively extreme, and yet cleansing and purification are enduringly popular activities at health spas, and seem to have some health benefits. Some of the gentler *shaman* palliation procedures may also have a useful place in daily health care, but the more strenuous *pancha karma* techniques should be carried out only under the supervision of a skilled and experienced Ayurvedic practitioner.

Unlike other CAM therapies that have been considered in previous chapters, Ayurveda does not generally overemphasize the therapeutic benefits of the patient-practitioner relationship, and has a strong self-care orientation. To be sure, Ayurvedic practitioners place a positive value on building a trusting relationship with their patients, but place a clear emphasis on self-responsibility in attaining optimal health. Practitioners of Ayurveda appear to act as both technicians and healers. While the Ayurvedic doctor performs the initial diagnosis and then makes recommendations for diet, herbal treatments, and lifestyle changes, the responsibility for carrying out the prescribed treatment resides primarily with the patient. Although historically Ayurveda included meditation as an important part of its science of MindBody integration, most practitioners of Ayurveda today, both in India and in the West, do not emphasize meditation, and tend to prescribe Ayurvedic preparations and procedures in the same way that Western medicine is practiced.

Insofar as Ayurveda constitutes an integrated orientation to healthy physical, mental, and spiritual practices, as it does in the Maharishi Ayur-Ved system, it would seem to be conducive to good health and mental and spiritual well-being. Outside the context of a commitment to a complete philosophical, physical, and spiritual system, it may be more difficult to integrate Ayurveda meaningfully into a comprehensive approach to health care in the West. Surely, a system of healing that is thousands of years in its evolution, spanning the array from physical disability to spiritual enlightenment, merits a prominent role in developing a true health care system of the twenty-first century.

CHAPTER 11

SPIRITUALITY AND HEALING

As Above . . . So Below

Religion and spirituality have been largely banished from modern science and medicine. In our zeal to free science from the constraints of religious dogma, we have neglected an important component of health and well-being, the spiritual factor.

With the emergence of CAM, however, spiritual and religious influences upon health have once again emerged as an appropriate domain for scientific inquiry.

It is ironic that spirituality should be treated as an alternative healing approach. Since earliest times and through all cultures, religion, medicine, and healing have always been closely connected. Throughout recorded history, community health care was typically delivered by religious figures, including medicine men, ministers, shamans, rabbis, priests, witch doctors, and holy men. Such healers were often the tribal or community leaders and the most educated members of the community. Even our modern health care delivery system traces its origins to the hospitals founded by the early Christian church.

Although spirituality and religion have again been recognized as important factors in health care, it's important to remember that these two elements are not identical. Spirituality is not synonymous with religiosity. One does not have to be religious to be spiritual, or vice versa. Broadly defined, spirituality is an inner sense of something greater than oneself, a recognition of a meaning to existence that transcends one's immediate circumstances. Religion, on the other hand, refers to the outward, concrete expression of spiritual impulses, in the form of a specific religion or practice.

Spirituality includes a broad range of characteristics, such as: a diminished focus on self; a feeling of love that leads to acts of compassion, empathy, gratitude; and the experience of inner peace. These characteristics are not only inherently enriching, but also eminently conducive to health and healing.

In spite of the modern separation of religion and spirituality from our secular life, Americans are essentially religious by nature. According to a 1997 survey of spiritual trends compiled by Duane Elgin and Coleen LeDrew of the Millennium Project, 96 percent of Americans believe in God or a universal spirit.

Today, faced by the limitations of modern medicine, and particularly its inability to adequately treat chronic illness, people are increasingly drawing upon inner resources to promote healing. In a 1994 survey by King of 203 adult inpatients of family practitioners in North Carolina and Pennsylvania, 77 percent felt that doctors should consider patients' spiritual needs.

In response to the recent inclusion of spirituality in medicine, modern scientific medicine is beginning to subject religious practices and spiritual beliefs to the same kind of scientific investigation that has been applied to other complementary and alternative treatment modalities. Epidemiological studies, or those involving large populations, and randomized clinical trials are now demonstrating that religion and spirituality can contribute to medical outcomes.

During a 1995 survey of studies on the effect of religion in healing, Dr. Dale Matthews of the Georgetown University School of Medicine found that scientific studies have shown religion to be beneficial to healing 81 percent of the time, neutral 15 percent of the time, and harmful 4 percent of the time. Any new pharmaceutical drug that offered such benefit-to-risk ratios would be an overnight success!

Medical professionals are beginning to acknowledge the need to include spiritual and religious concerns in clinical care, due to a growing body of promising research. A leading force in this movement is the National Institute for Healthcare Research, a private nonprofit organization in Rockville, Maryland, founded in 1991 by Dr. David Larson. NIHR has conducted reviews of medical research that have documented the positive benefits of religious commitment, and these reviews have attracted the attention of mainstream media. NIHR is also introducing spirituality into the curriculum of the nation's leading medical schools, and has organized several influential national conferences.

As a sign of the times, the front-page article in the February 1998 *Harvard Health Letter* focused on "Faith and Healing: Making a Place for Spirituality." Noting a major national trend among patients and practitioners, the article stated, "Today, the long-standing wall between medicine and religion is crumbling, due in part to the disillusionment of many Americans with what they see as high-tech, impersonal health care." There is a profound cultural shift toward spirituality, as evidenced in numerous national polls and such television series as *Touched by an Angel*, with its growing audience.

For many years, researchers have made some attempts to document the impact of spirituality and religion on health. However, careful, well-designed research on this subject is a relatively recent phenomenon. In 1997, Dr. Michael McCullough wrote that a review for the NIHR had found nearly thirty published studies on religion in peer-reviewed scientific literature, dating over the last twenty-five years. In these relatively recent studies, religious participation was found to be protective against death from respiratory disease, cancer, heart disease, suicide, and even stressful medical procedures. This protective effect was found in both men and women, who came from different religions, ages, ethnic groups, and countries. However, McCullough cautions that fewer than a dozen of the studies were designed rigorously enough to draw firm conclusions. Following are examples of some of the well-designed studies.

WHAT WORKS

- A study by Pressman in 1990 of elderly women who had undergone surgical repair of hip fractures found that those with strong religious beliefs were able to walk farther at discharge, and also showed lower levels of depressive symptoms.

- At the Duke University Medical Center, Dr. Harold Koenig, director of the Program on Religion, Aging, and Health, has conducted nearly a dozen studies. In a 1992 review, Dr. Koenig concluded that devout religiousness helps enhance health and well-being, and helps protect against both anxiety and depression.

- Another study by Dr. Koenig concluded that religious older adults have lower blood pressure and lower death rates from coronary heart disease than their nonreligious peers.

- After a six-month follow-up study of 200 older adults in 1995, Dr. Koenig found that people who scored high in religious coping were found to be less subject to depression.

- From the Dartmouth Medical School, a 1995 study by Dr. Thomas Oxman found that, among 232 older adults undergoing heart surgery, patients who were religious were three times less likely to have died six months after surgery than those who were not religious. Of 37 patients who described themselves as deeply religious, none died.

- Duke University researchers found an association between increased immune function and regular attendance at religious services. The investigation, reported in the October 1997 issue of the *International Journal of Psychiatry in Medicine,* involved 1,718 men and women over sixty-five, and reported that those who attended services at least once a week were about half as likely as nonattenders to have high blood levels of interleukin-6, a protein that regulates immune and inflammatory responses.

- Preliminary data from an ongoing study by the Institute of Noetic Sciences suggest that enhanced spiritual well-being may help women cope with and even survive breast cancer.

What Does Not Work

Religious beliefs can also have a negative impact. Religious dogma can be harmful when it fosters excessive guilt, perfectionistic expectations, fear, or lowered self-worth.

- At Bowling Green State University in Ohio, Dr. Kenneth Parga-
ment, a psychology professor, found that adherents to religions that
view humans as sinners in the hands of an angry God tend to have
elevated depression and anxiety.
- Prominent author Dr. Larry Dossey, who focuses his work on prayer
and health, acknowledges that prayer does not always work. As Dossey
states in *Be Careful What You Pray For,* "No therapy is 100% effective. We tell people that penicillin has a failure rate. . . . Should we have
a double standard on prayer? . . . There's a sense that prayer should be
perfect . . . but it isn't." Furthermore, Dossey notes that 5 percent of
Americans who pray sometimes pray for harm against other people.

Religious sects that rely solely upon prayer for health and eschew medical treatment, even in acute medical crises, are sometimes indirectly
responsible for the illnesses and deaths of their adherents. Such a highly
controversial stance can perhaps be bridged through some of the noninvasive CAM therapies.

How Religion and Spirituality
Influence Health

One practical health advantage of many religions is that they encourage
healthy lifestyles among their members. Proscriptions against gluttony,
drug use, smoking, alcohol use, and immoderate behaviors reinforce
health, as does the social communion among church members.

- Actively practicing Mormons develop fewer cases of cancer, cope
better emotionally and physically with the cancer that they do have,
and experience better outcomes than Mormons who are less religious, according to two 1982 studies done by Dr. John Gardner of
the University of Utah School of Medicine. Mormon church doctrines advocate abstention from tobacco and alcohol, and Mormons
have been found to have lower cancer rates at the sites associated
with tobacco and alcohol use.
- Seventh-Day Adventists, who are instructed not to use alcohol, consume pork, or smoke tobacco, are a notably healthy population. A

ten-year longitudinal study by Berkel in 1983 of 3,217 Seventh-Day Adventists in the Netherlands concluded that Adventist men live 8.9 years longer than the national norm, and Adventist women live 3.6 years longer. They have a 60 percent lower mortality rate from cancer, and a 66 percent lower mortality rate from heart disease.

- Religious commitment also has a strong influence in the prevention of substance abuse. In 1984, Dr. C. Kirk Hadaway of the Center for Urban Church Studies in Nashville, Tennessee, interviewed 600 adolescents in public schools in Atlanta and found that parents' church attendance, personal importance of religion, orthodoxy, and obedience to parents were all inversely related to adolescent use of alcohol, marijuana, and other drugs.

- Religion is also important in treating drug and alcohol abuse. Alcoholics Anonymous has a strong spiritual component, and a study funded by the National Institute of Drug Abuse found that heroin withdrawal was more effective among addicts who attended religiously based programs than for those who did not. Also, a 1996 study of smoking cessation programs for African-American smokers by Dr. Carolyn Voorhees at Johns Hopkins University School of Medicine found that a church-based smoking cessation program was more effective than a self-help intervention.

However, the health benefit of religion is apparently not all derived from healthy lifestyles. Much of the benefit appears to stem from the physical impact of positive belief systems and attitudes. Qualities such as faith, hope, forgiveness, and love have a demonstrable effect upon health and healing, even among people who do not attend religious services.

Faith

It is often observed that more heart attacks occur on Monday morning at nine o'clock than at any other time. Also, the per-day death rate in the United States drops by nearly 30 percent on Christmas Day, as reported by Dr. Dick Tibbits, of Florida Hospital and the Disney "Celebration" city project, in 1998. Beliefs and attitudes obviously play a role in such statistics. When expectations are positive, fewer people die.

Faith is a major source of positive expectations, and seems to have a powerful healing effect, perhaps by increasing resistance to stress.

- Based on a study by Justice in 1988, it was documented that among women who were about to undergo breast biopsies, those with the lowest stress hormone levels were those who utilized faith and prayer to cope with stress.
- From a 1993 study by Taylor of seventy-four patients with recurrent cancer, nearly half reported engaging in a search for meaning. In this study, the greater a patient's sense of meaning, the lower were the symptoms of distress.

People's beliefs about their health, and the possibility of recovery, have a strong influence upon the course of their hospitalizations. One of the most important individuals to articulate the profound difference between false hope and false pessimism regarding an invariant diagnosis was my longtime mentor and friend Norman Cousins. Although he expounded upon this theme in numerous books, his most succinct admonition is contained in his 1989 book *Head First: The Biology of Hope,* in which he wrote, "Don't deny the diagnosis . . . deny the verdict." That was, and is, a profoundly sagacious insight.

- In a 1996 study by Petrie and colleagues, conducted at two teaching hospitals in Auckland, New Zealand, researchers found that psychological factors are more important than medical factors during the recovery process following heart attack.

Beliefs of a patient's physician can also influence the course of disease and the outcome of treatment. A doctor's expectation of a drug's effectiveness can influence the outcome of therapy by 25 to 30 percent in either direction, according to a brief report in *Brain Mind Bulletin* in 1989. This is why studies of pharmaceuticals use double-blind methodology, with the physician not knowing whether he or she is giving a real drug or a placebo.

Placebo effect is, in fact, a very strong indicator of the healing power of a positive belief. For virtually any disease, approximately one-third of patients will improve when given a placebo.

Hope

In addition to faith, hope and optimism are strong potentiators of health and healing. Hope has been defined in a 1992 *Berkeley Wellness Letter* by Dr. Rick Snyder, a University of Kansas psychologist, as a "goal oriented attitude, a stance that a person assumes in the face of difficulty." By the same token, pessimism can have a profoundly negative impact upon health.

- Hope is such a significant ingredient in the healing prescription that it was described by Dr. William Buchholz in a 1990 opinion piece in the *Journal of the American Medical Association* as if it were a generic pharmaceutical. Dr. Buchholz warns that in an effort to avoid the appearance of false hope, doctors and nurses may generate false despair.
- A thirty-five-year longitudinal study by Peterson and associates of ninety-nine Harvard graduates found that optimism was linked with longer life and fewer illnesses, even when controlling for participants' physical and mental health at the initial assessment.
- People with a pessimistic attitude were found in a 1988 study by psychologist Dr. Christopher Peterson of the University of Michigan to have twice as many infectious illnesses, and to make twice as many visits to their doctors, as people who were more hopeful.
- Depression engendered by loss of hope places individuals at increased risk for suicide. In a 1991 review of studies of suicide, which included a spiritual variable, Dr. John Gartner of Loyola College and Dr. David Larson of Duke found that 81 percent of the time there was a positive correlation between spirituality and suicide reduction.
- An innovative 1998 study by Dr. Harold A. Koenig of the Duke University Medical Center focused on eighty-seven people over age sixty who were hospitalized for heart and other major problems. People who evidenced "intrinsic religiosity," or internal spiritual values independent of actual church attendance, were more resistant to depression and recovered more quickly.

In the absence of hope, many people become depressed, and clear links have been established between depression and both physical and mental illness as well as mortality. Estimated costs for the physical health care of depressed patients are approximately $8.9 million a year, compared to $3.8 million spent for their mental health care.

Establishing the legitimacy of appropriate hope and optimism may prove to be effective in terms of both clinical and cost benefits.

Forgiveness

Forgiveness is a practice that is encouraged by many spiritual and religious traditions. Confucius instructed, "Attack the evil that is within yourself, do not attack the evil that is in others." In the Bible, Jesus asked, "Why do you see the speck that is in your brother's eye, but do not notice the log that is in your own eye?" At the heart of forgiveness is the taking of responsibility for our own perceptions. When we forgive, we are recognizing that we can control our perceptions by taking a different view of the situation. Forgiveness has healing power in its ability to release from the mind the hostility and resentment that can grow out of past hurts.

At the Stanford University School of Medicine, Dr. Fred Luskin completed a significant doctoral thesis in 1997 which defined forgiveness as the experience of psychological peace that occurs when injured people transform their grievances against others. This transformation takes place by learning to take less personal offense, to attribute less blame to the offender, and to understand the personal harm that comes from unresolved anger. During 1999, this study is being replicated with different populations of adults to determine the range of effectiveness.

- Also at Stanford University, Dr. Luskin and Dr. Carl Thoesen conducted a successful 1997 study in which they trained fifty-five college students to forgive someone who had hurt them. After six weeks, the students in the treatment group were significantly less angry, showed greater self-efficacy, were more hopeful, and showed greater emotional self-management than their peers in the control group. Their improved mental health was maintained when they were tested ten weeks later.

Forgiveness has also been shown to be an effective healing intervention. In the presence of an unforgiving attitude of anger or resentment, our bodies manufacture potent stress-related chemicals, such as adrenaline, noradrenaline, and cortisol, which can accumulate in the bloodstream and produce a variety of symptoms. Forgiveness initiates a process of recovery, and helps to reduce these powerful chemicals.

- Noted Duke University cardiologist Dr. Redford Williams, author of *Anger Kills*, showed in 1993 that hostility is not only a barrier to happiness but can also lead to heart disease and other life-threatening illness. Hostility has been found to be as effective a predictor of heart disease as measurements of cholesterol and lipid levels.
- From the point of view of basic research, Dr. William Tiller of Stanford University found in 1996 that anger interfered with the immune system. Anger had deleterious effects on the immune substance salivary IgA, with the effects persisting for hours. Positive emotions produced an increase in salivary IgA.

Of all the positive emotional states, however, the one that may be most conducive to health and healing is love.

LOVE AND SOCIAL SUPPORT

Philosophers, poets, and some theologians attest that love is the very essence of spiritual experience. Every world religion teaches the importance of giving and receiving love. Now scientific research is beginning to verify the healing power of love.

- Parental love sets the scene for all of the love relationships in our lives. In the 1950s, in the Harvard Mastery of Stress Study, Harvard students rated their parents' degrees of love and caring. In a thirty-five-year follow-up of this study, Dr. Linda Russek and Dr. Gary Schwartz of the University of Arizona School of Medicine in Tucson found that individuals who had described their parents in positive terms in the 1950s were far less likely to have developed later illnesses, such as heart disease, high blood pressure, ulcers, and alcoholism. Ninety-five percent of the subjects who described their parents negatively had serious diseases in midlife, compared to 29 percent who described their parents positively.

To some extent, this finding is in contrast to the findings reported in my 1994 book *Sound Mind, Sound Body: A New Model of Lifelong Health*. This book focused on the common strategies developed by healthy and successful individuals with extremely demanding careers. Fifty-three individuals were interviewed, including David Rockefeller, Lindsay Wagner, Saul Zaentz, Laurel Burch, and George Lucas. Virtually all of them had accepted a commitment to adult spirituality as a way of giving back to society. Surprisingly, a majority of these individuals had suffered a major traumatic childhood event, and many of them identified one or both parents as the perpetrator of the trauma. Despite this trauma, or perhaps because of their successful adaptation to it, these individuals emerged as healthy, successful, and spiritually oriented adults. This phenomenon strongly suggests the vital importance of resolving childhood trauma.

One important reason love improves health is because it generally inspires support from other people. One of the main reasons that frequent attendance at religious services is associated with better health may be that church attendance promotes social support, and a sense of belonging, especially among older adults. In fact, older individuals are more involved in church groups than all other voluntary social groups combined, according to a 1995 report by Koenig.

Social support has been found to be a protective factor in preventing or alleviating many diseases.

- Epidemiologists found, in classic studies reported by Bruhn and colleagues in 1966 and later in 1978, that in the close-knit Italian-American community of Roseto, Pennsylvania, the death rate from heart attack was half of that of neighboring communities, and of the United States as a whole. While the residents of Roseto were generally overweight and sedentary, and had a high rate of cigarette smoking, they were apparently protected from heart disease by their very strong social support network. Over time, however, as the Rosetoans became more Americanized, individualistic, and mobile, their Old World values began to erode, their social support system broke down, and their rate of heart attacks increased.
- In another classic study, the 1979 Alameda County Study by Dr. Lisa Berkman and Dr. Leonard Syme of the University of California at Berkeley, social support was one of seven factors that was found to

have a positive benefit for health and longevity. People with many close social ties had a lower risk of death than those with few social ties. Moreover, people with close social ties and unhealthy lifestyle behaviors lived longer than those who had healthy behaviors but lacked close social ties.

- Even processes such as childbirth can be influenced by social support, according to 1980 research by Sosa. Among a group of women receiving social support, mean delivery time was 8.7 hours, compared with 19.3 hours for the group receiving standard treatment. Mothers who received social support had fewer complications during delivery and more readily bonded with their babies.

- Social isolation has been implicated as a risk factor for recurrent myocardial infarction and/or death. Dr. David Sobel and Dr. Robert Ornstein, in their excellent 1987 book *The Healing Brain*, report that 38 percent of patients without social support died following a heart attack, compared to 12 percent among those who had two or more sources of social support.

- In the classic Alameda County Study, a seventeen-year prospective follow-up study by Reynolds in 1990 disclosed that, among women, social isolation was a risk factor for the onset and progression of cancer.

- Other studies confirm that social support appears protective against cancer. A seventeen-year cohort study of 154 men and 185 women with cancer, by Reynolds in 1990, found that men with the fewest social contacts had a significantly shorter survival time, and women who reported they were more socially isolated had a greater incidence of cancer. A 1996 study by Maunsell of women with advanced breast cancer found that social support was associated with longer survival time.

Social support may promote health and healing in several ways. One way is by helping people resist unhealthy behaviors. Social support also improves health by decreasing stress.

Another aspect of love that increases health is active concern about the well-being of others, or altruism. Altruistic activities were reported to produce marked benefits in the personal health and well-being of the highly successful individuals described in my 1994 book *Sound Mind, Sound Body*. Other investigators have confirmed such findings.

- Research by Dr. Neal Krause in 1992 found that giving of oneself to help others enhances well-being and produces feelings of usefulness, especially among older adults.
- A study in 1992, by Dr. James House of the University of Michigan, found that volunteer work, more than any other activity, yielded a dramatic increase in life expectancy and improved health. Men who did no volunteer work were two and one-half times more likely to die than those who volunteered at least once a week.
- In an interview-based study by Hafen in 1996, people who showed the least evidence of altruism were relatively more likely to develop coronary disease.
- Altruistic behavior has a positive effect on immune response even when it is merely observed, rather than engaged in. In a 1985 Harvard University study, noted psychologist Dr. David McClelland found that when students were shown a film about Mother Teresa, they showed an immediate and significant increase in the immune antibody IgA. When students were shown a film about Attila the Hun, their antibody levels dropped.

As Dr. Bernie Siegel commented in 1991, "If I told patients to raise their blood levels or immune globulins or killer T cells, no one would know how. But if I can teach them to love themselves and others fully, the same change happens automatically. The truth is: Love heals." As simplistic and overstated as it may sound, research tends to support this assertion.

Love can be so powerful that it has healing effects even when it is shared with a pet. A number of recent studies indicate that pets can be powerful stimulators of health.

- Pets can help to lower blood pressure. At the University of Pennsylvania School of Veterinary Medicine, Dr. Aaron Katcher conducted a number of studies in 1980 in which he measured the blood pressure of dog owners while they were either reading a neutral text or enthusiastically greeting their pets. Blood pressure was significantly lower when they were interacting with their pets.
- In a 1988 study, Dr. Erika Friedmann at the University of Pennsylvania found a significant association between pet ownership and one-year survival in patients who were hospitalized for heart attacks

and other coronary diseases. Having a pet at home proved a stronger predictor of survival than having a spouse or having extensive family support.

- Psychologists Dr. Karen Allen and Dr. James Blascovich of the State University of New York at Buffalo found in a 1991 study that female dog owners performing stressful mental arithmetic experienced less stress when they were in the presence of their dog than when they were in the presence of either the researcher or their best female friend. Interestingly, when the female friend was present, the stress measures increased dramatically. Presumably, the women perceived their dogs as less threatening.

- During a program of animal-assisted therapy for the elderly, the Visiting Nurses Association of Eastern Montgomery County, Pennsylvania, brings dogs to visit elderly patients at retirement homes. Following a pet visit, patients show significant reductions in blood pressure and pulse rate. However, they do not exhibit the same reduction following a visit from a human, according to Dossey.

- According to a 1996 randomized clinical trial, Dr. Karen Allen and Dr. James Blascovich found that service dogs are a cost-effective source of social support and physical assistance for people with disabilities. One group of disabled people received trained service dogs and were compared to a control group. The group with dogs showed substantial improvements in self-esteem, internal locus of control, and psychological well-being. They also experienced increases in attendance at school and/or part-time employment, and experienced dramatic decreases in the number of paid and unpaid assistance hours.

Western philosophy has been characterized as footnotes to Plato. To me, the most profoundly insightful writing on the power of a respectful appreciation of nature and animals is in the book *The Outermost House* by Henry Beston. Inspired by Henry David Thoreau's writings, Beston purchased fifty acres of land in 1925 along the great outer dunes of Cape Cod. There he built his "outermost house" on the farthest reaches of the then-deserted Cape, and lived in solitary contemplation for a year. His reflections upon the relationship between nature, animals, and humankind provide a definitive and moving testimonial:

We need another and a wiser and perhaps a more mystical concept of animals. Remote from universal nature, and living by complicated artifice, man in civilization surveys the creature through the glass of his knowledge and sees thereby a feather magnified and the whole image in distortion. We patronize them for their incompleteness, for their tragic fate of having taken form so far below ourselves. And therein we err, and greatly err. For the animal shall not be measured by man. In a world older and more complete than ours they move finished and complete, gifted with extensions of the senses we have lost or never attained, living by voices we shall never hear. They are not brethren, they are not underlings; they are other nations, caught with ourselves in the net of life and time, fellow prisoners of the splendour and travail of the earth.

Animals are not to slaughter for food, to experiment upon when other more humane alternatives exist, or to imprison for entertainment. They are a unique and wondrous expression of consciousness, in a virtually infinite array of forms.

Experiencing communication with an animal often opens individuals to spiritual realms that are not accessible in our usual interactions with humans. Animals help us to recognize our connection with all of nature's creation. Loving animals enable people to glimpse a oneness with other life forms.

Prayer and Spiritual Healing

Prayer has been used as a means of healing throughout the ages and across all cultures. Even in our modern age, most Americans pray. In a 1990 Gallup poll, 76 percent of the Americans polled said that prayer was an important part of their daily lives.

Meditative prayer is practiced in many different forms. Within the Western world the stereotype of prayer consists of communicating to a cosmic white male parent figure. However, some faiths, such as Buddhism, do not address a personal God in prayer. Among other people, prayer is practiced simply as a state of being. Dr. Larry Dossey, who has examined extensive research on medicine and prayer, favors a broad definition of prayer as communication with the Absolute. He identifies two kinds of healing prayer in his 1997 writings: petitionary prayer, in which one prays for oneself; and intercessory prayer, in which one prays for someone else. Intercessory prayer includes distant prayer, in which the person being prayed for is not present. While there is a strong tradition of the use of healing prayers by priests, shamans, and other healers, ordinary people can be equally successful at intercessory prayer.

Healing power of prayer is widely accepted, even among conventional, allopathic physicians. A nationwide poll conducted by *MD* magazine in 1986 indicated that one-half of doctors polled believe that prayer helps patients, and two-thirds reported praying for a patient.

Skeptics often assert that prayer works only because of the placebo effect. However, in 1991, Dossey compiled a large number of controlled laboratory studies which show that prayer can produce beneficial changes that are not dependent upon the placebo response. Following are examples of research on prayer.

- In 1969, Dr. Platon Collip attempted to demonstrate that prayer on behalf of children with leukemia would improve their survival. In a triple-blind study, in which neither patients nor practitioners knew that a study was in progress, there was an almost threefold greater survival at fifteen months for the children who were prayed for, compared with those who were not prayed for. However, the methodology was flawed, and no sound replications have been published.
- Two major research reviews, compiled by Dr. Jerry Solfvin in 1984 and Dr. Daniel Benor in 1990, identified some 130 controlled studies of praying for various "targets" at a distance, nearly half of which show statistically significant results. Targets included a variety of cellular and biological systems, such as bacteria, fungi, yeast, algae, plants, protozoa, larvae, insects, chicks, mice, rats, gerbils, cats, and dogs, as well as enzyme activity and preparations of blood, nerve, and cancer cells, according to Braud in 1992. With people as the object of the distant prayers, research indicates that prayer appears to have affected such physiological parameters as eye movement, muscular movement, electrodermal activity, blood pressure, respiration, and brain rhythms.
- During 1988, Dr. Randolph Byrd, a cardiologist at the University of California School of Medicine in San Francisco, conducted an RCT of 393 patients in the Coronary Care Unit at San Francisco General

Hospital. One group was prayed for, and a control group was not. Neither the people praying, nor the patients, nor the physicians knew which patients received prayers. Over ten months, the group that was prayed for had fewer deaths, though there was not a statistically significant difference. Also, the prayer group required less ventilatory assistance, antibiotics, and diuretics. They also had a lower incidence of pulmonary edema, required less frequent CPR, and required less time in the hospital.

- In a large-scale double-blind Israeli study in 1994, Bentwich focused on male patients who had undergone hernia surgery. Patients who were prayed for showed improved recovery and wound appearance, had less fever after hospitalization, and experienced less pain.

Many of the methodological difficulties that plague studies on prayer can theoretically be addressed if nonhumans are used as subjects. Research on prayer with nonhuman subjects has largely been relegated to the field of parapsychology, or psi research. Parapsychology utilizes extremely careful methodology that parallels the best conventional laboratory science. Unfortunately, much of the work in this area is difficult to locate in the research databases because of differences in terminology. Psi researchers avoid using the word "prayer," and instead describe it as "distant intentionality." Rather than describing the subject as praying, psi studies may report that the subject "concentrated" or "applied mental effort." Nonetheless, several fascinating studies have been done that appear to confirm the effects reported in studies of prayer.

- With a 1997 literature review, researchers Dr. Marilyn Schlitz and Dr. William Braud identified more than 150 studies on distant healing or the positive effect of praying for people who are at a physical distance. In one type of study, researchers monitored the skin resistance of one person while another person in a separate room attempted to influence the subject's skin resistance, a sensitive measure of sweating in response to stress, by sending calming or activating thoughts. Such studies have been replicated in a number of laboratories.
- At the Harvard Medical School, Dr. Herbert Benson was one of the first medical researchers to study the health benefits of prayer and meditation. Early in his career, he identified what he came to call the

relaxation response, a scientifically definable state in which metabolism, breathing, and heart rate slow, blood pressure drops, and brain waves become less active. When he began working with the relaxation response, Benson did not have spirituality and religion in mind; however, he found that the response was most effectively elicited through different forms of prayer. By 1997, Benson became convinced that there is a strong spiritual component to meditation and relaxation. Benson now feels that a person's belief system, or what he calls the "faith factor," actually produces healing by itself.

- Similarly, Winzelberg and Luskin completed a pilot study in 1998 that investigated the effect of religious meditation on the physical and emotional manifestations of stress. Study participants were asked to meditate daily upon a favorite passage from the world's spiritual literature. This simple practice helped these people to better manage their stress.

THERAPEUTIC TOUCH

Touch was practiced as a healing modality in all the ancient cultures. Even though touch has always been an integral part of healing, modern taboos against physical contact, as well as time pressure, have prevented physicians from exploiting the full potential of touch. Touch and manipulation have become a specialized set of healing practices, reserved for use by nurses, massage and bodywork therapists, and licensed practitioners such as chiropractors and osteopaths.

Spiritual healers often practice "laying on of hands," in which the healer comes into physical contact with the patient. As we have seen, many spiritual healers also practice distant healing through prayer. Therapeutic touch represents a hybridization of these two approaches. It was developed in the early 1970s by Dolores Krieger, who was then a professor of nursing at New York University, along with Dora Kunz, a noted healer. Therapeutic touch (TT) draws on ancient concepts of healing, as well as modern Western approaches. Like many Eastern healing traditions, TT is based on the premise that the human body is surrounded by, and permeated with, an energy field that is connected with the universal life energy. By interacting with the patient's energy field, the practitioner helps to project universal energy into it.

Therapeutic touch does not actually involve physical contact. Holding the hands a short distance from the patient's body, the practitioner moves them through the patient's energy field without touching the patient.

Advocates of TT believe that the technique does not require a special gift, but that everyone has an inborn capacity for healing touch that can be developed through training. In itself, therapeutic touch does not have any religious content, and the patient is not required to believe in its efficacy in order for it to work.

Therapeutic touch has become very popular among professional nurses, and is now taught at some eighty colleges and universities in the United States. Typically, TT has been used in treating hospitalized patients, but is increasingly being delivered in an outpatient setting.

Benefits of TT are documented by an ever-growing body of research, particularly in the nursing literature. Also, among nonhuman subjects, therapeutic touch has been shown to speed wound healing in mice, to increase enzyme activity in test tube experiments, and to promote germination and growth of barley seeds, according to Ash in 1997.

- In controlled studies in 1973 and 1975 with human subjects, Dolores Krieger found that TT produced significant changes in hemoglobin levels in hospitalized patients.
- Nurse and psychologist Dr. Janet Quinn developed in 1984 a mock or placebo therapeutic touch technique in which the practitioner stands near the patient but does mental arithmetic instead of forming a healing intention. In a 1984 study, Quinn found that patients in a cardiovascular unit who received TT showed a significant reduction in anxiety, compared to patients receiving sham therapeutic touch when the nurse did not actually focus on healing the patient.
- As early as 1988, Meehan found that TT had a beneficial effect on postoperative pain. Patients who received the technique waited longer than controls before requesting pain medication.
- Based on a study in 1990, Dr. Daniel Wirth reported significant change in the healing rate of skin wounds in a carefully controlled double-blind study of TT.

Not all studies have yielded statistically significant or even positive results, when comparing TT with sham TT.

Therapeutic touch is part of a larger field, biofield healing, which is based on the premise that the human organism is surrounded and permeated by an energy field, such as that described as *qi* in China, or *prana* in India.

A number of modern biofield therapies are in use in medical settings in this country. At least four forms have been taught in medical institutions, namely Healing Science, Healing Touch, SHEN® Therapy, and Therapeutic Touch. These techniques are generally practiced by nurses, acupuncturists, and massage practitioners. Using the hands, practitioners are able to diagnose subtle changes in the patient's biofield, and then direct healing energy to it.

Since its inception, the Office of Alternative Medicine and now the National Center for Complementary and Alternative Medicine (NCCAM) has included these biofield therapies in research grant awards. At the Menninger Foundation, noted biofeedback researcher Dr. Steve Fahrion conducted an OAM-funded study in 1996 of the application of bioenergetic therapy for the treatment of basal cell carcinoma, the most common form of skin cancer. He found that four out of ten patients treated showed elimination or reduction of their tumors during the treatment period. Other patients showed no results, or equivocal results. Patients with three of the strongest and most balanced energy fields at initial assessment had the best outcomes.

WHAT'S IN THE WORKS

Spirituality is gaining increasing recognition as an important element of healing. In 1980, the World Health Organization added spiritual health to its definition of health care, so that the current WHO definition of health is "not just the absence of disease, but the optimal condition of body, mind, and spirit."

Most significant, in 1994 the American Psychiatric Association recognized the influence of spirituality and religion on psychological health when it added a new diagnostic code to the fourth edition of the *Diagnostic and Statistical Manual of Mental Disorders*, which cited "religious and spiritual difficulties" as a significant dimension of psychological well-being.

Science and biomedicine have until recently been wary of enlisting spirituality in research and clinical strategies. Recent changes in this attitude, however, are driven in part by a respect for the economic bottom line. Providing spiritual support in a clinical setting, attending to patients' spiritual needs, and acknowledging the value of religious participation and social interaction are all safe, efficacious, and cost-effective strategies.

It is indeed significant that a report commissioned by the National Institutes of Health, the 1993 *Report of the Panel on MindBody Interventions* by Drs. Jeanne Achterberg, Larry Dossey, and James Gordon, should make such a strong and urgent case for the recognition of nonlocal healing phenomena and other spiritual principles of healing.

Distant prayer and spiritual healing raise many questions that need to be addressed in future research. First of all, there is a serious need for both medical researchers and psi researchers to come together on common ground, in order to create a common language of research. Researchers also need to know whether any special skills are required for distant healing, whether such skills can be learned, and whether certain subjects are more responsive than others to the healing effects of prayer. Research also needs to look at the question of whether distant prayer can produce harmful as well as beneficial results.

In any case, it may be that distant healing cannot be optimally studied under controlled, double-blind conditions. Perhaps more flexible designs need to be developed which will recognize outcomes that have greater clinical relevance. Clearly, further work is needed to determine in what ways spiritual healing can be used as a complement to orthodox medical approaches.

Even more provocative are the questions raised by the very existence of the phenomenon of successful intercessory prayer on behalf of someone else. According to Dr. Jeanne Achterberg in 1993, well-designed laboratory studies have demonstrated that the mind is somehow able to bring about changes in faraway organisms. Distant healing challenges our current scientific explanatory models, and seems to call for a new view of reality. Not only may space be able to be overcome in distant healing phenomena, but so may time. Information and intention seem capable of being received by a distant target even before they have been transmitted by the sender.

Scientific resistance to research on distant healing is based in part on the absence of an underlying explanatory mechanism. However, a number of explanatory paradigms have been suggested. Writing in 1994, Dr.

Daniel Wirth offered several theoretical models by which distant healing might operate. These include the transfer of electromagnetic energy from healer to patient, an intuitive or direct information exchange, a state of consciousness that occurs in both healer and patient, and/or a process brought about through divine grace.

While Achterberg, Dossey, Gordon, and others propose various models drawn from modern physics as possible explanations of "nonlocal phenomena," occurrences that are simultaneous in time but physically distant, the answer may well lie beyond any science of which we can presently conceive. Ultimately, the challenge for researchers may be to cast their nets wide enough so that they may be able to capture the "footprints of God."

At the present time, Harvard's Dr. Herbert Benson is attempting to replicate the 1988 intercessory prayer study by Dr. Byrd. Seeking to correct some of the flaws in the original study's design, Benson and the late Dr. Richard Friedman designed a controlled, randomized, double-blind study of intercessory prayer, which is funded by the Sir John Templeton Foundation. Full details of the study have not been disclosed, but the researchers have said that the intercessors in this study will pray for two of three groups of coronary bypass patients. One group will know that it is being prayed for, while the other two groups will only know that one group is being prayed for, but will not know which group. This study will address two important questions: first, whether knowing that one is being prayed for is beneficial to health; and second, whether it is possible to influence health through pure thought, or prayer.

Writing in 1997, Dr. Larry Dossey remarked, "Modern medicine has become one of the most spiritually malnourished professions in our society." However, in calling for an integration of spirituality and medicine, we are by no means implying that religion and spiritual practices should be considered a replacement for conventional medicine.

In psychiatry and clinical psychology, when clinicians recognize that spiritual and religious issues, as well as so-called disorders of meaning, are appropriate areas for counseling and psychiatric intervention, this may lead to highly cost-effective treatment that will help prevent and heal both mental and physical ailments.

A final set of phenomena that must be acknowledged are the ostensible medical miracles. These are healings that defy the known course of disease. They are now being scrutinized by serious researchers. At

Lourdes, France, physicians have compiled some five thousand cases of supposedly miraculous healings, dating back to 1858. Sixty-five of the cases have been carefully reviewed and found to meet three stringent criteria, namely, that they represent (1) instantaneous alleviation of (2) an acute or chronic organic disease for which (3) there is no known cure. Consideration of this complex area is contained in my 1981 book *Longevity: Fulfilling Our Biological Potential*. Reductionistic approaches to reported miracles are an affront to both religion and science. Nonetheless, such well-documented occurrences cannot be dismissed.

Miracle cures may be attributed to the placebo effect, or perhaps may represent the intervention of some divine or higher force. A study by Dr. Richard Kalish of UCLA has identified a number of interesting associations between spontaneous remissions, miracle cures, and so-called voodoo death. In some ways these associations parallel the distinction between positive and negative placebo response, but they also serve to illustrate the powerful and unexplained influence that consciousness exerts on health and illness.

Throughout this book, there has been an emphasis upon not prematurely reducing any outcome, including miracle cures, to a reductionistic explanation. Such prematurity does a profound disservice to both spirituality and science. Nothing here should be interpreted as a futile attempt to explain away truly miraculous cures, nor to inhibit science from addressing such mysteries. Perhaps the apparent oxymoron of a scientific inquiry into miracles will take its place among the profound accomplishments of the modern era that at one time seemed impossible paradoxes, such as the horseless carriage and the wireless telegraph.

Prayer is not a substitute for effective medical care, but rather a complement to it. To date, research has not demonstrated any correlation between one's private religious beliefs and the effectiveness of prayer, so prayer may transcend personal beliefs and religions.

Science and well-designed experiments cannot yet explain how prayer works, nor can they determine whether it will work on a specific case-by-case basis. However, research has been able to demonstrate that it does have a powerful healing effect.

Finally, an appreciation of spiritual values can do much to heal our present dysfunctional attitudes toward terminal illness and death. Dying, in virtually all modern cultures, has been marginalized and medicalized. Approximately 80 percent of persons in the United States today die in institutions, where dying is compartmentalized as an unwelcome event in the context of conventional medical care. Modern medicine is a system in which death is interpreted too often as a failure of technical biomedicine, rather than as an inevitable part of life.

Dying is perhaps the most important spiritual event in each individual's life, yet death and the process of dying have been hidden from view, cloaked in denial and fear. Studies by Lynn in 1997 have documented that pain, feelings of isolation, and unconsciousness are common concomitants of the dying process for many Americans today. Many individuals throughout the world are too often deprived of the ability to experience the powerful spiritual and psychological transformation of their last days, hours, and minutes of life.

With the recognition of the nonlocal, unlimited, spiritual dimensions of consciousness, and with the embracing of these mysteries through caring and compassion, both doctors and patients may finally be able to accept death as an opportunity for a final transition marked by comfort, dignity, awareness, and love. Although researchers continue to investigate the links between spirituality, health, and longevity, people who already believe that spirituality can heal don't need scientific studies to convince them. Those who are skeptical may find the results intriguing, but science may never be able to fully assuage their doubts. Perhaps the twain shall never meet, but then again, perhaps they will.

CHAPTER 12

CAM INSURANCE

*Who Pays How Much
to Whom for What?*

Health-conscious Americans are flocking in ever-increasing numbers to CAM providers for at least a portion of their health care. There are many reasons for this trend, including disillusionment with the conventional treatment of chronic disease, concern over side effects, and disappointment with a biomedical model that views health and disease almost in terms of physical processes, without fully recognizing the role of the mind and spirit. Americans have also been influenced by exposure to other cultures' medical systems.

Conventional medicine received a wake-up call in 1993 from a *New England Journal of Medicine* article in which Dr. David Eisenberg of Harvard reported on his survey of the extraordinary extent of CAM use in the United States. To conventional medicine, the message was clear: CAM use is increasing, and is valued by consumers.

In 1997, John Weeks, a Seattle CAM integration consultant and editor in chief of *Alternative Medicine Integration and Coverage*, stated that "What may one day be recognized as the greatest popular movement in the United States in the second half of the twentieth century" was taking place right under the noses of the leaders of American medicine. American consumers, generally without the knowledge, and often despite the disapproval, of their physicians, HMOs, insurers, and employers, were seeking out alternatives to conventional medicine, and usually paying for it themselves.

According to the Eisenberg survey, the Americans who are most likely to use unconventional therapies tend to be highly educated, high-income, non-blacks who live in the western United States. Major users of these therapies generally fall between the ages of twenty-five and forty-nine, or are over sixty-five. These individuals are investing their own money because they have exhausted conventional options, and because they have been unable to obtain similar services from their conventional providers.

Most frequent users of CAM are also individuals who tend to require less medical care than average. This decreased need for care is very financially important to HMOs. When an HMO receives a fixed, or "capitated," amount of money per person per year, people who do not use medical services are profitable. This financial incentive to attract CAM users into managed care is a powerfully positive force supporting CAM.

Advocates of CAM suggest that CAM can help keep down medical costs. In addition, CAM may improve the quality of health care and encourage patients to assume more responsibility for their own health. Patients may feel more satisfied, and this may also reduce unnecessary office visits. Such arguments are now largely speculative, but do tend to be supported by limited findings.

However, there is only a small amount of high-quality research indicating that CAM will significantly lower health care costs. This observation is based on a definitive study of nineteen insurance and managed care providers who reimbursed for CAM as of January 1997. My colleagues and I conducted this study at the Stanford University School of Medicine, and are monitoring the trends revealed by it on an ongoing basis.

Incorporating CAM into the existing health care system may entail some compromises on the part of CAM therapies. CAM providers will probably need to align themselves more closely with the prevailing medical model if they wish to be reimbursed by third-party payers.

Following the 1990 Eisenberg study, subsequent surveys have provided health plans with information about what CAM products and services they should develop. In 1997, John Weeks reviewed a number of consumer surveys. He found that 20 to 35 percent of consumers had visited some kind of alternative practitioner during the previous two years.

Also in 1997, Dr. Eisenberg's updated survey indicated that CAM use had risen from 33.8 percent in 1990 to 42.1 percent in 1997. That means that nearly one out of every two individuals in the United States is now using CAM therapies, and there is every indication that this number is increasing daily.

Furthermore, the most active markets for CAM integration, including the Pacific Northwest, California, New England, and the upper Midwest, are the geographic areas where cultural trends tend to first emerge. Again, this fact is based on findings reported by Weeks in 1997.

Despite this surge of interest, CAM therapies are still much more widely used in Europe and Asia than in the United States. Fifty-six percent of Belgians use homeopathy, 48 percent of Swedes receive manipulative therapy, 24 percent of the British use herbal medicine, and 21 percent of the French use acupuncture. Japan's national health care sys-

Data Since Eisenberg on Use of Alternative Practitioners in 1990

Surveyor	Year	Market	Features	Percentage Seeing Alternative Provider
Eisenberg, et al.	1990	National	Phone survey of residents	10%
The Alternative Group	1994	Portland, OR	Phone survey of residents	35% (2 years)
Seattle–King County Dept. of Public Health	1995	King County, WA	Survey at public health clinics who saw N.D., D.C., L.Ac.	19% (1 year)
Oxford Health Plans	1995 1996	CT, NY, NJ	Phone survey of 750 plan members	33% (2 years)
Unified Physicians of Washington	1996	Seattle	Survey at a University District Women's Clinic	56% (1 year)
Presbyterian Healthcare System	1996	New Mexico	Phone survey of residents	33% (1 year)

Survey on CAM Interest Among HMO Members in an Active Market

	Chiropractic	Naturopathic	Acupuncture	Midwife*
Very Interested	30.3%	20.9%	14.0%	18.0%
Somewhat interested	25.7%	26.4%	25.2%	16.0%
Not interested	14.4%	16.1%	15.9%	6.4%
Not at all interested	29.6%	36.6%	44.9%	59.6%

*If female and not on Medicare.
SOURCE: Good Health Plan (Sisters of Providence Health System), Portland, Oregon.

tem covers 179 botanicals. Such findings suggest that the United States is lagging far behind other developed nations in its integration of CAM into mainstream health care.

Nonetheless, powerful forces are impelling the integration of CAM. One of the most powerful is consumer demand. Consumer interest in CAM therapies is coming to the attention of health plans at a time when consumer influence in plans' decision-making is increasing. Competition among health plans has led to a focus on the consumer, and plans that are pioneering CAM integration are doing so partly as a way of achieving visibility in the marketplace. Once a major health plan has set up a CAM program, others in the same geographic area feel it increasingly necessary to also offer CAM services. Patients are now considered "members" of HMOs, and industry standards require that health plans guarantee their members certain rights, including involvement in some decision-making processes.

Besides interest in consumer desires, commercial health plans are also embracing CAM because of scientific evidence of improved health outcomes from well-designed clinical trials.

In addition, the private business sector appears to be increasingly interested in CAM because of the results CAM produces. For the employer, medical care costs include not only the cost of the medical intervention itself, but also lost time and decreased total productivity. These considerations have a direct impact on the employer's bottom line. In 1996, according to a survey conducted by Business and Health, only 7 percent of employers were offering coverage of CAM therapies. However, by late 1997, a new survey by the same magazine found that 16 percent offered alternative medicine. For employers with more than five hundred employees, offerings jumped from 8 percent to an astounding 24 percent.

Another factor promoting CAM integration is that conventional medical practitioners do not appear to be opposed to incorporating CAM therapies into the conventional health care system. In a 1997 survey by Medalia of primary care providers in the Seattle area, 70 percent felt CAM integration would produce greater patient satisfaction, 39 percent felt it would yield more effective care, and 30 percent said it would result in more cost-effective care.

A 1998 comprehensive international literature search at the Stanford University School of Medicine, led by USC medical student Ms. Ariane Marie, found that 18 percent of physicians practice some form of CAM, 62 percent of physicians refer for CAM in general, and 57 percent believe in the efficacy of CAM. Among the most accepted types of CAM were diet, exercise, counseling, biofeedback, acupuncture, herbal medicine, and chiropractic. Too often, however, CAM proponents categorically accepted virtually all CAM interventions, while CAM opponents vehemently objected to virtually all CAM interventions. Neither position, it would seem, is objectively logical.

Other forces influencing the integration of CAM are influential private organizations and government agencies. Entities that have efforts under way to consider CAM therapies include the National Blue Cross Blue Shield Association beginning in 1996, Columbia HCA (in 1997), the American Public Health Association (in 1995), the American Association of Medical Colleges (in 1997), Kaiser Health Care (in 1997), the U.S. Bureau of Primary Health Care/Bureau of Health Professions (also in 1997), as well as other national private and governmental bodies. Coverage of CAM is becoming more frequent and decisions by such august organizations will continue to have a profound impact.

Additionally, various legislative mandates are stimulating the inclusion of CAM into the conventional health care system. At the national level, Senator Tom Harkin, Senator Orrin Hatch, and former senator Claiborne Pell have strongly supported the NCCAM with its research focus. Many states are mandating coverage of CAM. Forty-one states have mandates for provision of chiropractic services, eight for acupuncture, and three for naturopathic services as of 1997.

According to a study my colleagues and I conducted in 1997, these state mandates are as summarized below:

Because of the fluidity, complexity, and rapid growth of CAM integra-

State-Mandated Reimbursement for Alternative Providers

Providers	Number of States
Acupuncturists	8
Chiropractors	41
Dietitians	3
Massage therapists	1
Midwives	15
Naturopaths	3
Osteopaths	17
Physical therapists	10
Podiatrists	35

tion, no definitive list is available of insurers, HMOs, and hospitals that are offering or covering CAM. However, our research team at Stanford conducted a survey of hospitals with CAM centers, and of insurance and managed care companies that had or were developing policies to cover CAM. From this research, completed in 1998, we learned that several hospitals are collaborating with centers that offer CAM, or have a clinic that provides CAM within the hospital. Of the fourteen hospitals identified that have CAM programs, the most common types of CAM therapies offered were chiropractic, acupuncture, massage, and guided imagery at seven hospitals; tai chi offered at six hospitals; with other more unconventional therapies from Bach flower remedies to Feldenkreis movement exercises.

The table on pages 282–83 lists a number of the leading hospital CAM centers and describes the types of CAM offered. Few, if any, of these services are covered by insurance. For virtually all providers, the individual patient must pay out of pocket for these CAM services.

Following our 1997 CAM study, my colleagues Dr. John A. Astin, Dr. William L. Haskell, and I completed the second year of this three-year study in early 1999. During 1998, there were ten new managed care and insurance carriers that initiated CAM coverage. Survey results were analyzed for these ten new providers as well as the results of a cohort of eight insurers surveyed in both 1997 and 1998 to determine current trends. A majority of the insurers interviewed offer some coverage for the following: nutrition counseling, biofeedback, psychotherapy, acupuncture, preventive medicine, chiropractic, osteopathy, and physical therapy. All of the new managed care organizations and insurers said that market demand was their primary motivation for covering CAM. Factors determining whether insurers would offer coverage for additional therapies included potential cost-effectiveness, consumer interest, demonstrable clinical efficacy, and state mandates.

Among the most common obstacles listed to incorporating CAM into mainstream health care were lack of research on efficacy, economics, ignorance about CAM, provider competition and division, and lack of standards of practice. From our ongoing study, it is evident that consumer demand for CAM is motivating more managed care organizations and insurance companies to assess the benefits of incorporating CAM. Outcomes studies for both conventional and CAM therapies are needed to help create a health care system based upon treatments that work, whether they are conventional, complementary, or alternative.

HMOs appear to be increasingly integrating CAM into the therapies they cover. A 1995 survey reported by Goodwin of large national HMOs, undertaken by Decision Resources, a health consulting firm, found that 86 percent of HMOs covered chiropractic, 69 percent covered weight loss programs, 31 percent acupuncture, 28 percent relaxation therapy, 17 percent mental imagery therapy, and 14 percent massage therapy and hypnosis. However, the survey also found that some 46 percent of HMOs actively discouraged patients from using one or more alternative therapies.

In 1996, California-based Landmark Health Care conducted a survey of HMOs in states where there is substantial HMO presence. Marketing and medical directors at 70 percent of 156 HMOs reported an increasing request for alternative medicine, and 58 percent said they planned to increase their CAM offerings within two years. Acupuncture, chiropractic, and massage therapy were the top three therapies of interest to HMO plan members.

Through a literature review and information search, as well as telephone interviews with a definitive sample of eighteen insurers, our research team at Stanford ascertained in 1997 that a majority of the insurers interviewed offered some coverage for nutrition counseling, biofeedback, psychotherapy, acupuncture, preventive medicine, chiropractic, osteopathy, and/or physical therapy. Only a minority offered extensive coverage of CAM, with 22 percent offering sixteen to twenty therapies, 39 percent offering eleven to fifteen therapies, and 39 percent offering six to ten therapies. Smaller companies offered a greater number of CAM therapies than did larger ones.

Hospitals Associated with Centers for CAM

Name of Hospitals & Center	CAM Offered			
Stanford University Hospital UCSF/Stanford Health System Complementary Medicine Clinic	Acupuncture Biofeedback Comprehensive Evaluation and Complementary Medicine Counseling	Counseling for patients with serious illnesses: Cancer, Heart Disease, and AIDS	"Heart Health" classes and interventions Hypnosis Mindfulness Meditation	Therapeutic Cancer Support Groups Therapeutic massage Yoga
Columbia/HCA Grant Hospital & American Center, Chicago	Alexander Technique Ayurveda Bach Flower Counseling Biofeedback Body Centered Therapy Chiropractic	Conventional Therapy Educational Therapy Guided Imagery/ Visualization Homeopathy Hypnotherapy Massage/Shiatsu	Meditation/ Relaxation Midwifery/Doula Services Naprapathy, Naturopathy Nutrition Counseling Oriental Medicine	Psychoneuroimmunology Psychotherapy Reflexology Reiki, Skin Care Tai Chi Chuan Wellness Counseling Yoga
Ancilla Systems & Healing Art Center in Mishawaka, IN	Acupuncture Aromatherapy Art Therapy Ayurveda Biofeedback Energy Work, Flower Essence	Healing Touch Herbal Therapy Homeopathy Lymphedema Treatment Massage/Shiatsu	Meditation/ Visualization Mental Health Counseling Nutrition Conseling Reflexology Reiki	Spiritual/Conseling Stress Reduction Program Tai Chi Chuan Yoga
Franciscan Hospital Mount Airy & Franciscan Holistic Health Center in Cincinnati, OH	Acupuncture Aromatherapy Alexander Technique Art Therapy Biofeedback	Craniosacral Therapy Feldenkrais Method Guided Imagery Healing Touch Massage	Meditation Reflexology Self-Hypnosis Spiritual Counseling Tai Chi Chuan	Yoga Zero Balancing
Mercy Healthcare Arizona of Catholic Healthcare West & Arizona Center for Health and Medicine (closed in 1999)	Acupuncture Aromatherapy Biofield Healing Feldenkrais Method	Guided Imagery Herbal Therapy Homeopathy MindBody Medicine	Massage Nutritional Counseling Craniosacral Therapy	Spiritual Counseling Tai Chi Chuan Tragerwork Yoga
St. Vincent Hospital & Center for Complementary Medicine and Pain Management in Indianapolis, IN	Acupuncture Art Therapy Biofeedback Craniosacral Therapy	Energy Work Guided Imagery Herbal Imagery Hypnotherapy	Massage Meditation Nutritional Counseling	Mental Health Counseling Relaxation Methods Support Groups

Name of Hospitals & Center	CAM Offered			
University of Miami Hospital and Clinics & The Courtelis Center, Sylvester Comprehensive Cancer Center	Acupuncture Biofeedback Guided Imagery	Massage Meditation Mental Health Counseling	Nutrition Counseling Spiritual Counseling Physical Therapy	Self-Hypnosis Support Groups
California Pacific Medical Center & Institute for Health and Healing, San Francisco	Art/Movement Therapy Guided Imagery	Living Stories Project Psychoneuroim- munology	Stress Reduction Programs Support Groups	Tai Chi Chuan/ Qi Gong Yoga
St. Luke's Hospital in Cedar Rapids, IA, & Center for Health and Well-Being	Healing Touch Holistic Nurse Consultation	Massage Meditation	Reflexology Support Groups	Tai Chi Chuan Yoga
North Hawaii Community Hospital	Acupuncture Chiropractic	Healing/Therapeutic Touch	Massage Mental Health Counseling	Naturopathy
Deaconess Hospital & Division of Behavioral Medicine at Harvard in MA	Cognitive Therapy Exercise	Meditation Nutrition Counseling	Relaxation Methods Yoga	
Kaiser in Vallejo, CA, & Vallejo Alternative Medicine Clinic	Acupuncture	Acupressure	Meditation/ Relaxation	Support Groups
Imperial Point Medical Center & Center for Healing Arts in Fort Lauderdale, FL	Biofeedback	Guided Imagery/ Visualization	Relaxation Methods	Support Groups
Community Health Center of King County & Bastyr University in Seattle, WA	Acupuncture	Naturopathy	Nutrition Counseling	
Mercy Hospital & Medical Center and Wellspace Program in Chicago, IL	Feldenkrais Method	Meditation/ Visualization	Zero Balancing	

Coverage Reported by Insurers to Any Extent on Any Policy (number of insurers = 18)

Complementary Medical Practices	Number of Insurers
DIET, NUTRITION, AND LIFESTYLE CHANGES:	
Herbal Medicine	4
Nutrition Counseling	12
Ornish Program	6
MINDBODY CONTROL:	
Aromatherapy	0
Art Therapy	0
Biofeedback	16
Guided Imagery	5
Hypnotherapy	10
Martial Arts	0
Meditation	4
Psychotherapy	17
Qi Gong/Chi Kung	1
Support Groups	4
Yoga Therapy	2
ALTERNATIVE SYSTEMS:	
Acupuncture	17
Ayurveda	3
Homeopathy	8
Naturopathy	7
Tibetan Medicine	1
Chinese Medicine	4
Preventive Medicine	15
MANUAL HEALING:	
Acupressure	9
Alexander Technique	1
Chiropractic	18
Craniosacral	2
Massage Therapy	11
Naprapathy	1
Osteopathy	18
Physical Therapy	18
Reflexology	2
Reiki	1
Rolfing	2
Shiatsu	4
Tragerwork	2

As CAM integration accelerates, however, CAM is increasingly having to meet the standards applied to conventional medicine. One of these standards is credentialization. Accreditation standards for health plans place great emphasis on credentialing of health care providers. Through the credentialing process, the health plan assures its members that all its providers will meet certain minimum standards, which generally include licensing, education, and proof of malpractice insurance.

In light of credentialing requirements, the CAM practitioners who are the easiest for health plans to work with are those who belong to distinct, regulated, licensed professions. The next table summarizes the number of states that consider various therapists to be "licensed practitioners," according to the Stanford survey in 1997.

Licensing is based on educational criteria and usually requires passing an examination.

Several CAM professions are also now being covered by malpractice insurers, including licensed acupuncturists, naturopaths, massage practitioners, and licensed, direct-entry (non-nurse) midwives.

Other CAM therapies are more difficult to credential, such as yoga practitioners, body workers, or indigenous healers, who are not regulated

Therapies or Systems Designated as Having "Licensed Practitioners" by Number of States

CAM Therapy or System	Number of States
Acupuncture	33
Ayurvedic Medicine	0
Biofeedback	0
Chiropractic Medicine	50
Craniosacral Therapy	0
Herbal Medicine	0
Homeopathic Medicine	3
Massage Therapy	23
Midwifery	15
Naturopathic Medicine	11
Nutritionists or Dietitians	26
Osteopathy	50
Physical Therapy	50
Tibetan Medicine	0
Traditional Chinese Medicine	1

by states. Some plans require that practitioners in these areas be licensed in a conventional health profession, such as nursing, mental health counseling, or physical therapy.

One model that is used by health plans to provide alternative treatment is to offer CAM services through an external network of practitioners, which assumes the risk of providing the services. Networks have been widely used by health plans in the delivery of chiropractic services.

FORMS OF COVERAGE

CAM is currently covered by health plans in a variety of ways. Following are some of the various approaches to CAM coverage.

- *Comprehensive Plans.* Some insurers have developed major medical plans that specifically include coverage of CAM. These plans often cover visits to a variety of practitioners, including chiropractors, naturopaths, and acupuncturists.
- *Discounted CAM Services Through Credentialed Networks.* Some plans and purchasers have chosen to offer CAM services that do not put them at any risk, by developing programs for services that are not included in the benefits plan, and then offering them to their members at a discount of about 10 to 30 percent. There is a precedent for this approach in conventional care, where discount programs have been developed for such services as eye care or cosmetic surgery.
- *CAM Rider.* An even more popular method is to offer CAM services through a benefit rider. Chiropractic is the most commonly offered benefit, followed by acupuncture, naturopathy, and massage. Riders often allow direct access by the patient to the CAM service, without physician referral. An additional fee is charged for the rider. For example, a rider for chiropractic may run three to five dollars per member per month, depending on the benefit. Some riders require a higher-than-usual copayment by the member, often up to 50 percent.
- *Other Limited Benefit Forms.* In some health plans, coverage of CAM therapies is restricted to specific programs, such as the Ornish program for heart disease patients, which consists of a low-fat vegetarian diet, exercise, stress management, and group support. By

1990, Dr. Dean Ornish and his associates had demonstrated that patients following this program were able to control and even reverse atherosclerotic disease. Armed with their findings, the program's developers approached insurers, asking them to fund a national demonstration network of hospital-based sites. Mutual of Omaha committed up to $10,000 per patient to the program, far less than they would have paid for conventional care. At present, the Ornish program is offered in a small number of franchised centers nationwide. Such models have inspired other organizations to develop cost-effective CAM treatment programs for specific conditions.

However, despite the splashy press coverage of health plans that cover CAM, actual access to CAM coverage is currently quite limited. In addition, a majority of insurers do not offer CAM coverage for health promotion, disease prevention, or wellness enhancement. Instead, CAM is generally covered only if the treatment is deemed medically necessary for a specific diagnosis, and treatment is reimbursed only for a limited number of visits, and/or a dollar limit.

Medical necessity is also an important concept in controlling overutilization of services in any CAM policy, as it is in a policy covering conventional medicine. Thus, the criterion of medical necessity positions CAM therapies squarely in the context of conventional health care.

If CAM becomes better integrated into the health care system, it may lead to more cost-effective treatment in some areas. Comparative studies between conventional and CAM interventions for specific conditions need to be conducted with both clinical and cost outcomes. Advocates believe that the CAM approach can help the entire health care system move toward a focus on health maintenance and prevention, in the true spirit of reform.

REPRESENTATIVE
CAM PLANS AND EXPERIENCES

Insurance companies providing CAM coverage offer different arrays of CAM treatments, and have different reimbursement schedules. No centralized information is as yet available to the public for comparing various CAM plans.

Following, however, is a sampling of options available at the time of writing. This sample will indicate the variety of options.

Oxford Health Plan. In October 1996, Connecticut-based Oxford Health Plan attracted wide media interest with its historic announcement that it would be offering an alternative medicine benefit, the first of such magnitude to be offered by an HMO outside of a state mandate.

Oxford is a highly successful HMO with some two million members in the New York, New Jersey, and Connecticut markets. However, in early 1998, independently of its CAM offerings, Oxford underwent severe financial setbacks, and it remains uncertain how viable the company will be in the future of conventional or CAM coverage.

In market research before the initiation of the plan, a poll of large employers showed that 85 percent were interested in the CAM product. However, during the first eight months of 1997, only some forty thousand, or 2 percent, of Oxford's members had access to covered CAM services.

Oxford has created its own network of CAM providers, including chiropractors, acupuncturists, massage therapists, registered dietitians, clinical nutritionists, yoga instructors, and naturopathic doctors. CAM credentialing standards include N.D. or D.C. degrees, and state licensure for acupuncturists, as well as malpractice insurance. Providers in each field of practice must follow established standards-of-care guidelines, and have a minimum of two years of clinical experience, as well as continuing education courses. Quality assurance is monitored by member satisfaction surveys and routine checks of providers' treatment plans, visit patterns, and outcomes.

Commercial groups in New York, New Jersey, and Connecticut can purchase an additional alternative medicine rider from Oxford as an insured benefit. Patients have direct access to chiropractors, naturopaths in Connecticut, and acupuncturists, with no referral required from primary care providers. Members pay a copayment for chiropractic, acupuncture, and, in Connecticut, naturopathic services. Copayments are $10 or $15, depending on the plan, with maximums set at $2,000, $3,000, or $5,000.

Oxford Lifestyle Heart Program is also part of the CAM offerings. This is a natural treatment program for reversing coronary artery disease.

American Western Life. Although this company is no longer conducting business, it is of historical significance. American Western Life Insurance (AWLI) was a pioneer in the CAM insurance field. Its near-legendary Premier Wellness Plan, offered in six western states, was an integrated plan that offered both orthodox and alternative providers, and had over five thousand subscribers, a small percentage of AWLI's total business.

Members of the plan had a primary care physician, who could be any licensed professional. Credentialing required that they hold a certificate or license in good standing, and be graduates of an accredited school, with specific requirements depending on the modality of treatment.

Members under the Premier Wellness Plan were allowed one preventive visit per year. Other treatments, covered by the plan and considered medically necessary, were covered at 100 percent of negotiated fees, after a $20 member copayment. There was no limit on the number of treatments per year, or on the maximum monetary benefits per year for treatments that were deemed medically necessary. Exceptions to these unlimited benefits included outpatient prescriptions, which were covered 80 percent, up to a maximum of $30 per medicine, and natural medicinals, for which there was a $10 copayment per prescription, up to a maximum of $2,000 a year. There was a nutrition counseling maximum of two visits per year and $75 a year, and mental health benefits included six visits a year at $50 per visit copayment. Chelation therapy was covered at thirty visits per year and $50 per visit.

Coverage caps on prescriptions were instituted by AWLI after its experience with an earlier CAM plan, the Prevention Plus Plan, which had to be discontinued because of abuse of benefits. A majority of members were "maxing out" on the massage benefits, using their entire six massage visits a year. Providers were also reclassifying treatments under different benefits in order to provide additional services. For example, acupuncturists might be billing massage as acupressure, in order to increase the number of massage treatments that the patient could receive.

In addition to chiropractic, acupuncture seems to be the CAM therapy that has been most accepted by conventional health plans. Therefore, we will examine several plans that cover acupuncture in California.

Lifeguard Health Care. This Silicon Valley HMO announced in April 1997 that it would become the first California plan to offer acupuncture to its members.

Lifeguard's chief executive, Mark Hyde, said that the company decided to offer acupuncture partly because of demands from employers. Lifeguard had been providing a chiropractic option since 1993, for which some 86,000 of its 212,000 members had been paying slightly higher premiums. Lifeguard's acupuncture benefit was made available in the summer of 1997 to members who had already chosen the optional chiropractic package.

Blue Shield. Blue Shield of California is offering its Lifepath program, through which all of its 1.6 million members will be allowed a discount on a variety of CAM services. Under the Lifepath plan, members have access to a wide range of alternative services, including acupuncture, chiropractic, massage therapy, somatic education (movement awareness such as Alexander Technique or Feldenkrais), stress management programs using guided imagery, and fitness center, athletic club, and health spa facilities. Members are responsible for the entire cost of the service, paying the practitioner's advertised fees minus the discount, generally 25 percent.

For group purchasers, Blue Shield is also offering the option of paying an additional fee for an acupuncture rider benefit, through which employees will have access to acupuncture with a copayment of $10 to $15.

Health Net (Foundation Health Systems). Health Net of California is the second-largest California HMO, with over 2.5 million members, and began offering an acupuncture benefit as of January 1998. It is significant that Health Net is the largest part of the national company Foundation Health Systems (FHS), which is the fourth-largest integrated provider system in the United States. Since I am on the board of directors of Health Net, it has been a fascinating experience to see the evolution and integration of CAM from the perspective of a major health plan.

Health Net was one of the first HMOs to offer direct access to chiropractic care, beginning in 1990. Its chiropractic rider is offered to more than 600,000 of its 2.2 million members. Under the Health Net plan, the acupuncture benefit is also offered as a rider.

Health Net's acupuncture rider allows members direct access to an acupuncturist, who may also provide massage therapy and herbal remedies. A limited formulary of seventy herbals can be prescribed. Health Net's president at the time this CAM coverage was introduced, Dr. Arthur Southam, has emphasized the value of certain CAM therapies in treating intractable pain, and musculoskeletal problems.

Taking an even more innovative approach is the "WellRewards" program of Health Net, initiated in 1998. This program rewards healthy members by giving them discounts on vitamins, herbs, health club memberships, books and tapes, home fitness equipment, sporting goods, self-care medical supplies, and even veterinary services and pet care supplies. Modeled after airline mileage award programs, WellRewards is a major innovation for a health care system. WellRewards was begun in part to discourage healthy members from dropping out of the plan. The turnover rate for most plans tends to be as high as 20 to 30 percent annually, because of dissatisfaction and other factors. The WellRewards program, however, was designed to motivate loyalty among healthy members, who are the plan's most financially rewarding customers.

Kaiser. Kaiser Permanente, California's largest HMO, with 4.5 million members, was another early entry in announcing acupuncture benefits. However, Kaiser's acupuncture program is essentially limited to just a few sites.

Unlike Blue Shield and Health Net, Kaiser is offering acupuncture in-house, with the express intent of ascertaining whether this CAM therapy should be part of the HMO's standard of care in treating patients with chronic pain.

Acupuncture providers have been introduced into the Kaiser system by a number of strategies. One approach is to retrain conventional physicians to offer medical acupuncture. Another is to bring in licensed providers to work side by side with physicians.

Kaiser's alternative medicine clinic in Vallejo is considered a test project, combining acupuncture treatment and nutritional counseling with lessons in self-care acupressure. A similar clinic has also opened at Kaiser's Stockton facility.

In Washington, a state mandate program, which may soon influence other states, was established in 1995. A state law ruled that all plans had to include "every category of provider," such as acupuncturists, naturopaths, and the like. This controversial statute was overturned seventeen months later by a district court judge, but it stimulated significant activity among Washington insurers and health plans. Under this mandate, health plans scrambled to develop CAM programs. Following are two plan examples that were begun before the mandate was removed.

Blue Cross of Washington and Alaska. Before passage of the mandate, Blue Cross of Washington and Alaska had already begun to develop a natural medicine pilot plan, dubbed AlternaPath, covering only three types of providers: acupuncturists, naturopaths, and homeopaths. Services could include nutritional counseling, biofeedback, acupuncture, and acupressure, if delivered by these credentialed providers. Chiropractic had already been mandated. AlternaPath was not well received, and perhaps was doomed to failure from the start. The plan attracted high utilizers of both conventional and CAM services, and did not have well-designed maximum limits.

The new plan has more realistic limits. In the new plan, there is a benefit of up to $500 per year, with a 50 percent copayment required. Credentialing will require graduation from an accredited school and professional liability coverage. Coverage for health foods, vitamins, herbs, and homeopathic remedies will be discontinued or reduced under the new plan, and any herbs and vitamins that are still covered will require a medical condition necessitating such coverage.

Group Health Cooperative of Puget Sound (GHCPS). Widely respected, GHCPS, a Washington HMO, has extensive experience in offering CAM services and has demonstrated a willingness to share its process and results. Its benefit plan is not a rider, but offers CAM services to members as part of the core benefits, at no additional cost. Services covered include chiropractic, acupuncture, massage therapy, naturopathy, and home births by licensed midwives. Members are required to have referrals from their primary care providers. Approved CAM services are based on limited numbers of visits, and are approved only for certain conditions.

Early experience under this plan was reported at an American Association of Health Plans meeting in June 1997. Massage therapy presented the largest problem with utilization, and the plan has since developed a special program to help massage practitioners understand how to work in a managed care arena. Acupuncture and naturopathic services were deemed to have been helpful to at least some of the users, and the plan expected to explore an expansion of covered conditions.

Utilization of CAM services was less than had been anticipated, although it grew toward the end of the first year. It was clear, however, that the CAM program was not going to "break the bank" for Group Health.

A 1997 analysis of the Washington state mandate, published in *St. Anthony's Alternative Medicine Integration and Coverage,* noted that HMO executives generally felt that integrating CAM into HMOs proceeded with surprising success. The executives recognized a growing role for alternative medicine in managed care.

A noteworthy observation was that use of CAM services was not as high as anticipated. HMO executives expressed surprise at how low the first-year utilization had been. Reasons given for low utilization included members' lack of information, the requirement of physician referral, the existence of many conditions that were not covered, and the exclusion of a number of popular providers.

Actuaries had forecast cost increases up to 11 percent in nonmanaged care plans and 2 percent in managed care plans (which required physician referral), but actual added costs were less than 1 percent overall.

Actual Use of Alternative Medicine Providers vs. Percentage of Plan Members Indicating Interest

	Indemnity		Managed Care		% of Surveyed Members Expressing Interest	
	Policyholders Served	% of Total Policyholders	Members Served	% of Members Served	% Very Interested	% Somewhat Interested
Acupuncture	929	.31	73	.08	14	25.2
Naturopath	1,127	.37	48	.053	20.9	26.4
Massage	968	.32	89	.098	N/A	N/A
Total	3,024	1.00	210	.23	N/A	N/A

SOURCE: *Alternative Medicine Integration and Coverage,* June and July 1997

None of the Washington plans had determined whether CAM services replaced conventional services or simply added to them.

What's in the Works: Potentials and Challenges of CAM Coverage

Trends thus far generally indicate restriction of CAM services to a separate but unequal role in the health care system. For the most part, CAM therapies are not yet fully integrated into traditional health plans. Nor do the CAM treatments that are being delivered fully represent the whole-person-oriented approach of therapies such as chiropractic, naturopathy, traditional Chinese medicine, and homeopathy, which have constituted much of the essential core of CAM therapies in the uncontrolled marketplace.

Furthermore, the impact of managed care on CAM has not been entirely beneficial. Many CAM providers have expressed concern that benefits are too low, restricting the number of treatments and limiting the scope of practice of CAM practitioners. It appears as if some health plans may offer token or inadequate coverage of CAM therapies in order to attract new enrollees; however, these unwise restrictions can result in inadequate and ineffective treatment.

Furthermore, CAM providers often have little understanding of managed care and the concept of medical necessity. Some have overused laboratory tests, or overprescribed natural remedies. In general, CAM providers need to be familiarized with managed care, and need to help patients understand why certain therapies are not covered.

Rates paid to CAM providers by networks are often much lower than the rates they receive in the open market. Although participation in networks may attract new patients, CAM providers may find themselves in the position of having to cut corners.

CAM providers are also accustomed to treating patients within the context of a whole system of therapeutics, rather than through single interventions.

Incorporating CAM into the existing health care system may entail some compromises on the part of CAM therapies. Existing third-party payer insurance systems and HMOs evolved in the context of the prevailing biomedical model. Current management of health care service utilization is based on oversight of conventional diagnostic and therapeutic approaches. In 1995, Robert Padgug, director of health policies and government relations at Empire Blue Cross and Blue Shield, pointed out that the procedures and providers that are brought into the health care system will need to align themselves with the prevailing medical model if they wish to be reimbursed by third-party payers. This holds true even in other countries, where a more long-standing, open-minded attitude has prevailed toward CAM. National health insurance models of Canada, Great Britain, and Scandinavia, and the largely private mutual insurance form of coverage in Germany, France, Japan, and the Netherlands, seem to apply the same conventional medical model in managing provision of services.

Health plans that externalize CAM therapies through rider arrangements, and require referrals from primary care physicians, essentially treat CAM providers as specialists rather than as primary care practitioners. There is little opportunity in the context of managed care for CAM practitioners to provide preventive treatment.

For all these reasons, not all patients who go to CAM practitioners will rush to sign up with health plans that offer CAM coverage. Many may prefer to pay out of pocket.

In the future, to ensure the integration of CAM, several important issues must be thoroughly evaluated, including the future role of clinical research on CAM, the cost-effectiveness of CAM, the sources of funding for CAM research, malpractice liability for CAM interventions, terminology of CAM procedures, and the role of the consumer. These elements, to some extent, will determine the future of CAM integration into the current medical system, which is now dominated by managed care.

Although decisions about CAM coverage are partially based on demonstrated clinical efficacy, it is clear that some alternative therapies cannot be readily evaluated in large, randomized controlled trials. This is especially true of whole-system therapies that address each case on a highly individualized basis. As it stands at present, the gold standard of randomized, controlled clinical trials has only rarely been used to study CAM therapies. Nor is there any clear, compelling data on cost-effectiveness of CAM therapies, despite the common belief that integration of CAM therapies will help to control rising health care costs.

However, until strong evidence exists for the clinical effectiveness of CAM, cost-effectiveness cannot be meaningfully evaluated. Clinical research that demonstrates improved health outcomes from CAM therapies is thus the first order of business in the assessment of the potential for CAM integration.

Research on isolated CAM interventions does not do justice to the potential power of whole CAM systems as strategies for prevention and health maintenance, and for cost savings. This point has not been lost on the San Francisco–based Institute for Noetic Sciences, which has undertaken a values project to look at broad issues involved in health care reform. A primary concern of the researchers is that basic principles of wellness and holism not fall by the wayside as individual CAM therapies are added into the mainstream health care system.

One of the issues that plagues researchers who are attempting to study clinical and cost-effectiveness of CAM therapies is the lack of standardized insurance coding that allows CAM to be compared with conventional interventions. Often, in order to ensure coverage of a CAM treatment, practitioners misuse insurance codes so that they will qualify for payment by insurers. However, this sometimes makes it impossible to compare CAM therapies with conventional therapies. Developing codes specifically for CAM treatments would facilitate large studies on the effectiveness of specific CAM interventions.

Some preliminary steps have been taken in this area. Most significant, the American Medical Association asked the American Academy of Medical Acupuncturists to make a presentation on acupuncture coding issues in the spring of 1998. Work toward an appropriate coding for acupuncture is presently in progress. Also, the American Institute of Homeopathy (AIH) has initiated a formal process with the Health Care Financing Administration and the AMA to request new CPT codes for homeopathic treatment, although no action has been taken yet on the AIH request. A New Mexico company, Alternative Link, has developed a coding system for CAM therapies. In a 1997 pilot project, a network of CAM providers is using the new codes in providing services to employees of Highland Enterprises.

Funding for research on CAM therapies has historically been limited. Most alternative approaches are not patentable, and hence do not appeal as targets for funding to major corporations. Establishment of the NIH has been a critical step in facilitating the evaluation of CAM therapies. Appeals are also being made to private foundations, which have traditionally been reluctant to fund CAM research.

Early indications are that malpractice suits against CAM providers will be relatively rare, compared to those against conventional practitioners. Each CAM specialty has an individualized standard of care, and among some therapies, such as acupuncture, each style has its own standards. A more serious concern is for conventional physicians who are being put in the position of needing to refer their patients for CAM care. Worries about malpractice suits, unfortunately, might be the primary motivator for physicians to inquire into their patients' interest in CAM therapies. As CAM becomes more available, physicians need to consider the possibility that their patients may be taking unconventional treatments that may interact dangerously with allopathic drugs or procedures. In an important 1997 article in the *Annals of Internal Medicine,* Eisenberg strongly advises physicians against rubber-stamping referrals to alternative providers, and suggests that the referral process should be a cooperative undertaking between patient and physician.

Much of the controversy and uncertainty surrounding the integration of CAM therapies into the mainstream health care system can be summed up by an examination of the language that is used to describe these unconventional therapies. "Complementary" is a term prevalent in England, and carries the implication that unconventional therapies can coexist side by side with mainstream medicine. It seems to affirm that conventional medicine remains at the center of the health care system, and that the "other" therapies are merely additions, or complements. Another useful term advocated by Dr. Andrew Weil and the Foundation for Integrative Medicine is the designation "integrative," which denotes the evidence-based merger of conventional and alternative medicine.

For those who are paying for CAM treatments within the conventional health care system, however, the term "complementary" appears to imply an additional cost. "Alternative" sounds like a better word for those who are paying for CAM. For conventional medical providers, however, "alternative" suggests a loss of income, while the term appeals to consumers for the same reason.

Recently, Dr. Andrew Weil, founder of the Program in Integrative Medicine, has proposed the term "integrative medicine." While the term does not have much recognition among the public or the managed care industry at the present time, the concept of integration represents a step in the right direction.

An important lesson to be gained from the experience of the CAM integration movement is how important the role of the consumer can be. CAM benefits have been added to many health plans for the express purpose of attracting new consumers. Yet the question may still be raised whether delivering consumers should be the primary purpose of health plans, or whether there should not be more concern with delivering health. While many decisions as to the integration of CAM therapies have included scientific input, they have not been entirely based on scientific grounds.

This observation applies equally to allopathic therapies. Experimental procedures such as lung reduction surgery for emphysema, high-dose chemotherapy or bone marrow transplants, and many surgical procedures may not have been scientifically demonstrated to be safe and effective by the prevailing gold standard of randomized clinical trials. Coverage decisions are often driven more by consumer demand than by science.

Consumers may need to continue to exert pressure to bring CAM coverage into a more truly integrated position within the health care system. If the much-touted partnership with patients becomes a reality, integration may proceed toward fuller expression. Consumers who understand the value of integrating conventional and CAM therapies will need to make their voices heard if they want to see CAM offered not just as a side dish but as part of the main course in health care.

CHAPTER 13

WE'RE NOT IN KANSAS ANYMORE

Toward an Integrative Medicine

Entering the domain of complementary and alternative medicine is perhaps evocative of Dorothy's exclamation in *The Wizard of Oz:* "We're not in Kansas anymore!" Today, the world of CAM is a strange and exciting place, in which popular presumptions are sorely tested and eternal truths sometimes emerge. For many of us, CAM just is not what we're used to experiencing. Given its exotic nature, it is small wonder that people respond to CAM with both uncritical acceptance and total condemnation.

My focus throughout this book is on CAM practices that are currently used in the greatest frequency and have a reasonable basis in rigorous human clinical trials. As a result of these limiting criteria, this portrait of CAM is intentionally representative, not exhaustive or definitive. Many CAM areas such as chelation, cell infusion therapies, use of magnets, and many, many other of the over six hundred specific CAM practices cited by the NIH National Center for Complementary and Alternative Medicine have not been considered at all. However, as new evidence and data accumulate in the areas covered in the previous chapters and in these areas, they will be incorporated into future updated editions of this book.

Undoubtedly, many areas of CAM will remain controversial, but inexorably, unfounded opinions at both extremes will yield to scientific evaluation. Surely a common ground will emerge. When all is said and done, what works will no longer be polarized into conventional versus alternative, it will just be called good medicine. In the universal quest to end illness and suffering, there can be neither conventional nor alternative therapies, but only those therapies which are proven by the rigorous standards of science.

In addition, it is essential to bear in mind that a great deal of both conventional and CAM practices have little or no scientific underpinnings. Lacking an adequate scientific basis does not mean an intervention does not work, it simply means it is neither proven nor unproven. CAM effectiveness is real, and can be of help in many acute and chronic illnesses. There are limits and dangers to both CAM and conventional care which can be minimized when both approaches are harmoniously balanced and used appropriately. Most important, CAM practices may hold their greatest promise in the prevention of illness, facilitation of lifestyle change, and attainment of optimal health. However, concluding this foray into CAM is an occasion to reflect on several major themes, and to look toward the future.

Most important, let me again reiterate the prime directive throughout this book: "Think horses, not zebras!" Pay attention to the known, the documented, and the obvious before seeking the unproven, esoteric, questionable, and even dangerous. Be sure that well-researched conventional medicine does not already offer an effective, safe treatment before embarking on a search for an unresearched nonconventional course of treatment. By the same token, people should be equally sure that their illnesses cannot be overcome by simple modifications of lifestyle, such as eating better or managing stress, before engaging in potentially difficult courses of conventional medicine. Whether conventional or unconventional, medicine should be as safe, as effective, as mild, and as evidence-based as possible.

Conventional medicine is also undergoing a profound transformation in the basic research, clinical, and financial domains. Although the focus in this book has been on CAM, it is important to underscore such innovations in conventional medicine as the first large animal cloning of the sheep "Dolly" in Edinburgh during early 1997, which engendered so many scientific and ethical controversies with regard to human cloning. Therapeutic cocktails of protease inhibitors are now available that reduce HIV virus to near zero and in some cases actually arrest AIDS. Reductions in stroke damage by as much as 30 percent are now common practice through the administration of clot-busting recombinant drugs such as t-PA within three hours of a stroke. Promising true breakthroughs have come from researchers at Sweden's Karolinska Institute in using peripheral nerve grafts to restore limited movement in mice with severed spinal cords.

Clear evidence exists that intensive, lifestyle-based heart disease interventions do reduce the development and recurrence of cardiovascular complications as well as induce actual regression. Evidence has been discovered of a specific mutated gene, a beta-amyloid precursor, that induces Alzheimer's disease in laboratory animals and offers new insights into a potential intervention for this dreaded and increasingly common disease. Such a list could be extended virtually indefinitely, but is simply cited here to emphasize that conventional medicine is undergoing profound transformation. Great strides are being made in a vast array of areas. Conventional medicine is not an adversary, but an invaluable ally in combining conventional and CAM practices into a true health care system.

However, knowing which path to take may be challenging, particularly because so many of the CAM interventions have not yet been definitively proven by randomized, double-blind, human clinical trials. Randomized clinical trials, or RCTs, remain the gold standard for research, and all conventional and CAM interventions must eventually be evaluated by this standard. It is a profound misunderstanding of the scientific method to assert that CAM therapies are inherently incompatible with such an approach. Surely, CAM will demand an extension of current scientific methods to address subtle energies. Does "liver-heart-fire" in Chinese medicine equate to hypertension in conventional care? Many, many such issues remain unexplored. Before addressing the esoteric, it is essential to apply known methods of inquiry as extensively as possible. For both the clinician and researchers, "think horses, not zebras" is an appropriate admonition as well. Even so, we must not lose sight of the fact that because an intervention has not yet been proven in RCTs does not mean that it does not work. It simply means that it remains to be proven or disproven.

In considering the future of a true health care system, let us recall the perennial sagacity and irreverence of Mark Twain. Throughout his life, Twain maintained a skeptical view of both conventional and naturalistic medicine, perhaps because of his sickly childhood. His mother experimented upon him indiscriminately with patent medicines, faith healing, and other fashionable treatments. Twain wrote, "I can remember well when the cold water cure was first talked about. My mother used to stand me up naked in the back yard every morning and throw buckets of cold water on me, just to see what effect it would have. Personally, I had no curiosity upon the subject." However, Twain also spoke out passionately against the ongoing trend toward the enforced homogeneity of medicine, and always defended the right to medical freedom of choice. Like Twain, we must all hold both conventional medicine and alternative medicine to equally high standards of evidence, efficacy, rationality, and humanity.

There is nothing inherently more humanistic about CAM therapies than conventional medicine. CAM interventions are all too often practiced in the mechanistic, uncaring, reductionistic, and myopic manner that typically characterizes conventional medicine. In fact, there are thousands of superbly compassionate, humanistic allopathic doctors, just as there are thousands of caring CAM practitioners. In either case, these clinicians obtain significant, positive results with patients despite the lack of scientific verification. This is the "art" in the art and science of medicine.

It is not a clinician's philosophy of medicine that determines his or her level of compassion, nor commitment to the struggle against suffering. Similarly, a clinician's philosophy of medicine does not determine his or her level of skill as a practitioner. It is training, intelligence, and objectivity that determine excellence. To provide the best possible care, practitioners of both CAM and conventional medicine must address each patient compassionately and intelligently, with an understanding of that patient's entire condition. This condition includes symptoms and a diagnosis. But it may also include the lifestyle, spiritual, and emotional elements that comprise not just the case history, but the human being. Without recognizing the full dimension of the human being, both CAM and conventional care alike degenerate into reductionism, fragmentation, and a magic bullet orientation—whether the magic bullet is laser surgery or a Tibetan herbal formula.

SUCCESSFUL AGING AND CAM

Use of CAM therapies will be inexorably increased by the graying of planet Earth. Older adults use more CAM therapeutics at present, and that utilization will increase as the baby boomers enter middle age and beyond, continuing their 1960s legacy of independence, emphasis upon healthy lifestyles, and seeking beyond the conventional to enhance both the quality and quantity of their next fifty years. To work toward optimum health in life's later years, it is necessary for every individual to see himself or herself as actively involved in a lifelong journey. Managing our lifestyles and incorporating effective CAM practices is clearly one of the most effective means we have to improve health, successful aging, and longevity.

Nearly two thousand years ago, Virgil lamented in *Ecologue IX* that "Time bears away all things, even our minds." Despite the advances of medicine, remarkably little has changed since Virgil. More individuals attain the *average* life expectancy now than in the first century B.C., but the *maximum* life expectancy has not increased significantly since Virgil's era. Isocrates, the Athenian orator of 436–338 B.C., apparently lived to be ninety-eight. Philosopher and mathematician Pythagoras is believed to have lived to eighty (580–500 B.C.). In fact the apparent increase in average life expectency in the United States is due to reductions in infant mortality. If infant mortality is factored out, the average life expentancy has increased only 3.7 years since 1900! It also appears that the historical maximum life expectancy of 115 years remains approximately the same today.

In 1997, Jeanne Calment, the longest-living person for whom authenticated records existed, died after a brief illness in Paris at age 122. Such instances are an indication of a biological potential inherent in the human species as a whole. For more people to achieve this remarkable feat of healthy old age, we must remain ever aware of the lifestyle and the conventional and CAM influences that affect the health of people who evidence successful aging in each decade of life.

Recent basic genetic research has indicated that it may be possible to extend the absolute maximum lifespan, as well as the quality of those years. For now, a more modest but surely achievable goal is to extend the relatively healthy plateau of middle age into an individual's seventies or eighties.

Every major disease is age-dependent. It is evident that the progressive degeneration of aging, coupled with the development of increasingly severe, acute chronic disorders, places increased strain upon the organism, thus accelerating the overall degenerative process. It was the pioneering physician Sir William Osler who termed pneumonia "the old man's friend," referring to the final illness which brings a peaceful end to the weakening process of age. However, within a decade, breakthroughs in the human genome, conventional medicine, lifestyle change, and CAM will extend the boundaries of both the quality and quantity of human life and promote "successful aging" for future generations.

IT'S LIFESTYLE . . . LIFESTYLE . . . LIFESTYLE

More than ever, our culture has begun to recognize that general health, quality, and length of life may depend more on psychosocial and environmental factors than on the quality of the medical care system.

Successful aging involves an inextricable interaction between biochemical, psychosocial, socioeconomic, environmental, spiritual, and public policy influences. In the classic 1987 article "Human Aging: Usual and Successful" published in Science, Dr. John W. Rowe and Dr. Robert L. Kahn showed that biological aging was highly "plastic," and could be accelerated, slowed, and even reversed, predominantly by behavioral and psychosocial influences. With this seminal article, Rowe exhorted people not to confuse average aging with normal aging. It may be quite normal, he asserted, for people to be healthy and active in their eighties and nineties, even though the average person is not.

As the percentage of elderly people in the population continues to rise, and as life expectancy is extended, it will become increasingly important to manage the known lifestyle risks that lead to an institutionalized, incapacitated old age. It is clearly possible to make lifestyle changes that will extend life and prevent illness. This orientation is modern, but not new. Thousands of years ago, in The Yellow Emperor, Huang Ti stated, "Hence the sages did not treat those who were already ill; they instructed those who were not yet ill. . . ." Surely this perennial wisdom may be reinstated in the era of managed care.

Despite the sophistication of genetic, biochemical, and neuroendocrine research, it is becoming increasingly accepted that the single most accurate predictor of longevity is lifestyle. Many lifestyle factors determine longevity, but one particularly important predictor of longevity is work satisfaction. From a thirteen-year longitudinal study, Dr. Erdman Palmore has concluded that work satisfaction is the single best predictor of longevity among men aged sixty to sixty-nine.

Among other research findings relating lifestyle to longevity are that married couples tend to live longer than average, and that spiritually oriented people tend to be healthier than average. In fact, there is evidence of a "longevity syndrome," exemplified by characteristics such as feelings of well-being, high levels of physical and mental activity, creativity, and general enjoyment of life. Productivity, psychological adjustment, and overall life satisfaction are essential factors in increasing life expectancy. Shortsighted approaches to health care often exclude these lifestyle influences while overemphasizing the treatment of existing diseases.

"Why Can't a Woman Be More Like a Man?"

Actually, the hit 1950s song from *My Fair Lady* had it backwards. Closely related to the interaction between lifestyle and longevity is the fact that in virtually all modern societies, women tend to live longer than men. Prior to the early 1900s, the ratio of 106 male births to 100 female births compensated for the future toll of wars and occupational hazards on the male population. Currently, women actually do outnumber men on the planet.

Women use CAM therapies more than men. Historically, they have also adopted more positive lifestyles than men. Also, women are most often the decision-makers regarding what their spouse and families will access for their health care. Given this inordinate influence of women, it is vital to briefly consider the interaction between women's healthy lifestyles, CAM, and their continuing influence upon the future of integrative health care.

In a series of articles entitled "Why Do Women Live Longer than Men?," Dr. Ingrid Waldron of the University of Pennsylvania conducted an extensive inquiry into the possible biological basis for such a widespread difference. These articles contain an in-depth analysis of the role of influences such as greater male susceptibility to disease due to X-chromosome-linked recessive mutations; the role of female hormones such as estrogen, which does tend to prevent atherosclerosis in premenopausal women; effects of oral contraceptives; as well as cross-cultural studies of this mortality differential. From this extensive review, only the cross-cultural differentiation proved to be of significance. Higher male mortality is the norm in all of the ten modern postindustrial nations.

Genetic and hormonal factors are partially responsible for this male-to-female differential. However, the conclusions of Waldron's studies unequivocally underscore lifestyle as the major influence. Lifestyle factors emerge as the major determinants for each of the premature causes of death among males. These causes of death with clear behavioral components are responsible for one-third of the excess male mortality, and heart disease is responsible for an additional 40 percent of the excess deaths among males. Men may have higher death rates for heart disease in large part because they develop aggressive, competitive, coronary-prone behavior. Most significant, one-third of the sex differential in mortality is due to men's higher rates of suicide, fatal motor vehicle and other accidents, cirrhosis of the liver, respiratory cancers, and emphysema. Each of these causes of death is linked to lifestyles that are encouraged or accepted more in males than in females. Thus the self-destructive, macho behaviors expected of males in our society make a major contribution to their elevated mortality. What is evident in this and other research is not that women necessarily outlive men but rather that men do a better job of killing themselves prematurely.

At the UCLA School of Medicine, Dr. Charles E. Lewis and Mary Lewis have speculated on the potential impact of sexual equality on both male and female health. These researchers acknowledge that the major differences are related more to male and female behaviors and roles in society than to their genetics. As sex roles change, will those health-related behaviors that seem highly linked to sex also change? Will women gain equity in death rates for most diseases, as they already have for lung cancer due to increased smoking, especially among adolescent girls? Certainly, women will accumulate greater risks as they drive or fly greater distances and are subject to the stresses related to occupational responsibilities. Unfortunately, there is increasing evidence that women working in formerly male-dominated professions do begin to assume comparable risks with a resulting equalization of morbidity and mortality with men. Surely this is not the desirable outcome of equality for women or men.

Despite these dire trends, women have exerted and will continue to exert an increasingly dominant and positive influence upon themselves, their families, and the future of the integration of conventional and CAM therapies. Surely this is a true mirror image of Henry Higgins's chauvinistic admonition.

CAM and Lifestyle: An International Perspective

In a final foray into the area of "what works," it is instructive to note the factors that contribute to health in the most healthy cultures internationally. One of the most healthy modern cultures is that of Swedish nationals. Sweden is the country with the highest life expectancy in the world since the early 1960s.

From his research on Sweden, Dr. Richard F. Tomasson of the University of New Mexico suggests seven factors that would account for this: (1) Sweden's system of compulsory national health insurance; (2) the relative elevation of Sweden's lower socioeconomic class; (3) its highly structured and "tight" social order; (4) its extremely low infant mortality rate; (5) its low rates of violence; (6) its relatively low use of cigarettes and alcohol; and (7) its relatively low consumption of meat and sugar, and its high consumption of fish. Those factors all indicate the tremendous importance that lifestyle plays in achieving health and longevity.

Similarly, in America, certain subgroups known for their healthy lifestyles, including Mormons and Seventh-Day Adventists, also enjoy greater health and longevity than most Americans. Mormons in Utah have a 30 percent lower incidence of most cancers, and Seventh-Day Adventists have from 10 to 40 percent fewer hospital admissions for malignancies.

On the other hand, cultures that have begun to turn away from their traditional healthy lifestyles are increasingly suffering from chronic diseases. For decades, many of the Pacific Rim countries, including Japan, enjoyed a relative resistance to the modern pandemic of degenerative disease, apparently because of traditional dietary and lifestyle factors. However, as these cultures have increasingly adopted Western lifestyles, their resistance to these diseases has eroded. From 1983 to 1987, Japanese women had an alarming 59 percent increase in breast cancer rates.

During the same time, American women experienced a 28 percent increase. Other Westernized areas of Asia, such as Singapore, Thailand, and Hong Kong, have also seen dramatic increases. This same phenomenon has occurred in some Eastern European countries.

Breast cancer incidence is but one of a growing number of conditions with significant international variation. Many forms of complementary and alternative medical intervention will be discovered to be effective in different countries and traditions. It is incumbent upon researchers, clinicians, politicians, and the public to insist upon an integration of the best of CAM with the best of conventional care from all countries of the world for the betterment of all humankind.

Making Informed Choices

Peering into the future of the evolving health care systems throughout the world, certain trends are evident. For better or worse, managed care will increase. Neurosciences and the Human Genome Project will yield new insights into Alzheimer's, Parkinson's, dementia, and other inherited conditions of the elderly. Surely, the Internet will enable consumers, patients, and practitioners to access unprecedented information on both CAM and conventional care, and will stimulate self-responsibility for health. In addition, the limitations of surgery, hospitalizations, and medications will become increasingly evident. Ancient plagues and antibiotic-resistant microbes are emerging with renewed virulence.

As these forces evolve, individuals will have to make important choices about what type of health care to employ. Some may choose conventional care, some may choose CAM, and the majority will use both of these approaches. When Alice, adrift in Wonderland, queried the grinning Cheshire cat as to which road to take, he replied, "It all depends on which way you want to go!" A more prosaic variant of this dilemma is Yogi Berra's quip, "When you come to a fork in the road, take it!" For individuals seeking health care, the decision about which approach to take may seem overwhelming, especially during an acute crisis. To make a wise decision, an individual should become as informed as possible through books, articles, lectures, friends, the Internet, and discussions with practitioners.

In making well-informed decisions about CAM, it is vital that people do not allow themselves to believe that this approach is invariably safe. Many individuals are under the mistaken impression that something that is "natural" is always safe. Mushrooms are natural, but eating certain varieties can be fatal. Similarly, certain herbs may be therapeutic, others harmless, while some are potentially toxic. This underscores the necessity of working with an experienced practitioner, and educating yourself as much as is reasonably possible.

No therapy, CAM or conventional, is a guarantee against illness and death. In fact, extreme self-absorption, centered around health, is narcissistic and notably unhealthy, even though it is common. In *Worried Sick*, Dr. Arthur J. Barsky of the Harvard Medical School noted that Americans have become "prisoners of health, a society plagued by a sense of disease and malaise and a seemingly constant need for medical care." Attaining a state of health is considered by many to be tantamount to achieving not only freedom from disease but also moral virtue. In this context, health is not valued as a means of accomplishing fundamental personal goals, such as raising a family or helping others; it has become a substitute for them. Misguided individuals have replaced the religious quest of saving their souls with the secular quest of preserving their bodies. For many, the highest purpose of human activity is not to purify the soul but to purify the body. Outward appearance of perfect health is now the object of a sustained and deliberate endeavor to bathe in the Fountain of Youth.

In a world where dangers seem out of our control, we retreat to shore up our own physical integrity, to attempt to ensure survival by building resistance and stretching endurance. Again Barsky notes that "powerless to stem the seepage of toxic wastes into our drinking water, unable to avoid carcinogens in our vegetables, at the mercy of a psychopath who would assault us on the street, we check our blood pressure, fortify our diet, and carry weights with us as we jog." Faced with such a threatening external environment, we seek control over our internal environment in the name of health. We try to assert control in the one sphere of influence that remains ours—our bodies and our personal habits.

Nonetheless, we must learn to refrain from using CAM merely as a means to deny that we will all someday get old and die. We must not delude ourselves into thinking that CAM is a magical force that can protect us against all of the many factors that daily assault our health and longevity.

THINK HORSES, NOT ZEBRAS

Ultimately, health is the achieving of an optimal state of body, mind, spirit, and environment. This definition of health may encompass an Olympic athlete or a quadriplegic. It includes intervals of acute trauma and successful adaptation to chronic disease. It extends to people of all ages and cultures. It recognizes the value of individual practices, but does not abdicate social responsibility. It holds sway between life and death.

Current prescriptions for how to achieve health are a bewildering and often contradictory barrage of instant diets, panacea exercises, and CAM as well as conventional nostrums. For many people, an approach to achieving optimal health parallels the disease model. We seek something *outside* of ourselves as a solution.

When you enter into CAM therapies, they inevitably involve lifestyle change and the necessity of personal, internal introspection and transformation. Effectiveness of CAM therapies has a significant scientific underpinning in many instances, and can be of help in coping with both acute and chronic illness. However, the dimension of personal introspection and lifestyle change is not the exclusive domain of either CAM or conventional interventions per se. When CAM therapies are effective, they most often engender profound psychological and lifestyle changes. Change requires courage, and it requires paying attention to obvious habits and behaviors that we need to alter in our daily lives before seeking an external panacea. Pay attention to the obvious before seeking the external or esoteric. Think horses, not zebras!

Ultimately, however, there is no solution to the end of life, no matter how healthy you are. Remember the words of comedian Redd Foxx: "Health nuts are going to feel really dumb one day, lying in the hospital, dying of nothing!"

When you or someone you love is ill or even facing death, it is an essential time to reassess your life, embrace what is important, and let distractions fall away. Somehow, a crisis puts some people in touch with a deep inner resource, which in turn empowers them to do more with their lives than just strive for material perfection.

But is a crisis always necessary? What can we learn from those who have already embarked on such personal odysseys?

Focus on the immediate moment. See all the unnoticed miracles of every day. There are no guarantees that we will awaken to tomorrow's sunrise, or that we will revel in the brilliant colors of this evening's sunset.

Now that we are closer than ever to a deeper understanding of the inextricable interactions of mind and body, and between conventional and alternative medicine, it seems possible at last to bridge the gap between spiritual purpose and optimal health. Our direction is clear, but biomedical and genetic technology alone cannot provide the answers.

Buddhist scriptures formulated thousands of years ago advocated the journey inward, toward wisdom and enlightenment, to discover the essence of the soul. Twenty-first-century science will permit humankind to peer into intracellular space, and to chart the helical coils of the DNA molecule at the very heart of all life. Whether we are scientists or mystics, these perennial mysteries instill in us all an abiding sense of awe, humility, and compassion.

PART II

CAM THERAPIES FOR SPECIFIC CONDITIONS

In this section we summarize complementary and alternative treatments for specific conditions, organized by particular illness or ailment.

This information is not intended to replace the medical care of a physician or other licensed clinicians. All persons suffering from any of the following conditions should consult their physicians and licensed practitioners.

A detailed description of specific herbal indications, dosages, forms of preparation, contraindications, and cautions and warnings is given under the section for the condition most commonly treated with that herb.

GENERAL PRECAUTIONS

- Keep all conventional and CAM medications and supplements out of the reach of children.
- If you are planning a pregnancy, are pregnant, or are breast feeding, you should talk with your doctor before taking *any* supplements or herbs.
- Among the supplements currently on the market are a number of controversial substances whose health benefits have not been definitively proven by randomized clinical trials (RCTs).
- Not all CAM interventions are harmless. Some are dangerous when used inappropriately or to excess. Consumers should be cautious when selecting herbs. Since the herb industry is essentially unregulated, because the practice of botanical medicine is not formalized, and due to the fact that herbal medicine is not generally taught in the vast majority of medical and pharmacy schools, consumers have essentially been left to their own devices in determining how they will use botanical products. Some herbs themselves also have potentially harmful side effects, and should not be used without an understanding of the full range of their biological activity, and the advice of a physician.

- Some traditional Chinese medicine and Ayurvedic herbal preparations manufactured by companies in Asia are currently being imported
  into the United States. There is a lack of quality control in the manufacture of these products, resulting in questionable standards of purity,
  sanitation, and standardization. Many herbal compounds from China
  and India may be contaminated with biological materials, as well as
  with heavy metals, such as arsenic, mercury, or lead. However, some
  common Chinese and Ayurvedic preparations are now being produced by U.S. companies, and these are much safer.
- Herbal labels may be inaccurate. A finding published in the September 2, 1998, issue of the *Los Angeles Times* tested ten common
  over-the-counter (OTC) products lasbeled as St. John's wort. Out of
  the ten products, seven contained between 75 percent and 135 percent of the labeled hypericin and three contained no more than half
  of the amount stated on the label. Although this focused on St. John's
  wort, there is a similar unpublished study of wide variation in ginseng content, and it is likely that many other herbs and supplements
  may be inadequately or even inaccurately labeled.
- It is important to underscore that there are no long-term safety or
  efficacy studies on herbal preparations. Actually, there are also too
  few such studies on conventional pharmaceuticals.
- Grapefruit is a common food that increases the potency of many
  conventional medications, such as calcium channel blockers for high
  blood pressure, angina or chest pain, and arrhythmias; also Seldane,
  withdrawn from the market but formerly used for allergic rhinitis;
  and the benzodiazapenes commonly prescribed for anxiety and sleeplessness. Interaction effects of grapefruit or other common foods
  with herbs are not known. It would be prudent to avoid grapefruit
  while using herbs appropriate to any of the foregoing conditions.
- All herbal dosages and recommendations are based upon studies
  with adults. Safety and efficacy with children is completely unknown.
- Adults over sixty-five may have diminished liver or renal function
  and need to be particularly concerned about herbal or supplement
  excess and/or toxicity. Liver function assessments should be monitored periodically while taking herbals, supplements, as well as
  many conventional pharmaceuticals.
- Five excellent, ongoing sources for both public and professional information on alternative medicine are *Alternative Medicine Alert* from

American Health Consultant at (800) 688-2421; *Alternative Medicine Advisor* from Rebus Publishers (publishers of the Berkeley Wellness Letter and the Johns Hopkins Medical Letter) at (877) 212-1933; *Complementary Medicine for the Physician* from Churchill Livingstone Publishers; *The Integrative Medicine Consult* from Intergrative Medicine Communications at (617) 641-2300; and *Dr. Andrew Weil's Self Healing* from Thorne Communications at (617) 926-0200. For reliable information on herbals, the best source is the American Botanical Council, which published the *German Commission E Monographs,* in Austin, Texas, at (512) 926-4900; the *Encyclopedia of Natural Medicine* by Dr. Michael Murray and Dr. Joseph Pizzorno; and most important, the new *PDR for Herbal Medicines* from Physician's Desk Reference Publishers in Des Moines, Iowa. Finally, the best source of updates on insurance coverage, new clinics, and business opportunities is *The Integrator,* published by John Weeks in Seattle, Washington.

Acne

- In a 1995 RCT, researchers evaluated **Ayurvedic formulations** (which are herbal preparations from India's traditional system of natural medicine) used to treat acne vulgaris, which is a type of acne manifesting in blackheads, whiteheads, and inflammation, and not the more severe cystic form. Eighty-two patients were randomized into five groups. Four of the groups received different Ayurvedic preparations orally for six weeks, while one group received a placebo. One of the preparations, **Sunder Bati,** produced a significant reduction in acne lesions (see p. 243).
- A 1998 study of 280 people with acne vulgaris evaluated the traditional Ayurvedic formula **shanka bhasma.** Patients were assigned to groups based on *dosha* constitutions (see descriptions on pp. 232–35). At the end of the four-week study, the *vata* and *pitta* patients showed significant improvement, but the *kapha* patients did not. This study indicates that individualized treatment based on *doshas* may be a meaningful approach (see p. 244).

AIDS

- One published study focused on **relaxation combined with imagery** to affect immune system function, with potential applications in the treatment of cancer and AIDS (see p. 75).
- **Imagery** has important potential in multifactorial therapies for cancer, AIDS, and autoimmune diseases. This potential needs to be further explored (see p. 76).
- Among the claims made for the mineral **selenium** are that it prevents and treats AIDS-related pathology (see p. 101).
- Claims made for the hormone **DHEA** include that it combats AIDS, but that remains unproven. More than ten thousand scientific papers have been written about DHEA, and two international conferences have been held on DHEA research (see p. 108).
- **Astragalus,** which normalizes immune functions, is probably the most commonly used herb in China today, and has been used in the treatment of AIDS although its effectiveness is inconclusive (see p. 110).
- When used in conjunction with Western medicine, **traditional Chinese herbal medicine** (TCM) has become a popular, although unproven, approach in the United States for addressing certain life-threatening diseases, particularly cancer and AIDS (see p. 136).
- Among people with HIV and AIDS, **acupuncture and Chinese herbs** as adjuncts to conventional care, such as protease inhibitors, are considered the most promising alternative approaches. TCM reduces side effects of conventional medications and increases their efficacy (see p. 137).
- Controlled clinical trials of **Chinese herbs** need to be increased. Particular emphasis needs to be placed on testing herbs for conditions that often resist conventional treatment, such as AIDS (see p. 136).
- **Acupuncture** is a very popular complementary therapy for AIDS (see p. 136).
- In the treatment of HIV and AIDS, **acupuncture** has been demonstrated to increase total white blood cells and T-cell production. In a controversial program in Miami, acupuncture is purportedly increasing life span of AIDS patients and improving quality of life (see p. 146).

- **St. John's wort** is an herb that is currently of interest to AIDS researchers, who are analyzing the possible antiviral activity of one of its primary active compounds, hypericum (see p. 170).
- In a 1993 study in India, 129 asymptomatic HIV carriers were treated with individualized constitutional **homeopathic remedies,** and 12 became HIV-negative after three to sixteen months. A 1994 study in the Netherlands of homeopathic treatment of HIV and AIDS patients showed an improvement in CD4+ cells in 23 of 34 cases (see p. 191).
- Researchers are currently examining **naturopathic treatments** in people infected with HIV, and have found that herbal and nutritional therapies have produced improvement in some measures of immune functioning and slowed progression of AIDS (see p. 197).
- Significant work is being conducted to evaluate **combination therapies** (which is the use of alternative therapies in conjunction with conventional therapies) for AIDS (see p. 191).
- Therapeutic cocktails of **protease inhibitors** are now available that reduce HIV virus to zero and in some cases actually arrest AIDS (see p. 301).

Caution: Echinacea is an inappropriate herb for HIV and AIDS, since echinacea may promote the replication of T-cells, which is where the HIV virus resides (see p. 159).

ALCOHOLISM

- **Acupuncture,** particularly applied to the inner ear, has helped patients withdraw not only from opiates but also from alcohol and other addictive drugs (see p. 145).
- In a 1987 controlled study on hard-core alcoholics, a group that received **acupuncture** had half as many drinking episodes and admissions to detox centers as did a control group, which received sham acupuncture (see p. 145).
- Studies show **acupuncture** is successful in preventing relapse with severe alcoholics (see p. 145).
- **Milk thistle** extract has been proven in clinical studies to be effec-

tive for hepatitis, alcoholic cirrhosis, and liver damage from exposure to harmful chemicals (see p. 167).

- In a study of sixty-six patients, most of whom had alcohol-induced liver disease, thirty-one patients received a standardized **milk thistle preparation,** and showed significant improvement in liver enzyme levels (see p. 167).
- **Valerian** is a very safe herb, and unlike barbiturates and other conventional drugs for treating insomnia, it does not interact synergistically with alcohol (see p. 172). There is a potential interaction with other sedatives but there are few if any reported contraindications, warnings, or adverse effects.
- In **Ayurvedic medicine,** *pitta* types (described on pp. 232–35) are disturbed by consuming too much alcohol.
- A thirty-five-year study found that individuals who described **parents in positive terms** in the 1950s were far less likely to have developed later illnesses, such as alcoholism (see p. 260).
- One reason **Swedish citizens** may enjoy better health and one of the world's longest life expectancies is lower use of alcohol (see p. 307).

Caution: A study of beta-carotene found increased risk for lung cancer in people who smoked and also drank alcohol, or who smoked heavily; another study found neither harm nor benefit (see p. 98).

ALLERGIES

- **Hypnotherapy** is used to control allergies (see p. 69).
- **Astragalus** is probably the most commonly used herb today in China, and has applications for allergies (see p. 123).
- Irritable bowel syndrome patients on **allergy-free diets** reexperienced symptoms when allergens were reintroduced (see p. 191).
- Food allergy has been implicated in **otitis media,** a type of middle ear infection (see p. 193).
- A series of studies investigated a single remedy, **Galphimia glauca,** for hay fever. Nearly six hundred people were involved in the trials, which showed a statistically significant improvement in symptoms among people using homeopathy (see p. 204).

- A study of nasal allergies involving thirty-nine patients found statistically significant results in favor of a homeopathic remedy, **Galphimia glauca**. In a similar study, patients using other homeopathic remedies showed a statistically significant decrease in symptoms (see p. 204). A 1997 meta-analysis noted that five out of six studies of several different homeopathy remedies noted positive effects for several different remedies depending on differences in the specific allergy and symptoms.
- A study of the remedy **Similisan** in 1995 produced a statistically significant reduction in redness and itching among allergy patients (see p. 204).

Caution: Some studies suggest that melatonin can exacerbate allergies (see p. 112).

ALZHEIMER'S DISEASE

- A study of Alzheimer's patients indicated that **music therapy** enhanced memory of past events and improved mood (see p. 83).
- Human clinical studies of the antioxidant enzyme **SOD** are still at a very early stage, but some researchers claim it slows the aging process and has potential in treating Alzheimer's disease. SOD supplements are sold commercially in oral form, but consumers should be aware that oral SOD products are completely destroyed in the gut (see p. 105).
- Claims for the steroid hormone **DHEA** include alleviating Alzheimer's disease (see p. 108).
- *Ginkgo biloba* has been promoted for some time as a treatment for Alzheimer's disease, and recent studies indicate that it does have potential benefit in slowing progression of the disease (see p. 164). There is a reported cross-allergy with poison ivy.
- Evidence has been discovered of a specific **mutated gene,** a beta-amyloid precursor, that induces Alzheimer's disease in laboratory animals and offers new insights into a potential intervention for this dreaded and increasingly common disease (see p. 301).

ANXIETY

- Hypnotherapy is currently used in health care to modify feelings of pain, anxiety, and fear, and to gain acceptance of new behaviors (see p. 69).
- Imagery is used to prepare patients for medical procedures, to relieve pain and anxiety, and to soothe side effects that are aggravated by anxiety (see p. 72).
- Many patients have found **imagery** helpful, even if they were not cured, and have reported relief of anxiety and pain, better toleration of chemotherapy and radiation, and an increased sense of control (see p. 74).
- A study showed that **Qi Gong** exercises, involving physical movement and breathing techniques, were helpful for patients with reflex sympathetic dystrophy, a debilitating disease of the autonomic nervous system that often resists medical intervention. For these patients, Qi Gong significantly reduced pain and anxiety (see p. 81).
- Therapists use **music** for a number of purposes, including reduction of stress, anxiety, and social isolation (see p. 82).
- In the treatment of heart disease, **music** has been used as a pacemaker, helping patients to sustain normal heart rhythms. It also reduces anxiety in heart attack patients (see p. 82).
- Taking a holistic approach to the individual, traditional Indian **Ayurvedic medicine** maintains that all aspects of life contribute to health, including nutrition, hygiene, sleep, weather, and lifestyle, as well as physical, mental, and sexual activities. Emotional factors are also taken into consideration. Anger, fear, anxiety, and unhealthy relationships are believed to contribute to illness. A healthy emotional state is considered the very foundation of physical health (see p. 232).
- *Brahmi,* an Ayurvedic herb, is highly valued as an anti-anxiety compound (see p. 239).
- A study evaluated the effects of *pancha karma,* an Ayurvedic detoxification regimen (described on p. 240), on risk factors for heart disease in thirty-one adults. Patients who participated in a program of herbs, meditation, and moderate exercise were found to have an 80 percent increase in the ability of their blood vessels to dilate three months after the treatment, indicating improved function. Total

cholesterol was reduced in all the participants, with a reduced measure of free radical damage and significantly reduced anxiety (see p. 240).

- **Yoga** programs have shown the potential for helping to reduce heart disease by influencing such risk factors as blood pressure, anxiety, and unhealthy reaction to stress (see p. 247).
- As a result of over a dozen studies, it has been concluded that devout **religious belief** enhances health and well-being and helps protect against anxiety and depression (see p. 254). However, religious beliefs can have a negative impact. Religious dogma can be harmful when it fosters excessive guilt, perfectionistic expectations, fear, or lowered self-worth (see p. 254).
- A study found that patients in a cardiovascular unit who received **therapeutic touch,** a procedure involving the manipulation of the body's energy fields, showed a significant reduction in anxiety, compared to patients receiving mock therapeutic touch (see p. 269).
- Studies indicate that the herb **kava kava,** or "intoxicating pepper," may reduce anxiety and induce sleep. Kava should not be used with antidepressants, alcohol, muscle relaxants, tranquilizers such as Valium, or any other sedating pharmaceuticals used for the central nervous system. Kava can cause a skin reaction (dermatitis) or sensitivity to light. Rarely, hallucinations have been reported. If you use this herb for a long period of time, which is not advisable, your skin can become temporarily yellow. Your nails and your hair can react as well. If you overdose on kava you will have a strong urge to sleep and you might lose control of your voluntary muscles. Kava should not be used while driving a motor vehicle or operating heavy equipment, during pregnancy, or if you have a history of depression. The typical preparation is a crude extract of standardized kavalactone (30 percent) and the typical dose is 45–70 mg of kavalactone. Typical dosage is 250 mg of the standardized extract two or three times per day, preferably with meals. Do not take more than two 250 mg capsules in any four-hour period. Kava may relieve mild anxiety in less than an hour, but it can require up to eight weeks for any impact on severe anxiety. Take for a maximum of three months followed by abstaining for two to four weeks (see pp. 315–16).

ARTHRITIS

- Arthritis can be the result of common **lifestyle risks** such as smoking, overeating, or being too sedentary; some forms of arthritis can be prevented, arrested, or even reversed when patients stop making these lifestyle mistakes (see p. 32).
- **Exercise and movement,** which are used in many MindBody therapies, decrease the harmful effects of stress, and help prevent some of the diseases of aging (including arthritis). Some Eastern exercise disciplines, such as **yoga and tai chi,** address body and mind as an integral system (see p. 62).
- **Cognitive behavioral interventions** (education, training in coping skills and motivation techniques, and behavioral rehearsal) are very effective with patients suffering from chronic diseases such as arthritis, and are a viable addition to conventional treatment for arthritis (see pp. 67–69).
- Arthritis patients who participated in a lifestyle-based **pain management program** experienced an average 20 percent decline in pain, and a 40 percent reduction in doctor visits (see p. 68).
- **Qi Gong,** an ancient Chinese exercise involving physical movements and breathing exercises, has been studied in China for its impact on arthritis (see pp. 80–81).
- **Music therapy** (listening to and making music) has been found to raise the pain threshold of rheumatoid arthritis patients (see pp. 81–83).
- Hospitals and HMOs are increasingly including **MindBody** components in their managed care programs, and are successfully treating arthritis with this approach (see pp. 84–86).
- Injections of the antioxidant enzyme **SOD** are used in Europe to treat musculoskeletal inflammation and osteoarthritis. Bovine SOD, injected into the joint, has been found beneficial in treating osteoarthritis of the knee. However, treatment of rheumatoid arthritis has been disappointing (see p. 105).
- **Testosterone,** a hormone, has been studied as a treatment for rheumatoid arthritis, with equivocal results. Improvement was noted in rheumatoid arthritis symptoms; however, there was no significant effect on the disease (see p. 113).
- **Chinese herbal medicine** is the most dominant traditional Chi-

nese medicine (TCM) intervention worldwide, and several American companies are now making Chinese herbal formulas that can have positive impacts on diseases such as arthritis (see pp. 120–21).

- One of the most frequently used herbs in Japanese herbal medicine, **Bupleurum,** has been used in Japan for treating arthritis (see p. 123).
- An extract of **TCM anti-arthritis herb T-2** (*Tripterygium wilfordii*), was administered to seventy patients with rheumatoid arthritis of at least six months' duration, none of whom had responded to standard treatment. Herb T-2 produced positive results that were better than the results produced by a standard arthritis drug (see p. 135).
- In an arthritis study, 50 percent of osteoarthritis patients using **acupuncture** became much improved or symptom-free, compared to 31 percent of patients taking medication (see p. 143). In another arthritis study, 25 percent of patients scheduled for knee surgery were able to avoid surgery after a course of acupuncture (see p. 143).

    Caution: Among the most serious, occasional side effects of acupuncture are mild, transitory depression, anxiety, and fatigue (see p. 142).
- **Naturopathic medicine** in the form of nutritional supplements, botanicals, and physical medicine (electromagnetic field stimulation) has been found to have significant effects in the treatment of arthritis (see p. 186).
- **Glucosamine** is currently being investigated, in a large NCCAM-funded multicenter RCT, as an effective nutritional supplement. Considerable animal research indicates that glucosamine alone may arrest arthritic deterioration. There is less evidence supporting the addition of the supplements chondroitin or bromelain in conjunction with the glucosamine (see p. 186).
- Current research is addressing the effects of **homeopathic treatment** of osteoarthritis of the knee (see p. 195).
- **Homeopathy,** which is considered a complete medical system and is capable of addressing a wide array of health problems, has successfully treated arthritis (see p. 200).
- **Homeopathy** patients with rheumatoid arthritis have shown a sta-

tistically significant improvement in pain, stiffness, and grip strength, compared to a placebo (see p. 205).

- In homeopathy, **Rhus tox** is a commonly prescribed remedy for rheumatoid arthritis, but it is less commonly prescribed for osteoarthritis (see p. 207).
- **Ayurveda** is India's traditional system of natural medicine. In Vedic philosophy there are three essential, overriding qualities (or *doshas*) that are present in all things—*vata, pitta,* and *kapha* (described on pp. 232–35). *Vata* people most commonly have arthritis (see p. 234).
- **Ayurvedic herbs** are used both internally and externally to treat arthritis and muscle disorders (see p. 238).
- Ten medical conditions (including arthritis) were studied for effects of multiple **Maharishi Ayur-Ved interventions** (see p. 240) involving a nutritional program, individualized herbal preparations, and lifestyle guidelines. Seventy-nine percent of the patients showed improvement, 14 percent showed no change, and 7 percent became worse. All ten categories of medical condition showed significant improvement (see p. 240).
- An **Ayurvedic preparation** consisting of the herbs *Withania somnifera, Boswellia serrata, Cucurma longa,* and a zinc complex produced a significant reduction in pain in a study of arthritis (see p. 242).
- More than three-quarters of arthritis patients who were treated with **powdered ginger** achieved relief from pain and swelling, and all of the patients with muscular discomfort had pain relief. None of the patients reported adverse effects (see p. 242). Ginger is both an anti-inflammatory and an anti-coagulant and may induce excess bleeding.
- Patients receiving a special extract of **guggul** (the crude gum of the herb *Boswellia serrata*), known as H-15, were found to have reduced swelling and pain, compared with those who received placebo. Symptoms of rheumatoid arthritis were reduced in 50 to 60 percent of the patients (see pp. 241–44).

ASTHMA

- **Behavioral medicine** meets the needs of two groups of patients who are often not fully served by conventional medicine: patients with physical problems and patients with chronic conditions such as asthma (see pp. 67–68).
- A study of asthma patients found the use of **imagery** helped a significant number of subjects discontinue their medication entirely as compared with controls, although imagery did not have the same degree of influence on asthma symptoms (see p. 75).
- **Biofeedback,** a method of improving control over autonomic body functions, is used to treat 150 conditions, including asthma. In a fifteen-month study of asthmatics, biofeedback patients suffered fewer attacks and used less medicine (see pp. 76–77).
- Conditions that demonstrate an inconclusive reaction to the mineral **selenium** include asthma (see p. 101).
- Asthma patients using the nutrient **coenzyme Q_{10}** required less hospitalization, and episodes of pulmonary edema or cardiac asthma were significantly reduced. Research in this area is still in the early stages, and it remains uncertain (see p. 104).
- Conventional drug treatment often has side effects, so asthma patients sometimes seek alternative approaches. A study of T-cells showed that **herbal preparations** increased specific T-cell subset CD4, and increased CD8, which was suggested as the mechanism of action for inhibiting asthma (see pp. 130–31).
- Although **acupuncture** in America is most frequently used for pain, as early as 1979 the World Health Organization compiled a list of 104 conditions that acupuncture can treat, including asthma. In the United States, acupuncture is often used as a last resort for many of these conditions (see p. 142).
- There is some evidence that **acupuncture** may be of general value in treating asthma (see p. 148).
- In a UCLA study, bronchospasm in asthma patients whose illness averaged twenty-two years in duration was effectively controlled by **acupuncture** (see p. 148).
- Other clinical evidence indicates that **acupuncture** does seem to be effective in disorders such as asthma. The panel noted that

acupuncture may be safer and more effective than many accepted conventional treatments for asthma (see p. 150).

- A study yielded a 91 percent improvement of bronchial asthma with an **elimination diet** which systematically removes or eliminates potential allergens. Restricting an essential amino acid called **tryptophan** from the diet was found in a 1983 study to help improve asthma symptoms (see p. 186).

- A study of asthmatics showed that supplementation with 1,000 mg per day of the vitamin **ascorbic acid** for fourteen weeks produced less frequent and less severe asthma attacks (see p. 186).

- In a 1931 **nutritional therapy** study, treatment with hydrochloric acid before meals, and exclusion of food allergens, produced improvement in asthma patients. In a 1979 study, the herb *Tylophora indica* produced improvement in 135 patients with bronchial asthma (see p. 187).

- In studies, patients being treated with **homeopathy, physical medicine, counseling, and psychotherapy** showed significant improvement in asthma symptoms (see p. 187).

- Allergy patients treated with **homeopathy** achieved an improvement rate of 82 percent, compared to 38 percent of placebo patients (see p. 206).

- Based on research, there is some evidence that **homeopathy** is effective in treating allergy patients with highly dilute preparations of the original allergen (see p. 211).

- According to chiropractic theory, **chiropractic manipulation** has a general health-enhancing effect. Chiropractic has helped bronchial asthmatics (see p. 219).

- A small body of published clinical evidence suggests that **spinal manipulation** might be helpful for asthma (see p. 224).

- Ailments such as asthma are treated with yogic breathing and traditional Indian **Ayurvedic preparations,** including the herbs *Sida cordifolia* and *Tylophora asthmatica* (see p. 238).

- **Yoga** has proven beneficial in treating a variety of medical conditions including asthma. Yoga is also helpful for improving respiratory endurance and efficiency of breathing (see p. 246).

- A pilot study evaluated the effectiveness of multiple **Maharishi Ayur-Ved interventions** among a group of 126 adults with ten different chronic diseases, including asthma. Each participant received an individualized nutritional program, herbal preparations, and daily lifestyle guidelines. Seventy-nine percent showed improvement (see p. 240).

ATHEROSCLEROSIS

- According to literature, atherosclerosis patients treated with **Qi Gong** exercise showed improvements in memory, insomnia, dizziness, tinnitus (buzzing in ears), and numbness (see pp. 80–81).
- Since excess protein in general, and particularly excessive animal protein, is associated with increased risk of atherosclerosis, it is a good idea to reduce or **eliminate animal foods** from the diet (see p. 95).
- Humans cannot synthesize **carotenoids,** which are nutritious red pigments found in fruits and vegetables, so they must be derived from diet. However, they are not well absorbed. Carotenoids may help to protect LDL cholesterol from oxidation, thereby inhibiting atherosclerosis and heart attacks (see p. 97).
- A 1995 study of 605 heart attack patients documented the value of a **Mediterranean-type diet,** rich in alpha-linolenic acid, bread, root vegetables, green vegetables, fish, and fruit and low in meat, butter, and cream. After twenty-seven months, there were 73 percent fewer heart attacks and 70 percent fewer deaths (see p. 187).
- A study of 8,341 men with previous myocardial infarctions demonstrated the long-term benefits of **niacin,** a component of vitamin B. In a follow-up study, niacin supplementation was associated with an 11 percent reduction in mortality. In a 1985 study, supplementation with the alkaloid **L-carnitine** was found to increase exercise tolerance in patients with angina (see p. 187).
- A number of **herbal compounds** have been used to prevent atherosclerosis (see p. 238).
- **Guggul,** an herb, also identified as *Commiphora mukul,* has been used traditionally in Ayurvedic medicine for the last one thousand years for a variety of inflammatory problems, including osteoarthritis. There is considerable clinical evidence that *Guggul* lowers blood lipid or cholesterol levels and may protect against cardiovascular disease and atherosclerosis, and is also beneficial for the liver (see p. 244).

- An extensive inquiry was conducted into the possible biological basis for why women live longer than men. The in-depth analysis included an examination of the hormone **estrogen,** which tends to prevent atherosclerosis in premenopausal women (see pp. 305–306). Increasingly women are seeking naturally occurring estrogens, phytoestrogens, in such products as soy for an alternative to hormone replacement therapy (HRT).

ATTENTION DEFICIT DISORDER

- **Biofeedback,** a method of improving control over autonomic body functions, is used to treat about 150 conditions, including attention deficit disorder (see pp. 76–77).

BEDWETTING (SEE ENURESIS)

BIRTH DEFECTS

Caution: Beta-carotene accumulates in fat cells and has toxic effects. When taken at ten times the RDA, vitamin A has been associated with birth defects (see p. 97).

Caution: Pregnant women and nursing mothers should be cautious about Chinese herbs, and people taking other medicines should be alert for drug interactions. For utmost safety, anyone taking TCM herbs should tell his or her physician (see p. 124).

Caution: Ginger may not be safe for morning sickness nausea, because some components of ginger may have mutagenic effects, which could possibly cause birth defects (see p. 163).

BRONCHITIS

- In conventional medical facilities where traditional Chinese medicine (TCM) is offered, **TCM** may be the most reasonable first approach for bronchitis (see p. 125).

- In traditional Indian **Ayurvedic medicine,** most people have problems associated with their predominate *dosha. Kapha* people are more likely to suffer from bronchitis (see p. 234).
- **Maharishi Ayur-Ved interventions** can be effective in treating bronchitis (see p. 240).

BRUISES

- Chinese Americans most often use **traditional Chinese medicine** (TCM) for bruises (see p. 125).
- A study indicated that **acupuncture** provided short-term relief to 50 to 80 percent of patients with acute and chronic pain. Bruises responded well (see p. 143).
- **Arnica,** used internally and topically in homeopathy, is effective in reducing swelling and bruising. Do not drink more than two cups of arnica tea per day for more than three days. Typical preparation and dose are 1–2 tsp. per cup of boiling water of the dried herb, tincture diluted to one part. Homeopathic ointments of 15 percent arnica oil are for external use only (see pp. 315–16).
- **Comfrey** is often taken for bruises, but high dosages may obstruct blood flow to the liver (see pp. 172–173).

BUZZING IN THE EARS (SEE TINNITUS)

CANCER

- A study conducted by Dr. David Spiegel of the Stanford University School of Medicine documented that **hypnotherapy,** in conjunction with social support, doubled survival time for metastatic breast cancer patients (see p. 70).
- One study evaluated the use of **hypnotic imagery** with twenty-five breast cancer patients. Following this intervention, measures of depression and confusion were reduced, positive states were increased, and the percentage of natural killer cells in the blood was significantly increased (see p. 71).

- **Imagery** has been used in the adjunctive care of cancer patients. Patients were encouraged to imagine their immune system cells engulfing and devouring vulnerable cancer cells. Many patients have found it helpful (see pp. 73–74).
- A study examined **relaxation combined with imagery** to affect immune system function, with potential applications in the treatment of cancer (see p. 75).
- Benefits of **imagery and social support** were evaluated in a study of women with breast cancer. It was found that imagery and support groups had a small to modest positive effect on coping, attitudes, and support, but not on immune function (see p. 75). In a classic study, a seventeen-year prospective follow-up disclosed that, among women, social isolation was a risk factor for the onset and progression of cancer (see p. 262).
- **Qi Gong** exercise has been studied in China for its impact on cancer. Numerous papers have been presented at international conferences over twenty years. However, scientific literature is very limited in the United States (see p. 80).
- During a study, ninety-three patients with advanced cancer were treated with a combination of drugs and **Qi Gong** exercises, while a control group was treated with drugs alone. Eighty-one percent of the Qi Gong group showed an improvement in strength, 63 percent in appetite, and 33 percent were free from diarrhea compared to improvements of 10 percent, 10 percent, and 6 percent, respectively, in the other group (see p. 81).
- Hospitals and HMOs are increasingly including **MindBody** components in their managed care programs, including psychosocial support groups for cancer patients (see p. 85).
- Water-insoluble **fibers** (celluloses and hemicelluloses) protect against colon cancer by absorbing water, increasing stool volume, and speeding the passage of stool through the bowel. They also dilute the concentration of toxic bile acids, which can contribute to cancer (see pp. 91–92).
- To protect against heart disease or cancer, dosage levels of **vitamin E** may need to be twenty to thirty times greater than the RDAs (see p. 97).
- According to a study, low blood levels of **carotenoids** (nutritious red

pigments found in fruits and vegetables) are associated with cancer and coronary disease (see pp. 97–98).

- **Carotenoid lycopene** is ten times more potent than beta-carotene as an antioxidant, and apparently lowers rates of prostate cancer (see p. 98).
- Studies suggest that the nutrient **coenzyme Q$_{10}$** might be useful in protecting against breast cancer (see p. 103).
- **Coenzyme Q$_{10}$**'s antioxidant activity has led to suggestions that it might be beneficial in the treatment of cancer. In a study, none of the patients in the supplemented group died, contrary to the predicted or expected mortality. However, because a number of antioxidants were used, the results cannot be attributed to Q$_{10}$ alone (see p. 104).
- Claims for the hormone **DHEA** include that it combats some cancers. More than ten thousand scientific papers have been written about DHEA, and two international conferences have been held on DHEA research (see p. 108).
- Research has shown that low **DHEA** levels in the blood are associated with breast cancer (see p. 108).
- It has been claimed that the hormone **melatonin** is a powerful antioxidant that may reduce the risk of cancer, although that remains unproven (see p. 111).
- In a study, thirty patients with brain tumors received either radiation therapy alone, or radiation plus **melatonin.** Survival was higher in patients receiving the melatonin. Side effects of cancer immunotherapy, such as nausea from chemotherapy and radiation, were reduced with melatonin. In another study of patients with gastrointestinal cancer, immune functioning after surgery was improved by melatonin and immunotherapy (see pp. 111–12).
- Used in conjunction with Western medicine, traditional Chinese medicine (**TCM**) herbal preparations are now a popular approach for addressing certain troublesome diseases, particularly cancer (see p. 126).
- Traditional Chinese medicine (**TCM**) has no treatments that are used solely for cancer, but offers many formulas that help with various symptoms of cancer. Approximately 120 species of Chinese herbs are used to adjunctively treat cancer (see p. 126).

- **Acupuncture** is a very popular complementary therapy for cancer (see p. 138).
- In cancer therapy, **acupuncture** can help control nausea and other side effects of chemotherapy and radiation (see p. 146).
- **Herbs,** particularly **green tea,** are extensively used in the prevention of cancer (see pp. 152–77).
- **Naturopaths** often work with allopaths, traditional Western doctors, in treating cancer. (see p. 183) Green tea capsules may be taken in dosages of 100 mg to 300 mg daily. Green tea may be consumed as often as you like.
- Effects of **naturopathic** treatment of cancer appear to be promising (see pp. 183, 195).
- **Ayurvedic** traditional Indian medicine offers treatment for some forms of cancer (see p. 239).
- For years, researchers have attempted to document the impact of **spirituality and religion** on health. In recent studies, religious participation was found to prolong the lives of patients with cancer (see p. 253).
- Preliminary data from an ongoing study suggest that **enhanced spiritual well-being** may help women cope with and even survive breast cancer (see p. 254).
- **Practicing Mormons** develop fewer cases of cancer, cope better with the cancer they have, and experience better outcomes than Mormons who are less religious (see p. 255).
- A study of 3,217 **Seventh-Day Adventists** in the Netherlands concluded that Adventist men live 8.9 years longer than the national norm, Adventist women live 3.6 years longer, and they have a 60 percent lower mortality rate from cancer (see p. 256).
- **Support groups** have been demonstrated to have a very positive effect with cancer patients, and may extend life expectancy (see p. 262).
- **Pets** contribute to positive treatment of cancer as well as having a positive impact on a wide range of physical and mental disorders, especially with children and the elderly (see pp. 263–65).
- A noted **biofeedback** researcher conducted a study of the application of bioenergetic therapy for the treatment of basal cell carcinoma. Biofeedback is a training technique that claims to improve a person's control over autonomic body functions. He found that four

of ten patients showed elimination or reduction of their tumors (see p. 270).

Caution: Beta-carotene, as a supplement, may present health hazards for certain individuals (see p. 98).

Caution: A study indicated a 28 percent increase in lung cancer in smokers, ex-smokers and asbestos workers taking beta-carotene (see p. 98).

Caution: Chronic ingestion of 5,000 mcg a day of the mineral selenium has been reported to result in fingernail changes, hair loss, nausea, abdominal pain, diarrhea, nerve problems, fatigue, and irritability. Because vitamin E enhances the effects of selenium, it may increase this possible toxicity (see p. 100).

Caution: In a study, the steroid hormone DHEA was found to produce liver cancer in fourteen of sixteen rats. While this does not necessarily mean it would produce cancer in humans, if such a response were to occur in human research, DHEA would probably be banned by the FDA. DHEA is a hormone, and replacing any hormone that declines normally with aging must be carefully researched (see p. 109). DHEA levels in the blood are associated with increased body mass and impaired glucose tolerance (see p. 109). Serum levels of steroids should be monitored medically while taking DHEA supplements (see p. 110). Most important, there are a number of truly natural, completely safe ways to increase DHEA: stop smoking, reduce stress, exercise three to five times per week, take vitamin C, be sure your magnesium intake is adequate, and occasionally use Siberian ginseng (take 12–16 ml of fluid extract or 100–200 mg of standardized extract, one to three times per day).

CARDIOVASCULAR (HEART) DISEASE AND CHOLESTEROL

- **Hypnotherapy** is used to correct cardiac arrhythmias (see p. 69).
- **Biofeedback,** a training program used to improve autonomic body functions, is used to treat about 150 conditions including cardiac arrhythmias (see p. 77).
- **Plant-based, or phytonutrient, diets** contain disease-fighting

substances known as phytochemicals, and are rich in other nutrients. They are also low in fat and high in fiber, which helps prevent cardiovascular disease and helps remove dangerous toxins from the system (see p. 89). A high-fat diet increases risk of cardiovascular disease (see p. 92). It is widely accepted that modern high-fat, low-plant-content diets that accompanied industrialization have been associated with an increased incidence of degenerative diseases, including cardiovascular disease (see pp. 87–88).

- **Coenzyme Q$_{10}$**, a nutrient, protects against injury from tissue damage after heart attack or surgery (see p. 103).
- In a study of patients with multiple injuries, the antioxidant enzyme **SOD** helped mitigate cardiovascular and lung failure, and reduced intensive care treatment and inflammation (see pp. 105–106).
- Studies show that amino acid **L-carnitine** supplementation appears to reduce angina and ischemia, and improves exercise duration. In patients with myocardial infarction, it reduces infarction size, angina, cardiac death, and nonfatal infarction (see p. 107).
- **DHEA,** a steroid hormone, may replace other declining hormones in older women and protect against cardiac disease (see p. 109).
- **DHEA** reduces platelet aggregation in cardiovascular disease (see p. 110).
- In a study of the Chinese herbal medicine *Jianyanling*, statistically significant reductions in blood fats were found in the treatment group, which achieved significantly lower levels than the control group (see p. 132).
- **Garlic** is a popular substance for reducing cardiovascular risk factors. Garlic may lower blood pressure, triglyceride levels, and inflammation of the arteries, although the actual mechanism remains unknown. Usual dose is 300 mg taken 2 to 3 times per day. Garlic may enhance the blood-thinning effect of such frequently prescribed medications as Coumadin. However, several recent studies indicate that garlic has little or no effect on cholesterol levels and is not recommended for such use at this time (see pp. 161–62).
- **Hawthorn** is presently the plant medicine of choice in Europe for regulating heartbeat, angina, and congestive heart failure (CHF). It has a long history of use, with clinical evidence to support its cardiovascular benefits. Usual use of hawthorn is 360 mg daily with meals. It may take up to six weeks before the effects of hawthorn are

evident. Although hawthorn is relatively devoid of side effects, its use should be supervised by a physician, to avoid adverse effects. Heart disease should never be self-treated (see pp. 166–67).

- A number of **herbal compounds** have been used to prevent cardiovascular disease (see p. 238).

- *Guggul,* an herb from a small, thorny tree in India, has been used traditionally in Ayurvedic medicine for the last one thousand years for a variety of inflammatory problems. It also lowers cholesterol and triglyceride levels and helps maintain a healthy balance of HDL, the "good" cholesterol, to LDL, the "bad" cholesterol (the HDL/LDL ratio), thereby protecting against cardiovascular disease and atherosclerosis (see p. 241).

- **Cholestin** is a relatively new over-the-counter supplement made from rice fermented with a red yeast. The molecular structure of cholestin is virtually identical to the drug lovastatin. In 1999, the courts upheld the efficacy of cholestin to lower cholesterol and maintained it as an OTC rather than prescription substance.

- **Yoga** exercise is an essential component of a cardiovascular program to manage and reverse heart disease. Perhaps the only caution with yoga or other relaxation therapies is a possible hypotensive reaction, or transient drop in blood pressure when standing up too quickly (see p. 247).

- In a 1984 study, patients in a cardiovascular unit who received **therapeutic touch (TT),** a procedure involving the physical manipulation of a body's energy fields, showed a significant reduction in anxiety compared to patients receiving mock TT (see p. 269).

- **Lifestyle-based disease interventions** reduce development of and recurrence of cardiovascular problems (see p. 301).

Caution: In Germany, the cardiac catheterization rate is only 75 percent as high as that of the United States. Cardiac catheterization is a procedure used to help diagnose and treat heart trouble. Great Britain performs only one-third as many catheterizations as the United States. Similarly, the rate of coronary revascularization procedures is much lower outside the United States. Nonetheless, patients appear to fare well in these countries (see p. 48).

Caution: Patients taking the drug digitalis, a heart stimulant, can die of lethal heart arrhythmias (see pp. 51–52).

Caution: More than 400 IU of vitamin E per day may increase the risk of hemorrhagic stroke (see p. 97).

Caution: People who take thrombolytics, or medications that inhibit blood clotting, should not take vitamin E supplements without checking with their doctor (see p. 97). Herbal thrombolytics may cause excessive bleeding if combined with aspirin or prescription drugs such as Coumadin.

Caution: Active constituents of the herb ephedra are the alkaloids ephedrine and pseudoephedrine. These potent substances increase blood pressure and heart rate, and pose dangers for people with heart disease, high blood pressure, thyroid problems, and enlarged prostate, and for pregnant and lactating women (see p. 173).

Caution: Ginseng should not be used if you have high blood pressure, since it may diminish the effects of blood-pressure-lowering medications.

CARPAL TUNNEL SYNDROME

- In a 1990 study, all but one of thirty-six **acupuncture** patients attained excellent pain relief from carpal tunnel syndrome, which is a kind of chronic pain in the hands associated with repetitive motion. In a follow-up study, twenty-four patients showed 2.5 to 8.5 years of pain relief (see p. 144).

CERVICAL SPONDYLITIS

- From India, the herb **guggul** has been traditionally used for one thousand years to treat cervical spondylitis, a type of cervical inflammation and arthritis (see 244).

CHRONIC FATIGUE

- **Ginseng, Panaz Ginseng,** or *Crenshen* ("man root" in Chinese) is an "adaptogen" which can both stimulate and sedate and can serve a normalizing influence on energy levels. Studies indicate that ginseng increases energy, counteracts fatigue, and has a mild aphrodisiac effect (see p. 164).

Caution: Potential negative effects of ginseng excessive use or overdose include postmenopausal bleeding (stop using it), anxiety, high blood pressure, nervousness, insomnia, skin lesions, diarrhea, euphoria, and breast tenderness. It should not be used with any acute inflammatory disease, such as arthritis, and should not be used if you have hypertension. Vitamin C and other acids reduce absorption. Vitamin E and flaxseed oil increase effectiveness. Typical preparation and dose is 5 percent ginsenosides or between 200 and 500 mg per day (see pp. 315–16). Ginseng should be used in cycles of daily for two months, then abstain for two weeks.

CIRRHOSIS AND ALCOHOLIC LIVER DISEASE

- **Milk thistle** has been used since the eighteenth century to treat jaundice, and more recently hepatitis and cirrhosis, for increasing the production of bile used to break down fats, and detoxification of pollutants, toxins, and chemicals in the liver through promoting the production of antioxidant enzymes. It is a powerful antioxidant and liver protective as well as reparative since it seems to stimulate the growth of new liver cells. Usual dosage for supplements is 140 mg of 70 percent silymarin taken twice a day with meals. Milk thistle can result in loose stools at high doses. If symptoms persist, fiber compounds such as pectin, guar gum, psyllium, or oat bran may be used, to avoid this laxative side effect (see pp. 167–68).

COLDS/FLU

- Today, the top-selling remedy in France for flu is **Oscillococcinum,** a homeopathic medicine, representing 50 percent of the market. However, Oscillococcinum was not found to be effective in patients with severe flu (see p. 206).
- Some **phytochemicals,** nutrients found in fruits and vegetables, appear to be helpful for minor illnesses, such as colds (see p. 92).
- In conventional medical facilities where traditional Chinese medicine (**TCM**) is offered, it may be the most reasonable first approach for certain conditions, such as colds. Treatment with TCM generally produces positive changes within one to three months (see p. 125).

- Americans now use **herbs** for a variety of minor conditions, the most common being colds (see p. 155).
- **Echinacea purpurea** is an herb that is primarily used to prevent and treat the common cold, flu, and upper respiratory tract infections; to enhance immune system function; and to treat systemic *Candida* (a yeastlike fungi) infections. It is thought to be a transient immunostimulant. There is good clinical research support for its use in colds, flus, and upper respiratory infections, but research on other applications is more equivocal (see p. 159). When using echinacea to prevent cold and flu, or to relieve their symptoms, it should be taken in small doses every few hours, with a maximum length of treatment of six to eight successive weeks. Between any such treatment periods, you should abstain from taking any echinacea for at least two weeks. A typical preparation and dose is any one of the following three times a day: 0.5–1 g of the dried root, or a cup of tea made with that amount of dried root; 325–650 mg of the freeze-dried plant; 1–2 ml of *E. purpurea* juice stabilized in 22 percent ethanol alcohol; 2–4 ml (1–2 tsp.) of a 1:5 alcohol solution; 1–2 ml (0.5–1 tsp.) of a 1:1 fluid extract; 100–250 mg of the dry powdered extract of 6.5:1 or 3.5 percent echinacoside (see pp. 315–16). Among the cautions and contraindications are its use in patients with autoimmune disease; with tuberculosis, leukosis, collagenosis, or multiple sclerosis. Continuous use may result in immunosupression.
- Researchers have found that **ginseng** extract stimulates the immune system and helps prevent colds and flu (see p. 165).
- **Ephedra,** a twiggy herb, has proven valuable in treating colds (see p. 173). Ephedra can be dangerous for people with high blood pressure or heart disease (see p. 173). It may cause or worsen hypertension, arrythmias, stroke, pheochromocythoma, thyrotoxicosis, glaucoma, nervousness, anxiety, insomnia, palpitations, hyperglycemia, and can result in death.
- Influenza patients became symptom-free more quickly than a placebo group when treated with **botanicals and homeopathy** (see p. 194).
- Classical **homeopathy** is considered a complete medical system, capable of addressing a wide array of health problems, such as colds and flu (see pp. 200–203).

Caution: Echinacea should not be taken if you are pregnant or planning a pregnancy. It should not be taken if you have an autoimmune disease (such as multiple sclerosis or lupus). Echinacea may also interfere with drugs taken for immunosuppressive therapy, as well as treatments for HIV and tuberculosis, since echinacea does temporarily stimulate or enhance the immune system.

COLIC

- **Homeopathy** has always been considered particularly helpful for children. It is reported to resolve, gently and effectively, such problems as recurrent colic (see p. 201).
- A small body of published clinical evidence now suggests that **spinal manipulation** might be helpful for infantile colic (see p. 225). In a study cited in a 1994 issue of *Consumer Reports*, 316 babies with infant colic were treated with spinal manipulation, and almost all got better within two weeks. However, the study had several design flaws (see p. 225).

CONSTIPATION

- A study evaluated the effectiveness of multiple **Maharishi Ayur-Ved interventions** (see p. 240) among a group of 126 adults with ten chronic diseases, including constipation. Each received a nutritional program, herbal preparations, and daily lifestyle guidelines. Seventy-nine percent of participants showed improvement (see p. 240).

Caution: Consumers should be cautious in the use of teas whose labels imply that they promote weight loss, and should examine the list of ingredients carefully for laxatives. *Aloe barbadensis*, an herb, is a frequent ingredient and should not be taken during pregnancy or lactation and may cause intestinal cramps (see p. 175).

DEMENTIA AND/OR MEMORY LOSS

- Patients treated with **Qi Gong** exercise showed improvement in memory (see pp. 80–81).
- A 1993 randomized clinical trial (RCT) of Alzheimer's patients indicated that **music therapy** enhanced memory of past events and improved mood (see p. 83).
- Many modern pharmaceuticals have been derived from traditional Chinese medicine **(TCM) herbs.** Huperzine A, for example, derived from the herb *Huperzia serrata,* is used to treat senile dementia (see pp. 123–24).
- Commission E in Germany has approved the herb ***Ginkgo biloba*** for treatment of dementia-related memory deficits (see p. 163).
- In a twelve-week randomized clinical trial (RCT), **Ginsana** produced improvements in general physical condition, concentration, memory, and sleep, in sixty subjects aged twenty-two to eighty (see p. 165).
- Some forty neurological disorders are classified in traditional Indian **Ayurvedic medicine** as *vata* disorders (see p. 238). The herb *Centella asiatica* is valued as a memory enhancer. In the treatment of dementia, Ayurveda uses a number of herbal compounds as memory enhancers (see p. 238).

Caution: Ginkgo, an herb, can affect blood clotting if blood thinners (such as the drug Coumadin or warfarin) are also used. If you are taking such medications, talk with your doctor. If you have migraine headaches, ginkgo might increase their frequency. If you have any condition that diminishes your ability to absorb nutrients, you should discuss vitamin B_6 supplementation with your doctor. Gingko can induce decreased platelet activity, bleeding, cross-allergenicity with poison ivy; can cause cheilitis and gastrointestinal irritation. Do not use while pregnant or lactating.

DENTAL CRANIOMANDIBULAR DISORDER

- **Acupuncture** demonstrates positive results with dental craniomandibular disorder (see p. 148). For dental patients, this delicate joint of the jaw and skull is often the source of pain from such conditions as bruxism, or grinding the teeth.

DEPRESSION

- A study in 1985 revealed that patients who engaged in an eight-week program of **meditation** experienced less pain, anxiety, and depression than patients treated with conventional medications and physiotherapy (see p. 65).
- Results of a study suggest that **hypnotic imaging** may help in producing physical and psychological changes that will help patients deal with breast cancer by reducing depression (see p. 71).
- Research is still preliminary, but in Europe, steroid hormone **DHEA** products are being marketed for menopause-related depression (see p. 109).
- In a 1985 study, **acupuncture** compared favorably to treatment with conventional depression medications. After five weeks of acupuncture treatment, 70 percent of depression patients were cured or markedly improved, compared to 65 percent taking medication (see p. 148).
- Americans now use **herbs** mostly for a variety of minor conditions, the most common of which is depression (see pp. 154–55).
- Commission E in Germany has approved *Ginkgo biloba* extract for the symptomatic treatment of depression (see p. 163).
- Mental functioning of fifty patients with depression improved when treated with the commercial ginseng-based product **Ginsana,** a European brand of ginseng extract (see p. 165).
- **St. John's wort** is one of the powerhouses of contemporary herbal medicine. It has become very popular in the United States in a short period of time, and is used primarily to combat depression (see p. 169).

- In a 1988 study, twenty-three depressed subjects were placed on a **therapeutic diet** free of caffeine and sucrose for one or two weeks, then, challenged, in a blinded fashion, with caffeine and sucrose. When challenged, 50 percent responded with significant and sustained deterioration of their moods (see p. 189).
- In a study, twenty-four depressed elderly patients showed significant improvement on one gram of amino acid **L-acetylcarnitine** taken daily for one month, as compared with placebo (see p. 189).
- Among subjects in an **Ayurvedic** program, those who were highly adherent to the prescribed therapy showed a decrease in depression (see p. 241).
- A study of elderly women who had undergone surgical repair of hip fractures found that those with **strong religious beliefs** were able to walk farther at discharge, and also showed lower levels of depressive symptoms (see pp. 253–54).

Caution: Research on the hormone melatonin remains inconclusive, but some studies suggest that melatonin can deepen or induce depression (see p. 112).

Caution: Depression can be a side effect of acupuncture (see p. 142).

Caution: If you are taking St. John's wort, sunlight may cause a photosensitive reaction that can irritate and inflame the skin of light-skinned individuals. If you are taking any other antidepressants, discuss the use of St. John's wort with your doctor before using it. Do not take it if you are planning a pregnancy, during pregnancy, or when breast-feeding. In combination with common drugs such as Prozac (SSRI) or Nardil (MAO inhibitor), St. John's wort can result in fever, confusion, and muscle spasms. The standard MAO food warnings apply with St. John's wort. Typical preparation and dose are 300 mg of the standardized (0.3 percent) hypericin (thought to be the active agent), three times per day with meals, for a total of 900 mg per day. It may also be taken as two 450 mg tablets, two times per day. Or drink 1 to 2 cups per day of the dried herb tea boiled for ten minutes (see pp. 315–16). St. John's wort should be taken with meals to avoid stomach discomfort. At least four weeks should be allowed in order for blood levels to reach adequate concentrations to be effective.

DIABETES

- **Exercise** is now being called a "breakthrough" intervention in diabetes and is supported by decades of research from the National Institutes of Health. Patients who exercise may prevent or recover from diabetes (see p. 34).
- **Exercise and movement,** which are used in many MindBody therapies, decrease the harmful effects of stress and help prevent some of the diseases of aging, including diabetes (see p. 62).
- Research supporting **low-fat diets** is powerful and voluminous. Along with exercise, low-fat diets are also effective at controlling adult-onset diabetes (see p. 90).
- Eating a **plant-based diet** provides high levels of fiber. Water-soluble fibers, such as gums and pectins, protect against diabetes by binding in the gut with bile acids, thus preventing the reabsorption of these bile acids (see p. 91).
- Long valued in Asia as an adaptogen, the herb **ginseng** has become one of the top three herbal products in the United States. Use of ginseng includes the treatment of diabetes (see p. 164).
- **Botanicals, nutritional supplements, and counseling and psychotherapy** are effective treatments for diabetes millitus (see pp. 189–90).
- A number of **herbal compounds** have been used to treat diabetes (see p. 238).
- A 1989 pilot study evaluated the effectiveness of multiple **Maharishi Ayur-Ved interventions** (see p. 240) among 126 adults with ten chronic diseases, including diabetes. Each received an individualized nutritional program, herbal preparations, and daily lifestyle guidelines. Seventy-nine percent of the participants showed improvement (see p. 240).
- Presently, the aspect of **Ayurvedic medicine** that will probably be most investigated in the West is its potential for conversion of its herbal components into standardized drugs. Many Ayurvedic herbs are currently being examined for the treatment and prevention of diabetes (see p. 249).

Caution: Borderline chromium deficiency may help to trigger adult-onset diabetes, but is not the underlying cause of diabetes, so chromium cannot cure the disease (see p. 101). Chromium supplementation does present some dangers (see p. 101).

DIARRHEA

- In a study, ninety-three patients with advanced cancer were treated with a combination of drugs and **Qi Gong** exercises, while a control group was treated with drugs alone; 33 percent of the Qi Gong patients were free from diarrhea (see p. 81).
- Americans now use **herbs** mostly for a variety of minor conditions, one of the more common of which is diarrhea (see p. 155).
- A 1996 study showed that a **diet** based on medium-chain triglycerides reduced chronic diarrhea and malabsorption associated with HIV, compared with a long-chain-triglyceride-based diet (see p. 190).
- In a very small 1993 study, five AIDS patients with intractable diarrhea improved markedly after daily treatment of the colon (**colonic insufflations**) with medical ozone (see p. 191).
- **Homeopathy** has always been considered particularly helpful for children. It is reported to resolve, gently and effectively, such problems as diarrhea (see p. 201).
- From a 1994 study in *Pediatrics,* individualized **classical homeopathic treatment** using the 30C potency of different homeopathic remedies for childhood diarrhea has been successful (see p. 211). A series of three clinical studies conducted by noted homeopath Dr. Jennifer Jacobs demonstrated positive outcomes using different homeopathic remedies depending on the specific diarrhea symptoms.

Caution: The fat substitute olestra, according to some reports, interferes with the body's ability to absorb carotenoids, which are nutritious reddish pigments found in fruits and vegetables. One of the frequently reported side effects of preventing fat absorption is diarrhea (see p. 98).

Caution: Chronic ingestion of the amino acid selenium can cause diarrhea (see p. 100).

Caution: Large doses of L-carnitine may cause diarrhea (see p. 106).

Caution: Short-term adverse effects of herbal laxative use can include stomach cramps, nausea, vomiting, and diarrhea. With chronic use, laxative dependency can develop, causing sluggish bowel and even loss of colon function, accompanied by severe pain and constipation, which in some cases can require surgical removal of the colon. All laxatives, conventional or CAM, can cause excessive water and potassium loss if used for more than a few days. This risk is greatly increased if they are used with prescription diuretics or digitalis. Severe laxative abuse reactions include fainting, dehydration, and electrolyte disorders, which can lead to death (see p. 175).

DIVERTICULITIS

- Besides decreasing the risk of cardiovascular disease, a **low-fat diet** also decreases the risk of cancer, obesity, and diverticulitis, or pouches in the intestine, which can become inflamed or infected (see pp. 92–93).

DYSLEXIA

- **Ear acupuncture** (or auricular acupuncture) is based on the theory that the entire body can be affected by stimulating specific points on the outer ear. It is most often used for treating pain, dyslexia, and alcohol and drug addiction (see p. 141).

EAR INFECTION (SEE OTITIS MEDIA)

ECZEMA

- In a study, 14 of 20 eczema-afflicted children who completed a twelve-week **diet** excluding eggs and cow's milk responded favorably. In a birth cohort study, 1,265 children who received a diverse solid food diet during their first four months had a higher risk of developing eczema than those who did not (see p. 190).
- In a study of 40 adults with long-standing treatment-resistant skin

problems (refractory dermatitis), treatment with ten traditional **Chinese herbs** resulted in improvement in symptoms. Also, a 1981 study of seed extracts verified that its effectiveness in treating chronic eczema was comparable to corticoid drug therapy (see p. 190).

- A 1995 study showed that **autogenic training,** a form of relaxation by focusing on sensations of heaviness and warmth, and cognitive-behavioral treatment resulted in improved skin condition and less use of topical steroids (see p. 190).

- A 1989 pilot study evaluated the effectiveness of multiple **Maharishi Ayur-Ved interventions** (see p. 240) among 126 adults with ten chronic diseases including eczema. Each participant received an individualized nutritional program, herbal preparations, and daily lifestyle guidelines. Seventy-nine percent of the participants showed improvement (see p. 240).

ENURESIS

- A small body of published clinical evidence suggests that **spinal manipulation** might be helpful for childhood enuresis, or bedwetting, but it remains unproven (see p. 224).

EPILEPSY

- **Biofeedback,** a training program used to improve a person's control over autonomic body functions, is now used to treat about 150 conditions, including epilepsy (see p. 77).

EYE DISORDERS

- **Acupuncture** is used as a treatment for eye inflammation, according to a survey compiled by the World Health Organization (WHO). It is occasionally used as a last resort (see p. 142).

- **Bilberry,** which is known to include a wide number of powerful antioxidants, has been shown to be effective not only for arthritis but also for certain disorders of the eyes. Bilberry, or European blue-berry, was used by the Royal Air Force in World War II to improve night vision. There is no information at present indicating any serious side effects. There is evidence that 80–160 mg of bilberry three times per day may briefly improve night vision. Long-term use may mask serious underlying ocular diseases and should not be used without a complete ocular examination by an ophthalmologist (see pp. 315–16).

Fibromyalgia

- **Hypnotherapy** reduces muscle pain, fatigue, and sleep disturbances in fibromyalgia patients. In one study of patients with fibromyalgia, or painful benign cysts, by Hanerdos in 1991, eight sessions of hypnotism produced positive results (see p. 70).
- **MindBody** medicine is used to treat fibromyalgia. In Nashua, New Hampshire, the Matthew Thornton Health Plan has a very successful behavioral medicine pain program for patients with fibromyalgia (see p. 85).
- **Acupuncture** is used in the treatment of fibromyalgia. Dr. David J. Ramsay told the NIH in 1997 that acupuncture data was as strong as that supporting accepted Western medical therapies (see p. 149).
- **Homeopathy** can be effective in treating fibromyalgia. A 1989 study by Dr. Peter Fisher indicated that 25 percent more of the homeopathically treated fibromyalgia patients experienced pain relief than those receiving a placebo. Almost twice as many had improved sleep (see pp. 205, 211).
- **Spinal manipulation** may be helpful for fibromyalgia. A small body of published clinical evidence now suggests that spinal manipulation may be helpful for some patients (see p. 224).

Gastrointestinal (Stomach and Intestinal Disturbances)

- Gastritis can be successfully treated with **herbs.** In two studies of gastritis, Chinese herbs showed an ability to significantly improve symptoms. In one study, herbs used in combination with a pharmaceutical drug produced better results than the drug used alone (see p. 133).

- Gastritis responds to **homeopathic** treatment. In a 1966 study of the homeopathic remedy Nux vomica, forty-three of seventy-four patients responded positively to homeopathy compared to twenty-seven of seventy-three who received a placebo (see p. 209).
- *Pitta* people (**Ayurvedic medicine**) are more likely to suffer from gastritis. In addition, *pitta* people are more likely to have liver and gallbladder problems, hyperacidity, peptic ulcers, inflammatory disease, and skin problems (see pp. 232–35).
- **Aloe vera gel** has a healing effect upon the stomach and intestines, especially in the treatment of peptic ulcers and irritable bowel syndrome (IBS). Usual use is 100 mg of solid extract taken with at least 8 ounces of liquid, three times per day. There are no reported negative side effects even with indefinite periods of use (see pp. 315–16).

HAY FEVER

- Hay fever remedies in the United States include the drugs **ephedrine and pseudoephedrine.** Also, the herb ephedra, which is similar to these products, can be effective. However, each of these substances can have negative side effects (see pp. 173–74).
- Dutch researchers recently reported positive results in treating hay fever with **homeopathic** medicines. Five well-designed studies all indicated the efficacy of homeopathic remedies in hay fever treatment (see p. 203).
- **Homeopathic** treatment demonstrates efficacy in the treatment of hay fever. Several studies support this finding. In one study, approximately six hundred people were involved (see p. 204).
- **MAK-5,** a supplement containing several herbs, is used to treat hay fever. This substance, which is used in Ayurvedic medicine, has been reported to be effective in several double-blind trials (see p. 242).

HEADACHES

- **Behavioral medicine** is effective with headache patients. It is particularly effective for tension headaches, which are generally caused by a maladaptive reaction to stress (see pp. 67–68).
- **Biofeedback,** a training program used to improve a person's control over autonomic body functions, is used to treat headaches. Headache is one of about 150 conditions that appear to respond positively to biofeedback. It is often considered to be more scientific than other relaxation techniques (see pp. 76–77).
- **Acupuncture** is used as an effective treatment for headaches. In a 1984 study by Dr. Leng Loh of 48 migraine patients, 59 percent reported benefits from acupuncture, compared to 25 percent who benefited from drug therapy. Most recently in 1997, the National Institutes of Health indicated that acupuncture may be an effective treatment for headaches (see pp. 149–50).
- **Herbs** are often used as a treatment for headaches. According to a 1997 *Prevention* magazine survey, 22 percent of all medicinal herb use in America is used for the treatment of headaches. Herbs generally have a milder effect than pharmaceutical drugs, and often have fewer side effects (see p. 155).
- **Feverfew** is an herb in the daisy family that is frequently used in England for migraine prevention, arthritis treatment, as well as fever and menstrual problems (see p. 160). Usual dosage is to gradually increase up to 125 mg daily to prevent migraine headaches and upwards of 250 mg per day to prevent arthritic pain. Any feverfew product should be standardized to contain at least 0.4 percent parthenolide. Feverfew should not be used during pregnancy since it may stimulate uterine contractions and should not be used with anticoagulants such as Coumadin since feverfew acts as an anticoagulant. Although studies indicate that it can prevent and decrease the frequency and intensity of migraines, there is no evidence of a positive effect once a migraine is in onset.
- **Naturopathic** treatment of headaches can be effective. Headaches are one of the conditions naturopaths most commonly treat, using a wide, eclectic array of treatments including nutritional therapy, MindBody therapies, homeopathy, and herbal therapies (see p. 192).

- **Herbs** are used to treat migraine headaches. A 1988 study demonstrated reduced symptoms in migraine patients who used herbal medications (see p. 192).
- **Chiropractic** treatment of headaches may be effective, but results are equivocal. In a number of clinical studies, chiropractic was found to be at least as effective as medication and massage (see p. 223).
- *Brahmi* is valued in the treatment of headaches. This Ayurvedic herbal preparation is an anti-anxiety substance, and can be applied in conjunction with yoga and dietary therapy (see p. 239).
- **Maharishi Ayur-Ved interventions** (see p. 240) show significant success in the treatment of headaches. In a 1989 pilot study of 126 people who used these interventions for a variety of conditions, including headaches, 79 percent of the participants showed improvement, 14 percent showed no change, and 7 percent became worse. This suggests that the approach has merit (see p. 240).

Caution: Homeopathy appears not too effective for migraine headaches. Two well-controlled studies on the homeopathic treatment of migraines did not show that homeopathy was more effective than placebo. One study, conducted in 1997, was very well designed and showed no effect (see p. 208).

Caution: Effectiveness of chiropractic interventions for headache is promising, though not clearly effective, based on the findings to date. Relief of common headache would be significant if it resulted in long-term relief. Studies do not confirm that long-term relief occurs in the presence of chiropractic manipulation (see p. 223).

Caution: Approximately 10 percent of people using the herb feverfew may experience mouth ulcers. Other reported side effects are gastrointestinal upset, anxiety, and actually inducing headaches. Feverfew interacts with blood thinners, or anticoagulants, so consult with your doctor if you are using blood-thinning medications (see pp. 315–16).

HEART CONDITIONS

- **MindBody** therapies create a relaxed state in the treatment of heart diseases. Therefore, they can be of significant value. A wide array of

MindBody therapies have been applied to heart disease and appear to decrease the psychosocial stress that is related to many heart conditions (see p. 60).

- **Exercise and movement** reduce harmful effects of heart disease. They decrease the harmful effect of stress and help prevent some of the diseases of aging, including heart diseases (see p. 62).
- **Meditation** can be effective in the treatment of heart disease. Meditation appears to have a direct salutory effect upon breathing, and proper breathing is an important component in the reduction of stress, which is beneficial for the health of the heart (see p. 62).
- **Behavioral medicine** in the treatment of heart disease can have positive effects. Behavioral medicine is particularly effective for conditions that are primarily caused by stress and mood disorders, and for conditions that are strongly affected by stress and other psychological factors. These conditions include many types of heart disease (see pp. 67–68).
- **Hypnotherapy** is currently used in the treatment of heart disease to modify feelings of pain, anxiety, and fear, and to help patients accept new behaviors. A hypnotic state is similar to other forms of deep relaxation (see p. 69).
- **Imagery** can be effective for heart disease. In a 1994 controlled experiment, Dr. Christopher Sharpley used biofeedback-assisted imagery to train healthy volunteers to lower their heart rate activity while being exposed to stressors. Effects of this exercise were maintained twenty-eight weeks after the study had concluded (see p. 73).
- **Biofeedback** can help in the treatment of heart disease. Using various biological monitoring instruments, patients learn to consciously regulate the responses of the autonomic nervous system, including brain waves, muscle tension, blood flow, heart rate, and blood pressure (see p. 76).
- **Tai chi** exercises, in a 1992 study, improved heart rate and blood pressure as much as walking. In a 1995 study, elderly tai chi practitioners showed significantly improved cardiorespiratory function, compared to sedentary people (see p. 79).
- **Qi Gong** exercises are used in the treatment of heart disease. A twenty-year study in China, completed in 1993, reported benefits of lowered blood pressure. Patients using Qi Gong were 50 percent less likely to become ill or die from stroke (see pp. 80–81).

- **Music therapy** was used as a pacemaker, helping hearts to achieve normal heart rhythms, in two studies by Haas in 1980 and Bason in 1992. It also reduces anxiety in heart attack patients (see pp. 82–83).
- **MindBody** medicine is used in the treatment of heart disease. It has been used very effectively in a program developed by Dr. Dean Ornish that combines a vegetarian diet with yoga, meditation, group support, and moderate exercise. This program has halted progression of heart disease, as well as reversed it (see p. 84).
- **Diet,** in heart disease treatment, has been shown to be very effective as a means of preventing and correcting various cardiovascular conditions. Many studies support dietary therapy for heart disease. Most clinicians and researchers now agree that a low-fat diet is generally the best diet for the heart (see pp. 88–91).
- **Omega-3** protects against heart arrhythmias. It inhibits blood clotting and relaxes smooth muscles in blood vessel walls. The best source of this nutrient is flaxseed oil (see p. 93).
- **Vitamin E,** in the treatment of heart disease, can have powerful positive effects. Many studies show that vitamin E reduces clogging of the arteries, mitigates angina, and reduces coronary risk. A Harvard study of 135,000 health professionals found that those who took daily vitamin E supplements had one-fourth to one-third less coronary risk than those who didn't (see pp. 95–97).
- The nutrient **beta-carotene** can be effective in the treatment of heart disease. According to the Coronary Primary Prevention study, low blood levels of carotenoids are associated with coronary disease. In general, it is best to obtain beta carotene in its natural form from deeply colored yellow, red, and orange fruits and vegetables (see pp. 97–98).
- **Fiber** from whole oats, rice, and other grains helps prevent heart disease. At present, the United States government allows only four health claims to be made regarding the value of foodstuffs in preventing disease. One of these four claims is that soluble fiber from whole oats helps to prevent coronary problems (see p. 99).
- **Selenium,** a mineral, appears to have some value in the treatment of heart disease. In a 1994 Chinese study by Han, pregnant women at risk for high blood pressure showed reduction and prevention of hypertension. Epidemiological studies indicate that low selenium intake is associated with increased heart disease (see pp. 100–101).

- **Coenzyme Q_{10},** a nutrient, has shown promising results in the treatment of heart disease. It may protect against tissue damage in heart disease, and may help prevent heart disease through antioxidant action (see pp. 103–105).
- **L-carnitine** is an amino acid which may be of value for treating heart disease. Among the claims for L-carnitine are that it increases blood flow and enhances energy production during exercise. It appears to reduce angina and ischemia (see pp. 106–107).
- A 1995 study found low levels of the hormone **DHEA** in men with blocked arteries. Another study showed that DHEA supplementation reduced platelet aggregation, which occurs when blood cells stick together (see p. 110).
- **Melatonin** is a hormone that may be of some value in helping to prevent heart disease. It is a powerful antioxidant that helps to protect tissues. Some researchers believe that it may help retard the aging process (see pp. 110–12).
- **Chiropractic therapy** has been shown to be of value in improving overall health, and thereby improving cardiovascular function. However, most studies do not support the use of chiropractic manipulation as a specific modality for cardiovascular disorders, including hypertension. One study indicated chiropractic had no effect upon high blood pressure (see pp. 219, 224).
- **Garlic** may lower cholesterol, thin the blood, serve as a powerful antioxidant, lower blood pressure, and stimulate the immune system. Due to garlic's action on blood platelets, it is necessary to reduce doses of blood thinners and aspirin (see p. 161). Recent studies indicate that garlic may not actually lower cholesterol very much and may be of benefit to the heart by influencing other biological factors.
- **Herbs** are often used in the treatment of heart disease. **Hawthorn,** an herb, has been shown in several studies to be effective in relieving symptoms of heart disease such as angina. Hawthorn helps improve exercise tolerance, blood pressure, and anginal pain (see p. 166). High dosages can cause hypotension (too low blood pressure) and sedation.
- **Cascara sagrada (buckthorn), senna, and aloe** are not in widespread use, but in people with irregular heartbeat, these herbs can reduce blood levels of potassium and increase the effects of drugs

that regulate heart rhythms, such as lanoxin. Senna, cascara sagrada, and aloe are laxatives that can cause water and potassium loss. These are particularly risky if combined with prescription diuretics or digitalis. Consult with your doctor if you have any heart problems before taking any of these herbs (see p. 175).

- **Naturopathy** is employed in the treatment of heart disease. Atherosclerosis has been shown to respond to the eclectic approach of naturopathy, which includes dietary therapy, supplementation, and botanical medicines (see pp. 187–88).

- **Ayurvedic herbs** are used in the treatment of heart conditions. The goal of the Ayurvedic approach is to restore constitutional balance (see p. 238).

- *Guggul* is an herb found safe and effective for treating coronary heart disease. There is a long history of its positive effect on cardiovascular disease both through lowering cholesterol and as an antioxidant. Clinical studies recommend 25 mg of guggulsterone, three times per day. Usually the standardized supplement contains only 5 percent guggulsterone, which translates into an effective dosage of 500 mg three times per day with meals. In a 1988 Indian study, *guggul* produced reductions in blood cholesterol. It also appeared to cause a decrease in low-density lipoprotein, or LDL, levels. *Guggul* is considered to be an emenogogue, or agent that promotes menstruation, and should not be used during pregnancy (see pp. 243–44).

- **Ayurvedic medicine** treatment of heart disease appears to be promising. In a 1995 study, an Ayurvedic treatment provoked improvements in patients with refractory congestive heart failure (CHF) (see p. 243).

- **Lifestyle-based heart disease interventions** reduce development of complications. They also appear to induce regression in the blockages of the coronary arteries (see p. 301).

Caution: High doses of steroids used by athletes have been linked to heart disease, stroke, cardiomyopathy, and possibly cancer. Other adverse effects include liver toxicity, decreases in plasma testosterone, atrophy of the testes, prostate enlargement, impotence, decreased sperm count, breast enlargement in men, increased injury of muscles and tendons, increase in serum cholesterol, and decrease in high-density lipoproteins

(HDL), the "good" cholesterol. Psychological side effects can include euphoria, aggressiveness, irritability, nervous tension, changes in libido, mania, and psychosis (see p. 113).

Caution: Licorice can induce a rapid heartbeat. This can occur when there is excessive consumption over an extended period of time, which causes a sodium-potassium imbalance, with symptoms of fluid retention and rapid heartbeat (see pp. 122–23). There are potential negative interactions of high-dose licorice with antihypertensives, diuretics, diogoxin, and other digitalis derivatives (digitalic glycosides).

Caution: Ephedra increases heart rate. This herb, also known as *ma huang* in Chinese medicine, can be valuable in treating colds, but it has a stimulating effect, similar to that of caffeine.

HIGH BLOOD PRESSURE

- **Exercise** is effective against high blood pressure. It has been endorsed as beneficial by the National Institutes of Health, the A.M.A., and the United States Surgeon General (see p. 34).
- **MindBody exercises and movement** decrease the harmful effects of high blood pressure. They help to create a relaxed state, and decrease the negative effects of stress (see p. 62).
- **Meditation** reduces both systolic and diastolic blood pressure. This was shown in a study conducted by Cooper in 1978 (see p. 65) and a major 1997 study by Wenneberg and colleagues indicating blood pressure reductions with inner-city black men.
- **Behavioral medicine** helps high blood pressure patients. Components of cognitive behavioral interventions include education, training in coping skills, training in motivation techniques, behavioral rehearsal, and group support (see pp. 67–69).
- **Hypnotherapy** induces decreased blood pressure. Hypnosis creates reduced sympathetic nervous system activity, decreased blood pressure, slowed heart rate, and slower frequency brain waves. It can also bring about changes in thinking and behavior (see p. 69).
- **Imagery** is used to treat high blood pressure. It has been shown to reduce stress, help patients manage pain, reduce heart rate reactivity, and decrease resting heart rate. It can help patients enter an

altered state of consciousness, similar to that achieved by hypnosis (see p. 73).

- **Biofeedback,** a training program used to improve a patient's control over autonomic body functions, is sometimes used in the treatment of high blood pressure. It appeals to many patients because it encourages them to actively participate in their therapy. It also can significantly reduce treatment costs (see p. 77).
- **Tai chi** exercise improves heart rate and blood pressure. A 1992 study by Dr. Jin in Australia indicated that tai chi improved heart rate and blood pressure as much as brisk walking (see p. 79).
- **Qi Gong** exercises can help lower high blood pressure. A number of studies support the use of Qi Gong in treating cardiovascular disorders. In one study, patients using Qi Gong averaged a 10 percent drop in blood pressure (see p. 81).
- A diet centered on **plant foods,** or phytonutrients, presents less risk for high blood pressure patients. Animal fat has been shown to be the primary dietary factor in predisposing patients to cardiovascular risk. If and when animal fats are eaten, portions should be small (see p. 89).
- Women at risk for high blood pressure showed a reduction of hypertension when using the mineral **selenium.** This was demonstrated in a 1994 Chinese study by Han of pregnant women at risk for high blood pressure (see p. 100).
- **SOD** is an enzyme that has been investigated for its ability to protect against drops in blood pressure. This substance is a powerful antioxidant that may decrease the damage caused by oxygen deprivation to organs of the body (see pp. 105–106).
- **Licorice** reduces levels of potassium in the blood (see pp. 122–23).
- **Salvia,** an herb, has been applied in coronary artery disease and in other cases where there has been damage to body tissues, such as after a stroke. It promotes circulation in the small blood vessel beds, reduces blood pressure, and reduces cholesterol (see p. 123).
- **Garlic** has become one of the most popular substances for reducing cardiovascular risk factors. This medicinal application is partly based on a large number of clinical studies (see pp. 161–62).
- **Hawthorn** produces a mild reduction in blood pressure. Several studies indicate the healthful effects that this herb has upon the cardiovascular system (see p. 166).

- **Chiropractic** therapy can be of value in reducing high blood pressure, according to chiropractor Dr. Chester Wilk of Chicago (see p. 219).
- **Yoga** exercise can be effective in helping to reduce high blood pressure. It can induce a relaxed state in the autonomic nervous system (see p. 246).
- **Parental love** in a person's childhood can help protect against high blood pressure many years later. In a thirty-five-year study at the University of Arizona School of Medicine, doctors found that people who described their parents in positive terms during their middle-aged years were far less likely to suffer from a number of chronic conditions, including high blood pressure (see p. 260).
- **Pets** can help to lower blood pressure. In a 1988 study, researchers found that heart attack patients who had pets were even more likely to survive than patients who had a living spouse, or extensive family support (see pp. 263–64).
- **Prayer** can help to lower blood pressure. In numerous studies, Harvard's Dr. Herbert Benson has shown that prayer has a positive effect on many physical functions, including blood pressure (see pp. 267–68).

Caution: When combined with diuretics, such as lasix, or heart stimulants, such as lanoxin, licorice can cause muscle weakness and irregular heartbeats. Do not use licorice if you have high blood pressure or irregularities in heartbeats (see pp. 122–23).

Caution: Treatment with *Dasheng Jiangya* oral liquid, a Chinese herbal preparation, showed no significant effect upon high blood pressure, although it did appear to have other beneficial effects (see p. 132).

Caution: Ephedra is a powerful herb which can increase blood pressure to dangerous levels (see p. 173).

Caution: Two studies on chiropractic manipulation showed different results in its effect on high blood pressure. A 1985 study indicated that chiropractic manipulation did not improve blood pressure, but a 1988 study indicated that it did (see p. 224).

Impotence

- **Ginseng** has long been used to treat impotence. Ginseng is an adaptogenic herb that improves the function of the adrenal glands and enables the body to respond more favorably to stressors. It is also believed to increase circulation (see p. 164).
- **Saw palmetto** is an herb that is commonly used to treat prostate disorders, including those that contribute to impotence. Several inconclusive studies have indicated that saw palmetto may reduce the size of an enlarged prostate (see p. 168) but urinary flow is improved without a reduction in actual size.

Infertility

- **Traditional Chinese medicine** has successfully treated some cases of infertility. In one study, researchers using a combination of herbs elicited pregnancies in 32 percent of females, compared to 24 percent who were treated with standard medications (see p. 134).
- **Acupuncture** was as successful as hormone therapy in helping a group of women conceive, according to a 1992 study by Gerhard and Postneek (see p. 148).

Insomnia

- **Qi Gong** exercises helped patients with insomnia, according to a 1996 review of literature by Dr. Kenneth Sancier, President of the Qigong Institute in Menlo Park, California.
- **Melatonin,** a hormone, is among the most popular aids for overcoming insomnia. Researchers generally gave 2 mg of melatonin at bedtime. Research is still in the preliminary stages (see p. 111).
- **Herbs** are commonly used to treat insomnia. Insomnia is the sixth-most common condition for which herbs are used in America, accounting for 18 percent of all herb use, according to a 1997 *Prevention* magazine survey (see p. 155).
- **Valerian** is an herb that is frequently used for insomnia. In a German study, 72 percent of insomniacs who used valerian found relief from the condition. In another study, the herb helped 75 percent of

patients with insomnia. Valerian is used to relieve insomnia and restlessness and as a muscle relaxant, although researched evidence is fairly limited at the present time (see pp. 171–72).

- *Brahmi* is an Ayurvedic herb that appears to have some effectiveness in the treatment of insomnia. This herb, which is a mild sedative, is also reported to improve memory (see p. 238).

Caution: Some people are stimulated by the hormone melatonin and may have nightmares or hangovers. Also, a 1997 paper by the National Sleep Foundation claimed it may harm the reproductive system (see p. 00). Some studies suggest that melatonin can deepen or induce depression, lower luteinizing hormone (LH) levels, increase REM or dream sleep, and exacerbate allergies. Patients taking cortisone should avoid it. Also, some preliminary data suggest that melatonin may cause vasoconstriction (constriction of blood vessels), may inhibit fertility, may suppress the male sexual drive, and may produce hypothermia and retinal damage. As with any powerful hormone, melatonin should not be taken by pregnant women. Anyone considering taking melatonin for sleep disorders or jet lag should seek a medical opinion. Typical preparation and dose is 1–3 mg taken one hour before going to bed. Do not take more than 6 mg (see pp. 315–16).

Caution: As a tranquilizing herb, valerian may worsen depression. An overdose can cause muscle problems and liver toxicity. Valerian should not be taken in conjunction with antidepressants or sedatives, since it may enhance the effects of these drugs. In a few instances, valerian may cause mild, temporary stomach upset or nausea. There are many typical preparations, and any one of the following doses can be taken thirty to forty-five minutes before going to bed: 1–2 g of dried root (which can be taken as a tea); 4–6 ml of a 1:5 alcohol solution; 102 ml of fluid extract; 250–450 mg of powdered extract; or 150–300 mg of standardized (0.8 percent valeric acid) extract (see pp. 315–16).

IRRITABLE BOWEL SYNDROME (IBS)

- **Biofeedback,** a training program used to increase control over autonomic body functions, is now used to treat about 150 disorders, including irritable bowel syndrome (IBS) (see p. 77).
- **Naturopathic medicine** has been used to treat irritable bowel syn-

drome. Naturopaths often treat the disease in conjunction with medical doctors. Naturopaths focus relatively more upon the whole person than the disease condition. This can be helpful in the treatment of irritable bowel syndrome, which may have a number of causative factors. Among the treatments administered are dietary therapy, homeopathy, and psychotherapy (see pp. 191–92).

- **Homeopathy** is sometimes applied as a stand-alone therapy for irritable bowel syndrome (IBS). A large study using Asafoetida 3X found a statistically significant improvement in patients receiving the medication (see p. 209).
- **Ayurvedic medicine** is sometimes used to treat irritable bowel syndrome (IBS) (see pp. 238–39).

Ischemia

- **Transcendental meditation** elicited improvements in patients with ischemia, or poor circulation, due to coronary artery disease, in a 1997 study by Zamara (see p. 65).
- **L-carnitine,** an amino acid, has a protective effect among cardiac patients, according to a number of well-designed human studies. According to Bartels, Singh, and others, it appears to reduce angina and ischemia (see p. 107).

Kidney Stones

- **A plant-based, or phytonutrient, diet** appears to confer some degree of protection against the formation of kidney stones. Excessive protein intake, which can occur when high amounts of meat are eaten, appears to predispose people to kidney stone formation and impaired kidney function (see pp. 94–95).

Liver Disease

- **Licorice** is used in traditional Chinese medicine to treat many conditions, including hepatitis. It is present in about one-third of all

Chinese herbal preparations, and is thought to enhance the effectiveness of many herbal formulas (see p. 122).

- **Bupleurum,** one of the most frequently used herbs in Japanese herbal medicine, is often used to treat liver disease (see p. 123).
- **Ginseng,** an herb, is believed by some botanical researchers to be of value in helping to prevent liver toxicity (see p. 164).
- **Milk thistle** has a long history of use in the treatment and prevention of liver problems. It contains a substance called silymarin, which is used to treat toxic liver damage, and is used as a supportive treatment in chronic inflammatory liver disease and hepatic cirrhosis. It also stimulates formation of new liver cells (see p. 167).
- **Ayurvedic preparations** are sometimes used to treat liver disease (see p. 238).

Caution: Acetaminophen has been linked to sudden liver failure (see p. 55).

Caution: In large quantities, cinnamon can irritate the liver and should not be used by people with inflammatory liver disease (see p. 123).

Caution: Comfrey, an herb, contains pyrrolizidine alkaloids, which have been associated with death and illness among livestock that graze on them. They are particularly toxic to the liver, causing a blockage of the hepatic veins (veins in the liver), which can lead to fatal reactions. Comfrey cannot be recommended for internal use. Comfrey products for internal use may still be available in some stores, but have reportedly been removed from the market (see pp. 172–73).

Caution: Chaparral, an herb, may cause liver damage, but its liver toxicity is not well established (see pp. 174–75).

Lupus

- **DHEA,** the steroid hormone, may help improve symptoms of lupus in some people. In a 1995 study of twenty-five female lupus patients at the Stanford University Medical School, improvement was noted in energy, patients required less medication, and symptoms decreased (see p. 110).
- **Traditional Chinese medicine** has achieved some success in treating lupus. In a controlled study, Chinese herbs were adminis-

tered to twenty-seven lupus patients, along with prednisone. Prednisone alone was administered to a control group. The group using herbs responded more favorably (see pp. 134–35).

MEMORY DISORDERS

• **Gingko biloba,** an herb, is a commonly prescribed medication in both Germany and France for memory problems. Over twenty clinical studies have demonstrated its efficacy in relieving the symptoms of headaches, concentration difficulties, poor circulation to the extremities, cerebral vascular insufficiency, and impaired mental performance; it helps relieve presumed side effects of aging, such as short-term memory loss, vertigo, and lack of vigilance. It is also helpful in the treatment of senility, including Alzheimer's disease, cochlear deafness, tinnitus (or buzzing in the ears), senile macular degeneration and diabetic retinopathy, peripheral arterial insufficiency, arterial erectile disfunction, and idiopathic cyclic edema (or swelling). Also, preliminary indications exist for its use in the treatment of angina, congestive heart failure, asthma, urticaria (or hives), migraine, depression, and acute respiratory distress syndrome. Typical preparation and dose is a standardized extract of 24 percent flavanoid glycosides and 60 percent terpenoids with a dose of 40 mg, three times a day, or 60 mg twice a day with meals. It should be taken consistently for twelve weeks, although most people respond within two to three weeks (see p. 163).

Caution: No severe side effects generally occur, but ginkgo may cause occasional stomach/intestinal upset, headache, irritability, minor allergic skin reactions, restlessness, and possible bleeding, if used with blood-thinning agents such as aspirin or vitamin E.

MÉNIÈRE'S DISEASE

• **Acupuncture** is sometimes used to treat Ménière's disease, which consists of tinnitus or ringing in the ears, accompanied by vertigo, nausea, and vomiting. Attacks can last from a few hours up to 24 hours or more. Usually only one ear is affected. This disease is on the list released by the World Health Organization (WHO) of the 104 conditions that are most often treated effectively with acupuncture (see p. 142).

MENSTRUAL SYMPTOMS, MENOPAUSE, AND PMS

- **DHEA,** a steroid hormone, is used in Europe to combat menopause-related depression, and is being used with estrogen for hot flashes and other menopausal symptoms. DHEA also appears to be of value for postmenopausal women (see p. 109).
- *Tang kuei, tang quai,* or *dong quai,* is a traditional Chinese herb used as a treatment for menopausal symptoms. For utmost effectiveness, the herb is administered as part of a complete program, which includes other herbs. Typical preparations and doses taken three times a day are any one of the following: 1–2 g of dried root; 3–5 ml of a 1:5 alcohol solution; .5–2 ml of a 1:1 fluid extract (see pp. 315–16).
- **Herbs** are used to treat menopause in the United States and internationally. In a 1997 *Prevention* magazine study, menopause was the tenth-most common condition treated by herbs. Menopause accounted for 4 percent of all herbal use in America (see p. 155).
- A commonly applied herb for menstrual symptoms is **black cohosh,** which was originally used by Native Americans. This herb appears to improve the function of certain elements of the endocrine system (see pp.157, 158).
- **Feverfew** was used as early as Greco-Roman times for menstrual difficulties. A member of the daisy family, the herb has been studied primarily as a treatment for the prevention of migraines and treatment of arthritis pain (see p. 160).
- **Naturopathic medicine** appears to be effective in the treatment of menstrual symptoms. Among the primary components of naturopathy that are generally applied are dietary therapy, nutritional supplementation, botanical medication, and physical medicine including exercise. Considerable research supports this approach (see pp. 180–181).

Caution: For PMS, the herb *tang quai* can be taken from day fourteen until menstruation, but discontinue if heavy menstrual bleeding develops. It should not be taken during pregnancy, and can cause photosensitivity. Avoid during menstruation if you have fibroids. It may cause or aggravate bloating and diarrhea. Do not take with thrombolytic or blood thinning medications (see p. 315).

Caution: Commission E in Germany recommends the use of black cohosh for not more than six months. Potential side effects of black cohosh are heavy menstrual bleeding, headaches, dizziness, slow pulse, nausea, vomiting, and visual disturbances. For menopausal or PMS symptoms, the recommendation is 40 mg twice per day for a week to ten days prior to period. With menstrual cramps, take 40 mg three or four times per day as needed, preferably with meals. Overdose can result in extreme symptoms of all of these, as well as severe slow pulse, nausea, and vomiting. Typical preparation and doses are 10–15 drops of an alcohol solution one to two times daily, or 60 mg per day of the dry powder extract with meals. Capsules or tablets should be standardized to contain 2.5 percent triterpenes. More side effects occur with dry powder forms (see pp. 315–16). Allow up to eight weeks to determine benefits for menopausal problems, it should not be used for more than six months. Do not exceed these dosages.

Caution: See previous cautions on safe use of the steroid hormone DHEA, if it is used for menstrual symptoms.

Mononucleosis

- At the University of California Irvine Medical Center, See and colleagues examined cells infected with mononucleosis and found that the herb **echinacea** improved the immune function in these cells. This approach also worked in the cells of people with depressed immunity (see p. 160).

Nausea

- **Hypnotherapy** is documented to be effective in helping to control nausea following surgery, and the nausea associated with morning sickness (see p. 70).

- **Biofeedback,** a training program used to improve control over autonomic body functions, which is now commonly applied to about 150 conditions, is sometimes used to help control nausea. Research on biofeedback is quite extensive (see pp. 76–77).
- A large body of evidence indicates that **acupuncture** is effective for the treatment of nausea. Several well-designed studies indicate that acupuncture, as well as acupressure, controls nausea caused by recovery from surgery, seasickness, and chemotherapy (see pp. 145–46).
- **Feverfew,** an herb, was shown in one study not only to reduce frequency of migraines, but also to afford a significant reduction of nausea and vomiting during migraines (see p. 160).
- **Ginger** is widely used to treat nausea. A number of studies have been conducted, which indicate that ginger compares favorably with other antinausea substances, such as the drug scopolamine. Usual dose is 250 mg to 1 g several times per day (see p. 162).

Caution: High dosages of the mineral selenium can result in nausea (see p. 100).

Caution: When using a thrombolytic or blood thinning medication, such as Coumadin, ginger may amplify the drug's effect and cause bleeding disorders.

Caution: Ginger is not considered to be an appropriate treatment for the nausea caused by morning sickness, because some components of ginger may have mutagenic effects, which could possibly cause birth defects (see p. 163).

Caution: Short-term effects of some herbal laxatives can include nausea, as well as diarrhea, stomach cramps, and vomiting (see p. 175).

OBESITY

- A **plant-based, or phytonutrient, diet** appears to be the best dietary therapy for most people who are obese. This diet includes grains, fruits, vegetables, and legumes. A diet high in animal fat tends to predispose people to obesity (see pp. 89–90).
- **Ayurvedic medicine** is sometimes used to treat obesity. Herbal preparations are commonly used, among them guar gum and fennel (see p. 239).

Caution: See earlier cautions on excessive use of the herb ephedra, which is a common ingredient in weight-loss products. Ephedra is a powerful stimulant which can cause high blood pressure, strokes, and heart attacks.

OSTEOPOROSIS

* **Exercise** is important in preventing osteoporosis. This can consist of standard aerobic exercise and weight training, or of Eastern exercise disciplines, such as yoga and tai chi (see p. 62).
* A **plant-based diet** is helpful in preventing osteoporosis, according to the Physicians Committee for Responsible Medicine (see p. 89).
* One of only four claims for the medical value of foods is that **calcium** intake, particularly when consumed with magnesium, can slow the progression of osteoporosis. Most physicians agree that calcium supplementation helps people to receive the amounts of calcium needed to protect against osteoporosis. Consuming tofu and yams may help. Avoid carbonated drinks, especially root beer (see p. 99).
* **DHEA** is a steroid hormone that has been shown to help protect against osteoporosis. Research is still preliminary, but indications are that DHEA may reduce various problems that often occur in postmenopausal women, such as osteoporosis (see p. 109).

OTITIS MEDIA

* Infants who exclusively engaged in **breast-feeding** for at least four months had significantly fewer cases of otitis media or middle ear infections. This finding was derived from a large study in 1993 at the University of Arizona. Food allergy was also implicated in ear infections (see pp. 192–93).
* **Homeopathy** appears to be effective in helping to control ear infections in children. A 1996 study by Dr. K. H. Friese compared homeopathy with antibiotic therapy and found a decrease in pain, and fewer relapses, in children using homeopathy (see p. 210).
* A small body of evidence indicates that **spinal manipulation** may be of some value for people with otitis media. In a 1996 study, chi-

ropractic was found to have a significantly beneficial effect (see p. 225).

PAIN

- **Exercise** is helpful in reducing pain (see p. 34).
- In Germany, 77 percent of pain clinics employ **acupuncture** as part of their therapeutic regimen (see p. 48).
- **Relaxation techniques** appear to have a positive effect upon chronic pain. These techniques are generally MindBody therapies, such as imagery, hypnotherapy, tai chi, Qi Gong, and meditation (pp. 64–72, 78–81).
- **Biofeedback,** a method of improving control over autonomic body functions, is often used to treat chronic pain. Stress monitors allow patients to note their levels of stress. High levels of stress exacerbate pain (see pp. 76–77).
- **Music therapy** tends to decrease the perception of chronic pain, possibly by physically blocking the "gates of pain" that are primarily in the spinal cord (see pp. 81–83).
- In a study by Lin Chuanrong, **Chinese herbs** were administered to patients with cancer pain, along with chemotherapy. Pain relief was experienced by 68 percent of the people receiving herbs. A control group of patients receiving only chemotherapy did not fare as well; only 40 percent noted pain reduction (see p. 132).
- **Acupuncture** has long been used for chronic pain. As early as the late 1800s, it was considered among the best therapies for lower back pain. Current studies support this view (see pp. 143–44).
- **Naturopathic medicine** is often used in the treatment of chronic pain. Among the approaches that are applied are nutritional supplementation, physical medicine (including exercise), and counseling (see pp. 182–83).
- **Homeopathy** is effective for some forms of pain including childhood pains such as colic, ear infections, and teething. A review of studies conducted by Dutch professors found that homeopathy was effective against pain in eighteen of twenty studies (see p. 203).
- **Chiropractic therapy** is widely used to treat pain, particularly back pain and neck pain (which sometimes causes headaches). Chiro-

practic is considered by many to be the most effective therapy for pain in the lower back. Many studies support its efficacy (see pp. 220–23).

- Traditional Indian **Ayurvedic medicine** is sometimes used to treat painful conditions, including arthritis, sciatica, lower back pain, ulcers, and gastritis (see pp. 238–39).
- **Prayer** appears to be of benefit for pain patients. The act of prayer helps many people to relax. One study indicated that pain may be decreased in people who are prayed for by others (see pp. 267–68).
- Studies indicate that **therapeutic touch** decreases pain in postoperative patients. This approach is based on the theory that the human organism is surrounded by an energy field, such as that described as *qi* in China, or *prana* in India (see pp. 269–70).

Caution: Use of the mineral selenium, in excess, can cause abdominal pain in some people (see p. 100).

Caution: Among the most serious relatively common side effects of acupuncture are mild, transitory depression, anxiety, or fatigue (see p. 142).

Caution: Risks of chiropractic manipulation include increased pain, ruptured disks, and paralysis. Manipulation of the neck tends to produce the most serious injuries, including stroke and other neurological problems (see p. 220). Spinal manipulation is not recommended in the presence of such problems as fractures, rheumatoid arthritis, severe osteoporosis, bleeding disorders, and infection or inflammation of the spine. Manipulation of the neck can be relatively risky if the patient is taking oral contraceptives or blood-thinning medications, or has high blood pressure or other risk factors for stroke (see p. 224).

PARKINSON'S DISEASE

- Clinical research dating back to 1972 found the herb *Ginkgo biloba* to be effective in treating Parkinson's (see p. 130).
- Traditional Indian **Ayurvedic medicine** uses the herb *Mucuna pruriens* in treatment of Parkinson's. One study indicated that this approach was an effective, low-cost treatment (see p. 244).

Prostatic Hypertrophy (BPH) (Enlargement)

- **Saw palmetto,** an herb, may artificially decrease PSA (prostate specific antigen) levels. A baseline PSA is suggested prior to using saw palmetto. Inform your doctor if you are using it, since it may give false readings on a PSA test. Saw palmetto is commonly used to control benign prostatic hypertrophy (BPH) or enlargement of the prostate. Several studies have been done that indicate the herb is effective for reducing swelling of the prostate, frequent nighttime urination, and residual urine in the bladder. It is particularly helpful for men over fifty years old. Typical preparation and dose is in 160 mg doses taken two times per day for a total of 320 mg of standard liposterolic extract. Supplements should be standardized to contain 85 percent to 95 percent fatty acids and sterols (see pp. 168–69, 188–89). Side effects are relatively uncommon but may include mild abdominal discomfort, nausea, dizziness, headache, and rarely male breast enlargement. Lower the dose or stop taking saw palmetto if these side effects occur.
- A 1998 study in the special CAM issue of the *Journal of the American Medical Association* found that saw palmetto improved urinary flow in men with BPH. There are eighteen studies involving 2,939 men demonstrating that saw palmetto is as effective as the most frequent drug, Proscar, with fewer side effects (see p. 169).
- **Naturopathic medicine** is used to control prostatic hypertrophy. Among the two approaches most commonly applied are herbal medicines and nutritional supplements. Studies support both approaches (see p. 189).

Psoriasis

- Among the diseases that have responded to **Maharishi Ayur-Ved interventions** is psoriasis (see p. 240).

Respiratory Problems

- **Echinacea** is an herb used by many people in the treatment of respiratory tract infections. Clinical research supports this approach. Echinacea appears to enhance immunity (see p. 159).
- **Naturopathic medicine** is often used to treat respiratory infections. A number of modalities support the immune response to infection, including supplements, botanical medicines, and homeopathy (see pp.182–83, 194).
- **Homeopathy** can be effective in the treatment of people with upper respiratory infections, including children. In one study, children given homeopathic medicine required less antibiotic treatment (see p. 206).
- Some evidence supports the concept that **chiropractic** can be valuable for the treatment of respiratory infection (see p. 219).
- Traditional Indian **Ayurvedic medicine** is used in the treatment of respiratory infection. Herbs are generally administered, in conjunction with yogic breathing exercises (see p. 238).
- **Religious participation** has been credited as having a protective effect against many medical conditions, including respiratory tract infections (see p. 253).

Schizophrenia

- One study indicated that the herb *Ginkgo biloba* may be of some value to patients with schizophrenia. Significant improvement was noted during a thirteen-week period (see p. 131).

Sciatica

- Sciatica is one of 104 conditions most frequently treated with **acupuncture** (see p. 142).
- **Ayurvedic medicine** is sometimes used to treat sciatica. It is believed that *vata* people have a greater propensity to develop this condition (see p. 234).

SCLERODERMA

- **Superoxide dismutase,** or SOD, an antioxidant enzyme, can be useful in treating scleroderma, as well as other skin disorders. Research, however, is currently limited on this application (see p. 105).

SEXUAL DYSFUNCTION

- See Chronic Fatigue, Depression, Impotence, Infertility, and Prostatic Hypertrophy.

SINUSITIS

- **Traditional Chinese medicine** is used in the treatment of sinusitis or sinus infections. It is a reasonable first approach to take in conditions that are not life-threatening, such as sinusitis (see p. 125).
- Sinusitis is one of 104 conditions most frequently treated effectively with **acupuncture** (see p. 142).
- **Naturopathic medicine** is often used in the treatment of sinusitis. It may be used to decrease symptoms of the condition, to increase immune resistance, or to prevent sinusitis (see pp. 182–83).
- **Chiropractic therapy** has been employed to effectively treat sinusitis, although the evidence is not conclusive (see p. 219).
- Sinusitis was one of ten chronic conditions that was shown to be effectively treated with **Maharishi Ayur-Ved interventions** in a 1989 pilot study in the Netherlands (see p. 240).

SPRAINS

- **Traditional Chinese medicine** is the therapy of choice for sprains among Chinese Americans in San Francisco's Chinatown (see p. 125).
- A 1983 study indicated that **acupuncture** provides short-term relief to patients suffering from sprains (see p. 143).
- **Homeopathy** is very effective in the treatment of sprains, according

to two studies. A common, over-the-counter homeopathic preparation that was used is the commercial product Traumeel (see p. 206).

SUBSTANCE ABUSE

- **Biofeedback,** a method of improving control over autonomic body functions, is sometimes used to treat substance abuse (see pp. 76–77).
- **Traditional Chinese medicine,** particularly the use of herbs and acupuncture, is often used to treat substance abuse (see p. 136).
- One of the most popular therapies for substance abuse is **acupuncture.** A number of studies indicate the efficacy of this approach. Approximately 5 percent of all acupuncture patients worldwide are being treated for substance abuse (see pp. 144–45).
- **Ayurvedic medicine** has been used in the treatment of substance abuse. Among the multiple modalities that are generally applied are herbal medications, detoxification, diet, and yoga (see p. 239).
- **Religious commitment** has a strong influence on the prevention of and recovery from substance abuse, including the use of tobacco and alcohol (see p. 256).

TENDINITIS

- **Acupuncture** appears to be effective in the treatment of tendinitis, which is a chronic inflammation of the tendons, according to a panel convened by the National Institutes of Health in 1997 (see pp. 149–50).

THYROID DYSFUNCTION

- **Naturopathic medicine** is applied to the treatment of thyroid disorders in certain states; in other states, it is not legal. Homeopathy, which is often employed by naturopathic physicians, appears to be effective for some thyroid disorders (see p. 183).
- **Yoga** can be effective for controlling certain autonomic functions, such as thyroid function, if the approach is practiced diligently. Some Indian yogis are capable of regulating their own thyroid activity (see pp. 246–47).

Caution: Alkaloids pose dangers for people with thyroid dysfunction (see p. 173).

TINNITUS

- **Qi Gong** exercises are sometimes used to control the symptoms of tinnitus (or buzzing in the ears), according to a literature review by Dr. Kenneth Sancier of the Qigong Institute in Menlo Park, California, in 1996.

TONSILLITIS

- Germany's Commission E has approved the use of the herb ***Ginkgo biloba,*** or GBE, for tinnitus, ringing in the ears, of senile vascular origin. Ginkgo is known to increase circulation to the head (see p. 163).
- In **Ayurvedic medicine,** *kapha* people are considered to be most likely to suffer from tonsillitis (see p. 234).

TUBERCULOSIS

- **Naturopathic medicine** is sometimes applied in the treatment of tuberculosis, since the founder of naturopathy, Dr. Benedict Lust, reportedly cured himself of tuberculosis by using hydrotherapy, which is one element of naturopathy (see pp. 178–79).

ULCERS

- Among the conditions that have been treated with **Qi Gong** exercises are ulcers (see p. 80).
- **Bupleurum,** one of the most frequently used herbs in Japanese medicine, is used sometimes for treating ulcers, as well as other conditions (see p. 123).
- **Acupuncture** is occasionally used as a treatment for duodenal ulcers, and also for ulcerative colitis depending on a patient's specific symptoms (see pp. 142, 146).

- **Ayurvedic medicine** is used to treat ulcers. According to this approach, *pitta* people are most likely to suffer from ulcers. Herbs are usually used to treat the condition (see p. 234).

VAGINITIS

- Patients consuming eight ounces of yogurt daily had a threefold decrease in vaginitis, or vaginal infections, compared to those who consumed no yogurt. Yogurt contains *Lactobacillus acidophilus*, which helps to control *Candida* yeast infections (see p. 194).
- Women who used **Malaleuca alternifolia oil** were able to better control vaginal infections, including the common bacterial infection trichomonal vaginitis, according to a study performed in 1962 (see p. 194).

VARICOSE VEINS

- **Naturopathic physicians** are trained to perform a variety of minor surgical techniques, including sclerosing therapy for spider and varicose veins (see p. 181).
- **Horse chestnut** has long been used in Europe to treat circulatory problems of the legs, including overall poor circulation to the extremities, night cramps, and varicose veins. According to Dr. Phillippe O. Szapary of the University of Pennsylvania School of Medicine, horse chestnut appears to be as effective and safe as currently available conventional therapies such as compression stockings. The usual dosage is 75 mg two times per day with meals. Supplement should be standardized to contain 16–21 percent triterpine glycosides or "escin" units. It may be taken daily on a continuous basis with no known side effects except for occasional, temporary stomach upset. It should not be used by pregnant women without a physician overseeing its use (see pp. 315–16).

VERTIGO

- A 1998 randomized control study by Weiser and colleagues of 119 vertigo patients in the mainstream journal *Archives of Otolaryngology, Head and Neck Surgery* reported that a combination of four homeopathic remedies worked as well in treating vertigo as the usual conventional medication, betahistine hydrochloride.
- One 1986 RCT with a placebo control conducted by a team of French researchers indicated that **Ginko biloba** had a positive effect on alleviating vertigo.

YEAST INFECTIONS (SEE VAGINITIS)

SELECTED BIBLIOGRAPHY

NOTE: NIH-NCCAM pilot studies are not cited in the references because their results are preliminary and are not as yet published in peer review journals.

Chapter 1: THINK HORSES, NOT ZEBRAS

Abbot, N. C.; White, A. R.; and Ernst, E. (1996). Complementary Medicine. *Nature*, May 30, 381: 361.

Allukian, Myron (1990). Healthy People 2000 and Our Domestic Gulf Crisis. *The Nation's Health,* October, 2.

Angell, Marcia; and Kassirer, Jerome P. (1998). Editorial: Alternative medicine—The risks of untested and unregulated remedies. *New England Journal of Medicine,* 339(12): 839–41.

Barsky, Arthur J. (1989). Fitness Mania: The Body as Our Temple. *Harvard Medical Alumni Bulletin,* Spring, 11–15.

Berman, Brian M.; et al. (1995). Physicians' attitudes toward complementary or alternative medicine: A regional survey. *Journal of the American Board of Family Practice,* 8(5): 361–66.

Bero, Lisa, and Rennie, Drummond (1995). The Cochrane Collaboration: Preparing, maintaining, and disseminating systematic reviews of the effects of health care. *JAMA,* December 27, 274(24): 1935–38.

Blair, Steve N.; et al. (1989). Physical fitness and all-cause mortality. *JAMA,* 262(17): 2395–2401.

Blumberg, Daniel L.; et al. (1995). The physician and unconventional medicine. *Alternative Therapies,* July, 1(3): 31–35.

Blumenthal, David (1996). Quality of health care. Part 4: The origins of the quality-of-care debate. *New England Journal of Medicine,* October 10, 335(15): 1146–49.

Breo, Dennis L. (1992). Uwe Reinhardt, Ph.D.—The economist as health evangelist. *JAMA,* 268(10): 1332–36.

Breslow, Lester (1990). A health promotion primer for the 1990s. *Health Affairs,* Summer, 6–21.

Brody, Sam (1992). We Have Lost Our Humanity. *Newsweek,* September 7, 8.

Catalano, Ralph (1991). The health effects of economic insecurity. *American Journal of Public Health,* 81(9): 1148–52.

Chopra, Deepak (1993). *Ageless Body, Timeless Mind.* New York: Harmony Books.

Consumer Reports (1992). Pushing Drugs to Doctors. February, 87–94.

Couzin, Jennifer (1998). Beefed-Up NIH Center Probes Unconventional Therapies. *Science,* December 18, 282: 2175.

Crichton, Michael (1990). Greater Expectations. *Newsweek,* September 24, 58.

Davant, Charles, III (1996). When you hear hoofbeats, sniff the air. *Medical Economics,* October 14, 107–10.

Day, Kathleen (1997). Finding a Prescription for Economic Pain: Pharmacies Devote More Space to Alternative Remedies. *Washington Post,* January 16.

Eisenberg, David M. (1996). The Invisible Mainstream. *Harvard Medical Alumni Bulletin,* Summer, 20–25.

Eisenberg, David M.; et al. (1998). Trends in alternative medicine use in the United States, 1990–1997. *JAMA,* November 11, 280(18): 1569–75.

Ernst, Edzard; Resch, Karl-Ludwig; and White, Adrian R. (1995). Complementary medicine. What physicians think of it: A meta-analysis. *Arch Intern Med,* 155: 2405–8.

Ezzo, Jeanette; et al. (1998). Complementary medicine and the Cochrane Collaboration. *JAMA,* November 11, 280(18): 1628–30.

Ezzo, Jeanette; et al. (1998). Reviewing the reviews: The evidence base for contemporary medicine is weak. Unpublished poster session manuscript.

Farquhar, John W.; et al. (1990). Effects of communitywide education on cardiovascular disease risk factors. *JAMA,* 264(3): 359–65.

Fitzgerald, Faith T. (1994). The tyranny of health. *New England Journal of Medicine,* July 21, 196–98.

Foege, William H. (1990). The growing brown plague. *JAMA,* 264(12): 1580.

———. (1996). Preventive medicine and public health. *JAMA,* June 19, 275(23): 1846–47.

Fuchs, Victor R. (1992). The best health care system in the world? *JAMA,* 268(7): 916–17.

Goetzel, R. Z.; et al. (1992). Behind the scenes of a POS program. *Journal of Health Care Benefits*, March/April, 33–37.

Goldszmidt, Mark; et al. (1995). Complementary health care services: A survey of general practitioners' views. *Canadian Medical Association Journal*, 153: 29–35.

Hahn, Robert A.; et al. (1990). Excess deaths from nine chronic diseases in the United States, 1986. *JAMA*, 264(20): 2654–59.

Halpern, Charles R. (1992). The political economy of mind-body health. *American Journal of Health Promotion*, 6(4): 288–89.

Harkin, Tom (1991). Another pound of care. *JAMA*, 266(12): 1692–93.

———. (1995). Alternative Medicine. *U.S. News & World Report*, August 7, 7.

Herzlinger, Regina E. (1991). Healthy Competition. *Atlantic Monthly*, August, 69–81.

Hilts, Philip J. (1996). How Safe Are Tylenol and Advil? Helping Patients Sort Out Risks. *New York Times*, March 27, B8.

Himmel, Wolfgang; Schulte, Miriam; Kochen, Michael M. (1993). Complementary medicine: Are patients' expectations being met by their general practitioners? *British Journal of General Practice*, June, 43: 232–35.

Idler, Ellen (1988). Healthy aging. *Social Forces*, 66: 226–38.

Iglehart, John K. (1992). The American health care system. *New England Journal of Medicine*, September 3, 742–47.

JAMA (1998). Editorial: Alternative medicine—Learning from the past, examining the present, advancing to the future. November 11, 280(18): 1616–17.

Kienle, Gunver Sophia, and Kiene, Helmut (1996). Placebo effect and placebo concept: A critical methodological and conceptual analysis of reports on the magnitude of the placebo effect. *Alternative Therapies*, November, 2(6): 39–54.

Kirschstein, Ruth L. (1996). Unpublished letter circulated to OAM Center directors, June.

Kristein, M.; Arnold, C.; and Wynder, E. (1977). Health Economics and Preventive Care. *Science*, 195: 457–62.

Landmark Healthcare Inc. (1996). Health Maintenance Organizations and Alternative Medicine: A Closer Look. November.

LaValley, J. William, and Verhoef, Marja J. (1995). Integrating complementary medicine and health care services into practice. *Canadian Medical Association Journal*, July 1, 153(1): 45–49.

Lindberg, George D. (1992). National health care reform. *JAMA*, 267(18): 2521–24.

Locke, S. E., and Colligan, D. (1990). *The Healer Within*. New York: E. P. Dutton, 1986. Reprint: New York: New American Library. Spanish, Italian, Japanese, German editions.

Mandell, Harvey, and Spiro, Howard (1987). *When Doctors Get Sick.* New York: Plenum Press.

Marshall, Eliot (1990). Experts Clash over Cancer Data. *Science,* 250: 900–902.

———. (1994). The Politics of Alternative Medicine. *Science,* September 30, 265: 2000–2002.

McGinnis, J. M., and Foege, W. H. (1993). Actual causes of death in the United States. *JAMA,* 270: 2207–12.

McNaughton Collins, Mary, and Barry, Michael J. (1996). Controversies in prostate cancer screening: Analogies to the early lung cancer screening debate. *JAMA,* December 25, 276(24): 1976–79.

Moore, Thomas J. (1989). *Heart Failure: A Critical Inquiry into American Medicine and the Revolution in Heart Care.* New York: Random House.

Neu, Harold C. (1992). The Crisis in Antibiotic Resistance. *Science,* 257: 1064–72.

Nusselder, Wilma J.; et al. (1996). The elimination of selected chronic diseases in a population: The compression and expansion of morbidity. *American Journal of Public Health,* February, 86(2): 187–94.

Ornstein, Robert, and Sobel, David (1989). *Healthy Pleasures.* Reading, Mass.: Addison-Wesley.

Oullette-Kobasa, S.; Maddi, S.; and Kahn, S. (1982). Hardiness and health: A prospective study. *Journal of Personality and Social Psychology,* 42: 168–77.

Packer, Milton (1997). End of the oldest controversy in medicine. *New England Journal of Medicine,* 336(8): 575–76.

Payer, Lynn (1988). *Medicine and Culture: Varieties of Treatment in the United States, England, West Germany and France.* Los Angeles: Henry Holt.

———. (1992). *Disease Mongers: How Doctors, Drug Companies, and Insurers Are Making You Sick.* New York: John Wiley.

Pelletier, K. R.; et al. (1993). Healthy People–Healthy Business: Disease Prevention and Health Promotion Programs in Business and Industry. In *Introduction to Occupational Health and Safety.* Chicago: National Safety Council.

Pelletier, Kenneth (1979). *Holistic Medicine: From Stress to Optimal Health.* New York: Delacorte Press.

Perkin, Michael R.; Pearcy, Richard M.; and Fraser, Jocelyn S. (1994). A comparison of the attitudes shown by general practitioners, hospital doctors and medical students towards alternative medicine. *Journal of the Royal Society of Medicine,* September, 87(9): 523–25.

Rees, Michael K. (1997a). Alternative Medicine: Down the Slippery Slope. *Modern Medicine,* January, 65: 67–68.

———. (1997b). Clinical Trials: Do Surrogate End Points Translate into Real-Life Benefit? *Modern Medicine,* February, 65: 62–63.

Remen, Rachel Naomi (1988). Spirit: Resource for Healing. *Noetic Science Review,* Autumn, 5–9.

Rowe, John W., and Kahn, Robert L. (1987). Human Aging: Usual and Successful. *Science,* July 10, 146–49.

Sackett, David L.; et al. (1996). Evidence based medicine: What it is and what it isn't. *British Medical Journal,* January 13, 312: 71–72.

Schroeder, Steven A. (1992). On squeezing balloons. *New England Journal of Medicine,* 325(15): 1099–1100.

Seeman, Julia (1989). Toward a model of positive health. *American Psychologist,* August, 1099–1109.

Smith, Richard (1991). Where is the wisdom . . . ? The poverty of medical evidence. *British Medical Journal,* October 5, 1991, 303 (6806): 798–99.

Stradling, J. (1997). Sleep apnoea and the misuse of evidence-based medicine. *Lancet,* January 18, 349: 201–2.

Strawbridge, William J.; et al. (1996). Successful aging: Predictors and associated activities. *American Journal of Epidemiology,* 144(2): 135–40.

Strohman, Richard (1993). Ancient genomes, wise bodies, unhealthy people: Limits of a genetic paradigm in biology and medicine. *Perspectives in Biology and Medicine,* Autumn.

Sullivan, Louis W. (1990). Healthy people 2000. *New England Journal of Medicine,* 323(15): 1065–67.

————. (1991). Partners in prevention: A mobilization plan for implementing healthy people 2000. *American Journal of Health Promotion,* 5(4): 291–97.

Sultz, Harry (1991). Health policy: If you don't know where you're going, any road will take you. *American Journal of Public Health,* 81(4): 418–20.

UC Berkeley Wellness Letter (1997). Futile Attractions. March, 3.

United States Office of Technology Assessment of the United States Congress (1990). *Unconventional Cancer Treatments.* Washington, D.C.: US Government Printing Office (PB91-104 893).

Verhoef, M. J., and Sutherland, L. R. (1995). Alternative medicine and general practitioners. Opinions and behavior. *Canadian Family Physician,* June, 41: 1005–11.

Wechsler, Henry; et al. (1996). The physician's role in health promotion revisited—A survey of primary care practitioners. *New England Journal of Medicine,* April 11, 334(15): 996–98.

Wennberg, John (1997). Interview. *Medical Economics,* February 10, 40–56.

Chapter 2: SOUND MIND, SOUND BODY

Achterberg, J.; et al. (1992). Mind-Body Interventions. In *Alternative Medicine: Expanding Medical Horizons: A Report to the National Institutes of Health on Alternative Medical Systems and Practices in the United States.* Prepared under the auspices of the Workshop on Alternative Medicine,

Chantilly, Va. Washington, D.C.: Government Printing Office, 3–43.

Ader, R. (1981). *Psychoneuroimmunology.* New York-Academic Press.

Alexander, C. N.; et al. (1996). Trial of stress reduction for hypertension in older African Americans II. Sex and risk subgroup analysis. *Hypertension,* 28: 228–37.

Allen, K., and Blascovich, J. (1994). Effects of music on cardiovascular reactivity among surgeons. *JAMA,* 272(11): 882–84.

Bannerman, R. H.; et al. (1983). *Traditional Medicine and Health Care Coverage.* Geneva, Switzerland: World Health Organization.

Barnason, S.; et al. (1995). The effects of music interventions on anxiety in the patient after coronary artery bypass grafting. *Heart and Lung,* 24(2): 124–32.

Barraclough, J.; et al. (1992). Life events and breast cancer prognosis. *Behavioral Medicine Journal,* 304 (April 25): 1078–81.

Blankfield, R.; et al. (1995). Taped therapeutic suggestions and taped music as adjuncts in the care of coronary-artery-bypass patients. *American Journal of Clinical Hypnosis,* 37(3): 32–42.

Borysenko, Myrin (1987). Area review: Psychoneuroimmunology. *Annals of Behavioral Medicine,* 9: 3–9.

Caudill, M.; et al. (1991). Decreased clinic use by chronic pain patients: response to behavioral medicine intervention. *Journal of Chronic Pain,* 7: 305–10.

Chaves, J. (1994). Recent advances in the application of hypnosis to pain management. *American Journal of Clinical Hypnosis,* 37(2): 117–29.

Chesky, K. (1992). The effects of music and music vibration using the MVT (TM) on the relief of rheumatoid arthritis pain. University of North Texas, unpublished paper.

Cohen, Sheldon; Tyrell, David A. J.; and Smith, Andrew P. (1991). Psychological stress and susceptibility to the common cold. *New England Journal of Medicine,* 325(9): 606–12.

Cooper, M., and Aygen, M. (1978). Effect of meditation on blood cholesterol and blood pressure. *Journal of the Israel Medical Association,* 95: 1–2.

Cummings, N. A., and Bragman, J. I. (1988). Triaging the "somatizer" out of the medical system into the psychological system. In E. M. Stern and V. F. Stern, et al., *Psychotherapy and the Somatizing Patient.* New York: Hayward Press, 109–12.

Davison, Gerald C.; et al. (1991). Relaxation, reduction in angry articulated thoughts, and improvements in borderline hypertension and heart rate. *Journal of Behavioral Medicine,* 14(5): 453–68.

Debenedittis, G.; et al. (1989). Effects of hypnotic analgesia and hypnotizability on experimental ischemic pain. *Int. Journal Clin. Exp. Hypnosis,* 37: 55–69.

Dohrenwend, B., and Dohrenwend, B. (1974). *Stressful Life Events: Their Nature and Effects.* New York: Wiley.

Dorian, Barbara, and Taylor, C. Barr (1984). Stress factors in the development of coronary artery disease. *Journal of Occupational Medicine.* 26(10): 747–56.

Eppley, K. R.; et al. (1989). Differential effects of relaxation technique on trait anxiety: a meta-analysis. *Journal of Clinical Psychology,* 45: 957–74.

Fawzy, Fawzy I.; et al. (1990). A structured psychiatric intervention for cancer patients. *Arch. Gen. Psychiatry,* 47: 729–35.

Garlinkel, Marian S.; et al. (1998). Yoga-based interventional for carpal tunnel syndrome. *JAMA,* November 11, 280(18): 1601–3.

Goldberg, B. (1995). *Alternative Medicine: The Definitive Guide.* Puyallup, Wash.: Future Medicine Publishing, Inc., compiled by The Burton Goldberg Group.

Gong, L. S.; et al. (1981). Changes in heart rate and electrocardiogram during Taijiquan exercise: Analysis by telemetry in 100 subjects. *Chinese Medicine Journal,* 94: 589–92.

Gordon, M. (1972). Age and performance differences of male patients on modified Stanford hypnotic susceptibility scales. *Int. Journal of Clinical and Exp. Hypnosis,* 20(3): 152–55.

Gorman, James, and Locke, Steven (1989). Neural, Endocrine, and Immune Interactions. In H. I. Kaplan and B. J. Sadock, eds., *Comprehensive Textbook of Psychiatry,* 5th ed. New York: Grove & Stratton, 111–25.

Greenleaf, M., and Fisher, S. (1992). Hypnotizability and recovery from cardiac surgery. *American Journal of Clinical Hypnosis,* 35(2): 119–28.

Haanen, H. H.; et al. (1991). Controlled trial of hypnotherapy in the treatment of refractory fibromyalgia. *Journal of Rheumatology,* 18(1): 72–75.

Haas, F.; et al. (1986). Effects of perceived musical rhythm on respiratory pattern. *Journal of Applied Physiology,* 61: 1185–91.

Haskell, William L.; et al. (1994). Effects of Intensive Multiple Risk Factor Reduction on Coronary Atherosclerosis and Clinical Cardiac Events in Men and Women with Coronary Artery Disease. *Circulation,* 89: 975–90.

Hellman, C. J. C.; et al. (1990). A study of the effectiveness of two group behavioral medicine interventions for patients with psychosomatic complaints. *Behavioral Medicine,* Winter, 165–73.

Holroyd, J. (1980). Hypnosis treatment for smoking: an evaluative review. *Int. Journal of Clinical Exper. Hypnosis,* 28: 341–57.

Ikemi, Y.; et al. (1975). Psychosomatic consideration of cancer patients who have made a narrow escape from death. *Dynamic Psychiatry,* 31: 77–92.

JAMA (1996). NIH technology assessment panel on integration of behavioral and relaxation approaches into the treatment of chronic pain and insomnia. 276(4): 313–18.

Jin, P. (1992). Efficacy of tai chi, brisk walking, meditation, and reading in reducing mental and emotional stress. *Journal of Psychosomatic Research,* 36(4): 361–70.

Kabat-Zinn, J.; et al. (1985). The clinical use of mindfulness meditation for the self-regulation of chronic pain. *Journal of Behavioral Medicine,* 8(2): 163–91.

Kabat-Zinn, J.; Lipworth, L.; Burney, R.; and Sellers, W. (1987). Four-year follow-up of a meditation-based program for the self-regulation of chronic pain: Treatment outcomes and compliance. *Clinical Journal of Pain,* 2: 159–73.

Kaplan, G., and Camacho, T. (1983). Perceived health and mortality: A nine-year follow-up of the human population laboratory cohort. *American Journal of Epidemiology,* 117: 292–304.

Keefe, F., and Caldwell, D. (1997). Cognitive behavioral control of arthritis. *Medical Clinics of North America,* 81(1): 277–89.

Kiecolt-Glaser, Janice K.; et al. (1996). Psychosocial enhancement of immuno-competence in a geriatric population. *Health Psychology,* 4(1): 24–41.

Lai, J-S.; et al. (1995). Two-year trends in cardiorespiratory function among older tai chi chuan practitioners and sedentary subjects. *Journal of the American Geriatric Society,* 43: 1222–27.

Lee, R. H. (1992). *Scientific Investigations into Chinese Qi-Gong.* San Clemente, Calif.: China Healthways Institute.

Leserman, J.; et al. (1989). The efficacy of the relaxation response in preparing for cardiac surgery. *Behavioral Medicine,* 15: 111–17.

Levitan, A. A. (1997). Hypnotherapy: a unique medical tool. *Complementary Medicine for the Physician,* 2(4): 25, 31–32.

Locke, S. E. (1976–82). *Mind and Immunity: Behavioral Immunology.* New York: Institute for the Advancement of Health, 1983, annotated bibliography.

Locke, S. E., and Gorman, J. R. (1989). Behavior and immunity. In H. I. Kaplan and B. J. Sadock, eds., *Comprehensive Textbook of Psychiatry,* 5th ed. New York: Grove & Stratton, 1240–49.

Locke, Steven E.; et al. (1984). Life-change stress psychiatric symptoms, and natural killer cell activity. *Psychosomatic Medicine,* 46(5): 441–53.

Lord, T., and Garner, J. (1993). Effects of music on Alzheimer patients. *Perceptual and Motor Skills,* 76(2): 451–55.

Lorig, K.; et al. (1993). Evidence suggesting that health education for self-management in patients with chronic arthritis has sustained health benefits while reducing health care costs. *Arthritis and Rheumatism,* 36(4): 439–46.

Luskin, F. M.; et al. (1998). A review of Mind/Body therapies in the treatment of cardiovascular disease with implications for the elderly: Part I. *Alternative Therapies in Health and Medicine,* May, 4(3): 46–61.

Marx, Jean L. (1985). The Immune System "Belongs in the Body." *Science,* 227: 1190–92.

McGrady, A.; et al. (1996). Biofeedback assisted relaxation in insulin dependent diabetes: a replication and extension study. *Ann. of Behavioral Medicine*, 18(3): 185–89.

Mechanic, D. (1977). Illness behavior, social adaptation, and the management of illness: A comparison of educational and medical models. *Journal of Nervous and Mental Disorders*, 165: 70–87.

Miller, Andrew H. (1989). *Depressive Disorders and Immunity*. Washington, D.C.: American Psychiatric Press.

Mossey, J., and Shapiro, E. (1982). Self-rated health: A predictor of mortality among the elderly. *American Journal of Public Health*, 72: 800–808.

Murphy, M., and Donovan, S. (1989). *The Physical and Psychological Effects of Meditation: A Review of Contemporary Meditation Research with a Comprehensive Bibliography, 1931–1988*. San Rafael, Calif.: Esalen Institute of Exceptional Functioning.

Nakao, M.; et al. (1997). Clinical effects of blood pressure biofeedback treatment on hypertension by auto-shaping. *Psychosomatic Medicine*, 59: 331–38.

Orme-Johnson, D. W. (1987). Medical care utilization and the Transcendental Meditation Program. *Psychosomatic Medicine*, 49: 493–507.

Orme-Johnson, D. W., and Farrow, F. T. (1977). *Scientific Research on the Transcendental Meditation Program: College Papers*, Vols. 1–5. Los Angeles: MERU Press.

Ornish, D.; et al. (1993). Can lifestyle changes reverse coronary heart disease? *Lancet*, 336: 129–33.

Parkes, C.; Benjamin, B.; and Fitzgerald, R. (1969). Broken heart: A study of increased mortality among widowers. *British Medical Journal*, 1: 740–43.

Pelletier, K. (1979). *Holistic Medicine: From Stress to Optimum Health*. New York: Delta.

———. (1992). *Mind as Healer, Mind as Slayer: A Holistic Approach to Preventing Stress Disorders*. New York: Delta.

———. (1985). Holistic Medicine. *The World Book Encyclopedia—Volume H*. Chicago: World Book—A Scott Fetzer Company.

———. (1994). *Sound Mind, Sound Body*. New York: Fireside.

Pelletier, K. R., and Herzing, D. L. (1988). Psychoneuroimmunology: Toward a MindBody model—A critical review. *Advances: Journal of the Institute for the Advancement of Health*, 5(1): 1–30.

Peper, E., and Tibbets, V. (1992). Fifteen-month follow-up with asthmatics utilizing EMG/incentive inspirometer feedback. *Biofeedback and Self-Regulation*, 17(2): 143–51.

Pilisuk, M., and Parks, K. (1985). Health and social support: Caring relationships and immunological protection. In M. Pilisuk and S. Hiller, eds., *The Healing Web: Social Networks and Human Survival*. Boston: University of New England Press.

Prinsley, D. (1986). Music therapy in geriatric care. *Australian Nurses Journal,* 15: 48–49.

Riccio, C.; et al. (1990). Adding purpose to the repetition exercise of elderly women through imagery. *American Journal of Occupational Therapy,* 44(8): 714–19.

Rider, M., and Achterberg, J. (1989). Effect of music assisted imagery on neutrophils and lymphocytes. *Biofeedback and Self-Regulation,* 14(3): 247–57.

Rider, M.; et al. (1990). Effect of immune system imagery on secretory IgA. *Biofeedback and Self-Regulation,* 15(4): 317–32.

Sancier, K. (1996). Medical Applications of Qigong. *Alternative Therapies,* 2(1): 40–46.

Schnall, Peter L.; et al. (1990). The relationship between "job strain," workplace diastolic blood pressure, and left ventricular mass index. *JAMA,* April 11, 263(14): 1929–35.

Schneider, R.; et al. (1995). A randomized controlled trial of stress reduction for hypertension in older African Americans. *Hypertension,* 26(5): 820–27.

Schorr, J. (1993). Music and pattern change in chronic pain. *Advances in Nursing Science,* 15(4): 27–36.

Scogin, F.; et al. (1992). Progressive and imaginal relaxation training for elderly persons with subjective anxiety. *Psychology and Aging,* 17(3): 419–24.

Sharpley, C. (1994). Maintenance and generalizability of laboratory based heart rate reactivity control training. *Journal of Behavioral Medicine,* 17(3): 309–29.

Sheng-han, X. (1994). Psychophysiological reactions associated with qigong therapy. *Chinese Medical Journal,* 107(3): 230–33.

Smith, G.; et al. (1985). Psychologic modulation of the human immune response to varicella zoster. *Archives of Internal Medicine,* 145: 2110–12.

Smyth, Joshua M.; et al. (1999). Effect of writing about stressful experiences of symptom reduction in patients with asthma or rheumatoid arthritis: A randomized trial. *JAMA,* 281(14): 1304–10.

Spanos, N.; et al. (1993). Hypnotic suggestion and placebo for the treatment of chronic headache in a university volunteer sample. *Cognitive Therapy and Res.,* 17(2): 191–205.

Spiegel, D.; et al. (1993). Predictors of smoking abstinence following a single-session restructuring intervention with self-hypnosis. *American Journal of Psychiatry,* 150(7): 1090–97.

Spiegel, David (1999). Healing words: Emotional expression and disease outcome. *JAMA,* 281(14,): 1328–29.

Spiegel, David; et al. (1989). Effect of psychosocial treatment on survival of patients with metastatic breast cancer. *Lancet,* October 14, 1: 888–91.

Stein, M.; Miller, A. H.; and Trestmen, R. L. (1991). Depression, the immune system, and health and illness: Findings in search of meaning. *Archives of General Psychiatry,* 48: 171–77.

Stockdale, L. (1991). The effects of audiotaped guided imagery relaxation exercises on anxiety levels in male automatic implantable cardioverter defibrillator recipients. *Dissertation Abstracts Int.*, 51(9): 4270–B.

Strain, J. J. Cost effectiveness from a psychiatric consultation-liaison intervention with elderly hip fracture patients. *American Journal of Psychology*, 148: 1044–99.

Taylor, S. E. (1989). *Positive Illusions: Creative Self-Deception and the Healthy Mind.* New York: Basic Books.

Thornby, M. A.; et al. (1995). Effect of distractive auditory stimuli on exercise tolerance in patients with COPD. *Chest*, 107: 1213–17.

Tse, S-K., and Baily, D. (1992). Tai chi and postural control in the well elderly. *American Journal of Occupational Therapy*, 46(4): 295–300.

Wang (1993). Effects of qigong on preventing stroke and alleviating the multiple-cerebro-cardiovascular risk factors; a follow-up report on 242 hypertensive cases over 30 years. *Proceedings, Second World Conference for Academic Exchange of Medical Qigong*, Beijing, China, 123–24.

Weinstein, E., and Au, P. (1991). Use of hypnosis before and during angioplasty. *American Journal of Clinical Hypnosis*, 34(1): 29–37.

Wenneberg, S.R.; et al (1997). A controlled study of the effects of the Transcendental Meditation program on cardiovascular reactivity and ambulatory blood pressure. International Journal of Neuroscience, Jan., 89 (1–2): 15–28.

Wolf, S.; et al. (1996). Reducing frailty and falls in older persons: an investigation of tai chi and computerized balance training. *Journal of American Geriatric Society*, 44: 489–97.

Wolfson, L.; et al. (1996). Balance and strength training in older adults: intervention gains and tai chi maintenance. *Journal of American Geriatric Society*, May, 44: 498–506.

Yeung, Alan C.; et al. (1991). The effect of atherosclerosis on the vasomotor response of coronary arteries to mental stress. *New England Journal of Medicine*, 325(22): 1551–80.

Zamarra, J.; et al. (1996). Usefulness of the transcendental meditation program in the treatment of patients with coronary artery disease. *American Journal of Cardiology*, 77(10): 867–70.

Zimmerman, L.; et al. (1989). Effects of music in patients who had chronic cancer pain. *W. Journal of Nursing Research*, 11: 298–309.

Chapter 3: FOOD FOR THOUGHT

ADA Reports (1988). Position of the American Dietetic Association: Vegetarian diets—Technical support paper. *Journal of the American Dietetic Association*, 88: 3.

Albanes, D.; et al. (1995). Effects of alpha-tocopherol and beta-carotene supplements on cancer incidence in the Alpha-Tocopherol Beta-Carotene Cancer
Prevention Study. *American Journal of Clinical Nutrition,* 62: 1927s–1430s.

Abraham, A. S.; Brooks, B. A.; and Eylath, U. (1992). The effects of chromium
supplementation on serum glucose and lipids in patients with and without non-
insulin-dependent diabetes. *Metabolism: Clinical and Exp.,* 41(7): 768–71.

Anderson, R. A.; et al. (1991). Supplemental chromium effects on glucose,
insulin, glucagon and urinary chromium losses in subjects consuming controlled low chromium diets. *American Journal of Clinical Nutrition,* 54:
909–16.

Barni, S.; et al. (1995). A randomized study of low dose subcutaneous inter-
leukin-2 plus melatonin versus supportive care alone in metastatic colorectal
cancer patients progressing under 5-fluorouracil and folates. *Oncology,* 52(3):
243–45.

Barrett-Connor, E., and Ferrara, A. (1991). Dehydroepiandrosterone, dehydroepiandrosterone sulfate, obesity, waist-hip ratio and noninsulin-dependent
diabetes in postmenopausal women: The Rancho Bernardo Study. *Journal of
Clinical Endocrinology and Metabolism,* 81: 59–64.

Bartels, G. L.; et al. (1996). Anti-ischaemic efficacy of L-propionylcarnitine—a
promising novel metabolic approach to ischaemia? *European Heart Journal,*
17(3): 414–20.

Birch, R.; Noble, D.; and Greenhaff, P. L. (1994). The influence of dietary creatine supplementation on performance during repeated bouts of maximal iso-
kinetic cycling in man. *European Journal of Applied Physiology and
Occupational Physiology,* 69(3): 268–76.

Booji, A.; et al. (1996). Androgens as adjuvant treatment in postmenopausal
female patients with rheumatoid arthritis. *Annals of the Rheumatic Diseases,*
55(11): 811–15.

Burke, L. M.; Pyne, D. B.; and Telford, R. D. (1996). Effect of oral creatine supplementation on single-effort sprint performance in elite swimmers. *International Journal of Sports Nutrition,* 6(3): 222–33.

Batrum, R. R.; Clifford, C. K.; and Lanza, E. (1988). NCI Dietary Guidelines
Revisited. *American Journal of Clinical Nutrition,* 48: 888–95.

Cacciatore, L.; et al. (1991). The therapeutic effect of L-carnitine in patients
with exercise-induced stable angina: a controlled study. *Drugs Under Experimental and Clinical Research,* 17(4): 225+35.

Casson, P. R.; et al. (1995). Replacement of dehydro-epiandrosterone enhances
T-lymphocyte insulin binding in postmenopausal women. *Fertility and Steril-
ity,* 63(5): 1027–31.

Chello, M.; et al. (1994). Protection by coenzyme Q_{10} from myocardial reperfusion injury during coronary artery bypass grafting. *American Thoracic
Surgery,* 58(5): 1427–32.

Chello, M.; et al. (1996). Protection by coenzyme Q_{10} of tissue reperfusion injury during abdominal aortic cross-clamping. *Journal of Cardiovascular Surgery*, 37(3): 229–35.

Clancy, S. P.; et al. (1994). Effects of chromium picolinate supplementation on body composition, strength and urinary chromium loss in football players. *International Journal of Sports Nutrition*, 4:142–53.

Clark. L. C.; et al. (1996). Effects of selenium supplementation for cancer prevention in patients with carcinoma of the skin. A randomized controlled trial. Nutritional Prevention of Cancer Study Group. *JAMA*, 276(24): 1957–63.

Commission on Dietary Supplement Labels (1997). *Commission on Dietary Supplement Labels Report to the President, the Congress, and the Secretary of the Department of Health and Human Services,* June, draft report.

Consumer Reports (1997). A Supplement Worth Watching: Vitamin E Hasn't Lost Its Glow. March, 70.

Cooper, K. H. (1996). *Advanced Nutritional Therapies*. Nashville, Tenn.: Thomas Nelson Publications.

Dawson, D.; Encel, N.; and Lushington, K. (1995). Improving adaptation to simulated night shift: Time exposure to bright light versus daytime melatonin administration. *Sleep*, 18(1): 11–21.

Decombaz, J.; et al. (1993). Effect of L-carnitine on submaximal exercise metabolism after depletion of muscle glycogen. *Med. Science Sports Exerc.*, 25: 733–40.

Delmas-Beauvieux, M. C.; et al. (1996). The enzymatic antioxidant system in blood and glutathione status in human immunodeficiency virus (HIV)-infected patients: Effects of supplementation with selenium or beta-carotene. *American Journal of Clinical Nutrition*, 64(1): 101–7.

Flohe, L. (1988). Superoxide dismutase for therapeutic use: Clinical experience, dead ends and hopes. *Molecular and Cellular Biochem.*, 84(2): 123–31.

Folkard, S.; Arendt, J.; and Clark, M. (1993). Can melatonin improve shift workers' tolerance of the night shift. Some preliminary findings. *Chronobiology International*, 10(5): 315–20.

Folkers, K., and Simonsen, R. (1995). Two successful double-blind trials with coenzyme Q_{10} on muscular dystrophies and neurogenic atrophies. *Biochemica et Biophysica Acta*, 1271(1): 281–86.

Gardner, Christopher D., and Kraemer, Helena C. (1995). Monounsaturated versus polyunsaturated dietary fat and serum lipids. *Arteriosclerosis, Thrombosis, and Vascular Biology*, November, 15(11): 1917–18.

Giovannucci, E., and Ascherio, A. (1995). Intake of carotenoids and retinol in relation to risk of prostate cancer. *Journal of Nutrition Cancer Institute*, 87(23): 1767–76.

Gordon, A.; et al. (1995). Creatine supplementation in chronic heart failure increases muscle creatine phosphate and muscle performance. *Cardiovascular Research*, 30(3): 413–18.

Greenhaff, P. L.; et al. (1993). Influence of oral creatine supplementation of muscle torque during repeated bouts of maximal voluntary exercise in man. *Clinical Science*, 84(5): 565–71.

Hall, G. M.; et al. (1996). A randomized trial of testosterone therapy in males with rheumatoid arthritis. *British Journal of Rheumatology*, 35(6): 568–73.

Han, L., and Zhour, S. M. (1994). Selenium supplement in the prevention of pregnancy induced hypertension. *Chinese Medical Journal*, 107(11): 870–71.

Hennekens, C. H.; et al. (1996). Lack of effect of long term supplementation with beta-carotene on the incidence of malignant neoplasms and cardiovascular disease. *New England Journal of Medicine*, 334: 1145–49.

Herrington, D.; et al. (1995). DHEA and coronary atherosclerosis. *Ann. of New York Acad. Science*, 774: 271–80.

Iliceto, S.; et al. (1995). Effects of L-carnitine administration on left ventricular remodeling after acute anterior myocardial infarction: The L-Carnitine Ecocardiografia Digitalizzata Infarto Miocardico (CEDIM) Trial. *Journal of the American College of Cardiology*, 26(2): 380–87.

Kasper, C.; et al. (1994). L-carnitine supplementation and running performance. *Med. Science Sports Exerc.*, 26: §39 (abstract).

Lampertico, M., and Comis, S. (1993). Italian multicenter study on the efficacy and safety of coenzyme Q_{10} as adjuvant therapy in heart failure. *Clinical Investigations*, 71(8 Suppl): §129–§33.

Lissoni, P.; et al. (1994). A randomized study with the pineal hormone melatonin versus supportive care alone in patients with brain metastases due to solid neoplasms. *Cancer*, 73(3): 699–701.

Lissoni, P.; et al. (1995). Immune effects of preoperative immunotherapy with high-dose subcutaneous interleukin-2 versus neuroimmunotherapy with low-dose interleukin-2 plus the neurohormone melatonin in gastrointestinal tract tumor patients. *Journal of Biol. Regulators & Homeostatic Agents*, 9(1): 31–33.

Lissoni, P.; et al. (1996). Increased survival time in brain glioblastomas by a radioneuroendocrine strategy with radiotherapy plus melatonin compared to radiotherapy alone. *Oncology*, 53(1): 43–46.

Lockwood, K.; et al. (1994). Apparent partial remission of breast cancer in "high risk" patients supplemented with nutritional antioxidants, essential fatty acids and coenzyme Q_{10}. *Molecular Aspects of Medicine*, 15 Supple: §231–§40.

Lukaski, H. C.; et al. (1996). Chromium supplementation and resistance training: Effects on body composition, strength, and trace element status of men. *American Journal of Clinical Nutrition*, 63: 954–65.

McGovern, G. (1977). *Dietary Goals for the United States*. A report of the Select Committee on Nutrition and Human Needs, U.S. Senate, December, Washington, D.C.: Government Printing Office.

Marzi, I.; et al. (1993). Value of superoxide dismutase for prevention of multiple organ failure after multiple trauma. *Journal of Trauma*, 35(1): 110–20.

Meydani, S. N.; et al. (1997). Vitamin E supplementation and in vivo immune response in healthy elderly subjects. *JAMA*, 277(17): 1380–86.

Modern Medicine (1997a). Another Weight-Loss Therapy: Chromium Supplements Help Patients Shed Pounds. 65: 11–12.

———. (1997b). Sleep Foundation Is Critical of Melatonin. 65: 4.

Morales, A. J.; et al. (1994). Effects of replacement dose of dehydroepiandrosterone in men and women of advancing age. *Journal of Clinical Endocrinol. Metabolism,* 78(6): 1360–67. Note: Published erratum appears in *Journal of Clinical Endocrinol. Metabolism* 1995: 80(9): 2799.

Morisco, C.; Trimarco, B.; and Condorelli, M. (1993). Effect of coenzyme Q_{10} therapy in patients with congestive heart failure: A long term multicenter randomized study. *Clinical Investigations,* 71(8 Suppl): §134–§36.

Muizelaar, J. P.; et al. (1993). Improving the outcome of severe head injury with the oxygen radical scavenger polyethylene glycol-conjugated superoxide dismutase: A phase II trial. *Journal of Neurosurgery,* 78(3): 375–82.

Natali, A.; et al. (1993). Effects of acute hypercarnitinemia during increased fatty substrate oxidation in man. *Metabolism,* 42: 594–600.

Otto, R.; et al. (1987). The effect of L-carnitine supplementation on endurance exercise. *Medical Science Sports Exerc.,* 19: §68 (abstract).

Oyono-Enguelle, S.; et al. (1988). Prolonged submaximal exercise and L-carnitine in humans. *European Journal of Applied Physiology,* 58: 53–61.

Peeke, P. (1997). Nutrition and Dietary Supplements (commissioned literature review).

Pelletier, K. (1979). *Holistic Medicine: From Stress to Optimum Health.* New York: Delacorte and Delta.

Petrie, K.; et al. (1989). Effect of melatonin on jet lag after long haul flights. *British Medical Journal,* 298 (6675): 705–7.

Petrie, K.; et al. (1993). A double-blind trial of melatonin as a treatment for jet lag in international cabin crew. *Biological Psychiatry,* 33(7): 526–30.

Phillips, R. L. (1975). Role of lifestyle and dietary habits in risk of cancer among Seventh Day Adventists. *Cancer Research* (Suppl), 35: 3515–22.

Pollak, R.; et al. (1993). A randomized double-blind trial of the use of human recombinant superoxide dismutase in renal transplantation. *Transplantation,* 55(1): 57–60.

Press, R. I.; Geller, J.; and Evans, G. W. (1990). The effect of chromium picolinate on serum cholesterol and apolipoprotein fractions in human subjects. *West Journal of Medicine,* 152: 41–45.

Regelson, W., and Colman, C. (1996). *The Super-Hormone Promise.* New York: Simon & Schuster.

Reiter, R. J. (1995). Functional pleitropy of the neurohormone melatonin: Antioxidant protection and neuroendocrine regulation. *Front in Neuroendocrine*, 16(4): 383–415.

Singh, R. B.; et al. (1996). A randomized, double-blind, placebo controlled trial of L-carnitine in suspected acute myocardial infarction. *Postgrad. Medical Journal*, 72(843): 45–50.

Stephens, N. G.; et al. (1996). Randomized controlled trial of vitamin E in patients with coronary disease: Cambridge Heart Antioxidant Study (CHAOS). *Lancet*, 347:781–86.

The Surgeon General's Report on Nutrition and Health (1988). Washington, D.C.: U.S. Department of Health and Human Services.

Taggart, D. P.; et al. (1996). Effects of short-term supplementation with coenzyme Q_{10} on myocardial protection during cardiac operations. *Ann. Thoracic Surgery*, 61(3): 829–33.

Trevisan, M.; et al. (1990). Consumption of olive oil, butter and vegetable oils and coronary heart disease risk factors. The Research Group ATS-RF2 of the Italian National Research Council, *JAMA*, 263(5): 688–92.

UC Berkeley Wellness Letter (1996). DHEA—The Promise of Youth and Health. January, 1–2.

———. Better Beta-Carotene Advice. May, 4.

van Noord, P. A.; et al. (1993). Selenium and the risk of postmenopausal breast cancer in the DOM cohort. *Breast Cancer Research and Treatment*, 25(1): 11–19.

van Poppel, G., and Goldbohm, A. (1995). Epidemiologic evidence for beta-carotene and cancer prevention. *American Journal of Clinical Nutrition*, 62:1393s–11402s.

van Vollenhoven, R. F.; Englemen, E. G.; and McGuire, J. L. (1995). Dehydroepiandrosterone in systemic lupus erythematosus. Results of a double-blind, placebo controlled, randomized clinical trial. *Arthritis & Rheumatism*, 38(12): 1826–31.

Warner, H. R. (1994). Superoxide dismutase, aging, and degenerative disease. *Free Radical Biology and Medicine*, 17(3): 249–58.

Willett, Walter C. (1994). Diet and Health: What Should We Eat? *Science*, April 22, 264: 532–37.

Zimmerman, M. (1996). Is DHEA an antidote to aging? *NFM's Nutrition Science News*, October, 30–34.

Chapter 4: TRADITIONAL CHINESE MEDICINE

Adachi, I. (1989). Role of supporting therapy of Juzenthaiho-to (JTT) in advanced breast cancer patients. *Gan To Kagaku Ryoho (Japanese Journal of Cancer and Chemotherapy)*, 16(4 Pt 2-2): 1533–37.

Bensoussan, Alan; et al. (1998). Treatment of irritable bowel syndrome with Chinese herbal medicine. *JAMA*, November 11, 280(18): 1585–89.

Cao, Tiemei; et al. (1994). Treatment of 124 cases of hyperlipidemia with Ehuang Jiangzhi Tablet. *Chinese Journal of Integrated Traditional and Western Medicine*, 14(3): 167–68.

Cardini, Francesco, and Weixin, Huang (1998). Moxibustion for correction of breech presentation. *JAMA*, November 11, 280(18): 1580–84.

Chen, Xiaoping; et al. (1994). Effects of Zhibai Dihuang Pill on male immunologic infertility and associated humoral immunity. *Journal of Traditional Chinese Medicine*, 35(10): 610–11.

Chen, Xiaoping; et al. (1995). Guyin Decoction in the treatment of immunosterility and its effects on humoral immunity. *Journal of Traditional Chinese Medicine*, 15(4): 259–61.

Chu, D. (1990). A fractionated extract of *Astragalus membranaceus* potentiates lymphokine-activated killer cell cytotoxicity generated by low-dose recombinant interleukin-2. *Chung Hsi I Chieh Ho Tsa Chih (Chinese Journal of Modern Developments in Traditional Medicine)*, 10(1): 34–36.

Collinge, W. (1996). *The American Holistic Health Association Complete Guide to Alternative Medicine.* New York: Warner Books.

Dharmananda, S. (1996). The current status of Chinese medicine in the U.S. *START Group Manuscripts*, Portland, Ore.

———. (1997). Controlled Clinical Trials of Chinese Herbal Medicines: A Review (unpublished, commissioned review).

Haguenauer, J.P.; et al. (1986). [Treatment of equilibrium disorders with Ginkgo biloba extract: A multicenter, double-blind drug vs. placebo study] [French]. *Presse Med*, 15: 1569–77.

Hong-Yen, Hsu (1988). The study of scientific Chinese herbal preparation. *Oriental Healing Arts International Bulletin*, 13(2): 105–25.

———. (1989). The safety of Chinese medicinal herbs. *Int. Journal of Oriental Medicine*, 14(1): 5–43.

Hsiao, W. C. L.; et al. (1996). Medicine in China. *New England Journal of Medicine*, August, 89: 430–32.

Ko, R. J. (1998). Hidden toxic ingredients in Asian patent medicines. *New England Journal of Medicine*, 339: 847.

LeBars, P. L. (1997). A placebo-controlled double-blind, randomized trial of an extract of *Ginkgo biloba* for dementia. *JAMA*, 278(16): 1327–32.

396   Selected Bibliography

Lee, R. (1975). Interaction Between Chinese and Western Medicine in Hong Kong: Modernization and Professional Inequality in Chinese Cultures. In Kleinman, et al., eds., *Medicine in Chinese Cultures: Comparative Studies of Health Care in Chinese and Other Societies*. Washington, D.C.: John E. Fogerty International.

Lerner, M. (1996). *Choices in Healing*. Cambridge, Mass.: MIT Press.

Li, Hongfen; et al. (1996). Clinical effects of Chinese medicine in treating asthma. *Chinese Journal of Integrated Traditional and Western Medicine*, 2(2): 125–26.

Lin, Chuanrong; et al. (1996). An observation on combined use of chemotherapy and traditional Chinese medicine to relieve cancer pain. *Journal of Traditional Chinese Mediciine*, 16(4): 267–69.

Liu, G-Q. (1995). Chinese natural products and new drugs. *Pharmaceutical News*, 2(2): 10–12.

Lu, Decheng; et al. (1994). Effects of Jianyanling on serum lipids, apolipoprotein, and lipoprotein. *Chinese Journal of Integrated Traditional and Western Medicine*, 14(3): 142–44.

Lu, Youzhi; et al. (1994). Treatment of 27 cases of systemic lupus erythematosus with combined Chinese herbal drugs and corticosteroids. *Journal of Clinical Dermatology*, 23(6): 326–27.

Luo, Hechun; et al. (1997). Clinical study on shuxuening combined with antipsychotics in treating chronic schizophrenia. *Chinese Journal of Integrated Traditional and Western Medicine*, 3(3): 191–94.

Pearl, W. S.; et al. (1995). Use of Chinese therapies among Chinese patients seeking emergency department care. *Ann. of Emergency Medicine*, 26(6): 735–38.

Qiu, Xiaoguang, and Pu, Qing-tian (1994). Treatment of mammary dysplasia with herbal drugs. *Liaoning Journal of Traditional Chinese Medicine*, 21(11): 509–10.

Shao, Changrong; et al. (1996). The research on the prevention and treatment of bronchial asthma by Chuanxiong Antiasthma Mixture. *Chinese Journal of Integrated Traditional and Western Medicine*, 2(2): 91–94.

Shi, Pei-heng; et al. (1994). Clinical and experimental studies of No. 90 Dasheng Jiangya Oral Liquid in treating hypertension. *Chinese Journal of Integrated Traditional and Western Medicine*, 14(3): 145–47.

Skolnick, A. A. (1997). Old Chinese herbal medicine used for fever yields possible new Alzheimer's disease therapy. *JAMA*, 277(10): 776.

Stemmler, C. (1997). Integrated medicine: Combining Western and Eastern tools in primary care (interview). *Complementary Medicine for the Physician*, 2(5): 1, 38–40.

Tao, X.; et al. (1991). Effect of an extract of the Chinese herbal remedy Tripterygium Wilfordii Hook F on human immune responsiveness. *Arthritis and Rheumatism*, 34: 1274–81.

Tian, Qiong; et al. (1994). Treatment of hepatocellular carcinoma with Dilong Capsule and intra-arterial chemotherapy. *Chinese Journal of Clinical Oncology*, 21(6): 445.

Wang, Xuemei, and Xie, Zhufan (1996). A clinical study on the effect of reinforcement of kidney on senile brain function. *Journal of Traditional Chinese Medicine*, 17(2): 92–95.

Workshop on Alternative Medicine, Chantilly, Va. (1992). Herbal Medicine. In *Alternative Medicine: Expanding Medical Horizons: A Report to the National Institutes of Health on Alternative Medical Systems and Practices in the United States*. Washington, D.C.: Government Printing Office, September 14–16, 183–206.

Wu, Dian; et al. (1995). Effects of the clearing-heat and nourishing-stomach method in the treatment of chronic gastritis with positive Campylobacter pylori. *Journal of Traditional Chinese Medicine*, 15(1): 28–30.

Yamada, H. (1989). Chemical characterization and biological activity of the immunologically active substances in Juzen-taiho-to (Japanese kampo prescription). *Gan To Kagaku Ryoho (Japanese Journal of Cancer and Chemotherapy)*, 164(4 Pt 2-2): 1500–1505.

You, Deshi; et al. (1994). Treatment of 46 cases of verrucous gastritis with integrated traditional Chinese and Western medicine. *Chinese Journal of Integrated Traditional and Western Medicine*, 14(3): 150–51.

Xie, Zhu-fan, and Li, Ning (1995). Methodological analysis of clinical articles on therapy evaluation published in *Chinese Journal of Integrated Traditional and Western Medicine* (in Chinese), 1982–1994. *CJIM*, 1(4): 301–6.

Chapter 5: ACUPUNCTURE

Aglietti, L.; et al. (1990). A pilot study of metoclopramide, dexamethasone, diphenhydramine and acupuncture in women treated with cisplatin. *Cancer Chemothera. Pharmacology*, 26: 239–40.

Ahonen, E.; et al. (1983). Acupuncture and physiotherapy in the treatment of myogenic headache patients. Pain relief and EMG activity. *Advanced Pain Research Therapy*, 5: 572–76.

Barsoum, G.; Perry, E. P.; and Fraser, L. A. (1990). Postoperative nausea is relieved by acupressure. *Journal of Royal Society of Medicine*, 83: 86–89.

Berman, Brian M. (1995). Efficacy of traditional Chinese acupuncture in the treatment of symptomatic knee osteoarthritis: A pilot study. *Osteoarthritis and Cartilage*, 3: 139–42.

Birch, S. (1995). Testing the clinical specificity of needle sites in controlled clinical trials of acupuncture. *Proc. Soc. Acupuncture Research*, 2: 274–94.

Birch, Stephen, and Hammerschlag, Richard (1996). *Acupuncture Efficacy: A Summary of Controlled Clinical Trials*. The National Academy of Acupuncture and Oriental Medicine, August.

Blom, M.; Davidson, L.; and Angmar-Mansson, B. (1992). The effect of acupuncture on salivary flow rates in patients with xerostomia. *Oral Surgery, Oral Medicine, Oral Pathology*, 73: 293–98.

Bratteberg, G. (1983). Acupuncture therapy for tennis elbow. *Pain*, 16: 285–88.

Bullock, M.; Culliton, P.; and Olander, R. (1989). Controlled trial of acupuncture for severe recidivist alcoholism. *Lancet*, 1: 1435–39.

Bullock, M. L.; et al. (1987). Acupuncture treatment of alcoholic recidivism: A pilot study. *Alcoholism: Clin. Exp. Res.*, 11: 292–95.

Cahn, A. M.; et al. (1978). Acupuncture in gastroscopy. *Lancet*, 1: 182–83.

Cardini, F., and Marcolongo, A. (1993). Moxibustion for correction of breech presentation: A clinical study with retrospective control. *American Journal of Chinese Medicine*, 21: 133–38.

Christensen, B. V.; et al. (1992). Acupuncture treatment of severe knee osteoarthrosis: A long-term study. *Acta Anaesthesia Scand.*, 36: 519–25.

Christensen, P. A.; et al. (1989). Electro-acupuncture and postoperative pain. *British Journal of Anaesthesia*, 62: 258–62.

Clavel, F.; et al. (1985). Helping people to stop smoking: Randomized comparison of groups being treated with acupuncture and nicotine gum with control group. *British Medical Journal*, 291: 1538–39.

Coan, R.; Wong, G.; and Coan, P. L. (1982). The acupuncture treatment of neck pain: A randomized controlled study. *American Journal of Chinese Medicine*, 9: 326–32.

Coan, R. M.; et al. (1980). The acupuncture treatment of low back pain: A randomized controlled treatment. *American Journal of Chinese Medicine*, 8: 181–89.

Consumer Reports (1994). Acupuncture. January, 4–9.

De Aloysio, D., and Penacchioni, P. (1992). Morning sickness control in early pregnancy by Neiguan point acupressure. *Obstet. Gynecol.*, 80: 852–54.

Deluze, C.; et al. (1992). Electro-acupuncture in fibromyalgia: Results of a controlled trial. *British Medical Journal*, 305: 1249–52.

DeVernejoul, P.; et al. (1985). Study of acupuncture meridians using radioactive tracers (in French). *Bulletin de L'Academie Nationale de Medicine*, October 22, 1071–75.

Dickens, W., and Lewith, G. T. (1989). A single-blind, controlled and randomized clinical trial to evaluate the effect of acupuncture in the treatment of trapezio-metacarpal osteoarthritis. *Complementary Medicine Research*, 3: 5–8.

Dundee, J. W.; et al. (1989). Effect of stimulation of the P6 antiemetic point on postoperative nausea and vomiting. *British Journal of Anaesthesia,* 63: 612–18.

Dundee, J. W., and Yang, J. (1990). Prolongation of the antiemetic effect of P6 acupuncture by acupressure in patients having cancer chemotherapy. *Journal of Royal Society of Medicine,* 83: 360–62.

Ehrlich, D., and Haber, R. (1992). Influence of acupuncture on physical performance capacity and haemodynamic parameters. *Int. Journal of Sports Medicine,* 13: 486–91.

Ellis, N.; Briggs, R.; and Dowson, D. (1990). The effect of acupuncture on nocturnal urinary frequency and incontinence in the elderly. *Complementary Medicine Research,* 4: 16–17.

Eskinazi, D. P. (1996). NIH Technology Assessment Workshop on Alternative Medicine: Acupuncture. *Journal of Alternative Complementary Medicine,* 2: 1–256.

Fox, E. J., and Melzack, R. (1976). Transcutaneous electrical stimulation and acupuncture: Comparison of treatment for low back pain. *Pain,* 2: 141–48.

Fung, K. P.; Chow, O. K. W.; and So, S. Y. (1986). Attenuation of exercise-induced asthma by acupuncture. *Lancet,* 2: 1419–22.

Gerhard, I., and Postneek, F. (1992). Auricular acupuncture in the treatment of female infertility. *Gynecol. Endocrinol.,* 6: 171–81.

Ghaly, R. G.; Fitzpatrick, K. T. J.; and Dundee, J. W. (1987). Antiemetic studies with traditional Chinese acupuncture: A comparison of manual needling with electrical stimulation and commonly used antiemetics. *Anaesthesia,* 42: 1108–10.

Gunn, C. C.; et al. (1980). Dry needling of muscle motor points for chronic low back pain. *Spine,* 5: 279–91.

Haker, E., and Lundeberg, T. (1990). Acupuncture treatment in epicondylalgia: A comparative study of two acupuncture techniques. *Clinical Journal of Pain,* 6: 221–26.

Hansen, P. E., and Hansen, J. H. (1983). Acupuncture treatment of chronic facial pain—a controlled cross-over trial. *Headache,* 23: 66–69.

Hao, J.; et al. (1995). Electric acupuncture treatment of peripheral nerve injury. *Journal of Traditional Chinese Medicine,* 15: 114–17.

Helms, J. (1993). *Physicians and Acupuncture in the 1990s.* Report for the Subcommittee on Labor, Health and Human Services, and Education of the Appropriations Committee, U.S. Senate, June, 24. American Academy of Medical Acupuncture Review, 5: 1–6.

Helms, J. M. (1987). Acupuncture for the management of primary dysmenorrhea. *Obstet. Gynecol.,* 69: 51–56.

———. (1995). *Acupuncture Energetics: A Clinical Approach for Physicians.* Berkeley, Calif.: Medical Acupuncture Publishers.

Hesse, J.; Mogelvang, B.; and Simonsen, H. (1994). Acupuncture versus meto-prolol in migraine prophylaxis: a randomized trial of trigger point inactivation. *Journal of Internal Medicine*, 235: 451–56.

Ho, R. T.; et al. (1990). Electroacupuncture and postoperative emesis. *Anaesthesia*, 45: 327–29.

Holden, Constance (1997). Thumbs Up for Acupuncture. *Science*, November, 278(14): 1231.

Holder, J. (1991). *New Auricular Therapy Formula to Increase Retention of the Chemically Dependent in Residential Treatment.* Research study funded by the State of Florida, Department of Health and Rehabilitative Services.

Hu, S.; et al. (1995). P6 acupressure reduces symptoms of vection-induced motion sickness. *Aviation Space Environment Medicine*, 66: 631–34.

Hyde, E. (1989). Acupressure therapy for morning sickness: A controlled clinical trial. *Journal of Nurse-Midwifery*, 34: 171–78.

Jobst, K.; et al. (1986). Controlled trial of acupuncture for disabling breathlessness. *Lancet*, 2: 1416–19.

Johansson, A.; et al. (1991). Acupuncture in treatment of facial muscular pain. *Acta Odontol Scand.*, 49: 153–58.

Johansson, K.; et al. (1993). Can sensory stimulation improve the functional outcome in stroke patients? *Neurology*, 43: 2189–92.

Junnila, S. Y. T. (1982). Acupuncture superior to Piroxicam™ in the treatment of osteoarthritis. *American Journal of Acupuncture*, 10: 341–46.

Kaptchuk, T. J. (1983). *The Web That Has No Weaver*. New York: Congdon and Weed, pp. 4–6.

Laitinen, J. (1976). Acupuncture and transcutaneous electric stimulation in the treatment of chronic sacrolumbalgia and ischialgia. *American Journal of Chinese Medicine*, 4: 169–75.

Lao, Lixing; et al. (1995). Efficacy of Chinese acupuncture on postoperative oral surgery pain. *Oral Surgery, Oral Medicine, Oral Pathology*, April, 79: 423–28.

Lee, Y. H.; et al. (1992). Acupuncture in the treatment of renal colic. *Journal of Urology*, 147: 16–18.

Lipton, D. S.; Brewington, V.; and Smith, M. (1994). Acupuncture for crack-cocaine detoxification: Experimental evaluation of efficacy. *Journal of Substance Abuse Treatment*, 11: 205–15.

List, T., and Helkimo, M. (1992). Acupuncture and occlusal point therapy in the treatment of craniomandibular disorders. Part II. A one-year follow-up study. *Acta Odontol. Scand.*, 50: 375–85.

Loh, L.; et al. (1984). Acupuncture versus medical treatment for migraine and muscle tension headaches. *Journal of Neurological Neurosurgery Psychiatry*, 47: 333–37.

Loy, T. T. (1983). Treatment of cervical spondylosis—electroacupuncture versus physiotherapy. *Medical Journal of Australia*, 2:32–34.

Luo, J.; Jia, Y.; and Zhan, L. (1985). Electroacupuncture vs. amitriptyline in the treatment of depressive states. *Journal of Traditional Chinese Medicine*, 5: 3–8.

Lytle, C. D. (1993). *An Overview of Acupuncture*. Washington, D.C.: Center for Devices and Radiological Health, U.S. Department of Health and Human Services, Public Health Service, Food and Drug Administration.

MacDonald, A. J. R.; et al. (1983). Superficial acupuncture in the relief of chronic low back pain. *Ann. Roy. Coll. Surg. Eng.*, 65: 44–46.

Margolin, A.; et al. (1993). Acupuncture for the treatment of cocaine dependence in methadone-maintained patients. *American Journal of Addiction*, 2: 194–201.

Martelete, M., and Fiori, A. M. C. (1985). Comparative study of the analgesic effect of transcutaneous nerve stimulation (TNS), electroacupuncture (EA) and meperidine in the treatment of postoperative pain. *Acupuncture Electro-Therapy Research Int. Journal*, 10: 183–93.

Molsberger, A., and Hille, E. (1994). The analgesic effect of acupuncture in chronic tennis elbow pain. *British Journal of Rheumatology*, 33: 1162.

Naeser, M. A.; et al. (1992). Real versus sham acupuncture in the treatment of paralysis in acute stroke patients: A CT scan lesion site study. *Journal of Neurological Rehabilitation*, 6: 163–73.

NIH Consensus Development Conference on Acupuncture (1997). November 3–5, William H. Natcher Conference Center, National Institutes of Health, Bethesda, Md.

Petrie, J. P., and Langley, G. B. (1983). Acupuncture in the treatment of chronic cervical pain: A pilot study. *Clin. Exp. Rheumatology*, 1: 333–36.

Pomeranz, B. (1986). Scientific Basis of Acupuncture. In Stux and Pomeranz, et al., *Acupuncture: Textbook and Atlas*. Berlin: Springer-Verlag.

Raustia, A. M.; Pohjola, R. T., and Virtanen, K. K. (1985). Acupuncture compared with stomatognathic treatment for TMJ dysfunction. Part I: A randomized study. *Journal of Prosth. Dent.*, 54: 581–85.

Sallstrom, S.; et al. (1996). Acupuncture in the treatment of stroke patients in the subacute stage: A randomized, controlled study. *Phys. Ther.*, 4: 193–97.

Shlay, Judith C.; et al.; for the Terry Beirn Community Programs for Clinical Research on AIDS. (1998). Acupuncture and amitriptyline for pain due to HIV-related peripheral neuropathy. *JAMA*, November 11, 280(18):1590–95.

Sung, Y. F.; et al. (1977). Comparison of the effects of acupuncture and codeine on postoperative dental pain. *Anesth. Analg.—Curr. Res.*, 56: 473–78.

Tashkin, D. P.; et al. (1977). Comparison of real and simulated acupuncture and isoproterenol in methacholine-induced asthma. *Annals Allergy*, 39: 379–87.

Thomas, M.; Eriksson, S. V.; and Lundeberg, T. (1991). A comparative study of diazepam and acupuncture in patients with osteoarthritis pain: A placebo controlled study. *American Journal of Chinese Medicine*, 19: 95–100.

Vincent, C. A. (1989). A controlled trial of the treatment of migraine by acupuncture. *Clinical Journal of Pain*, 5: 305–12.

———. (1990). The treatment of tension headache by acupuncture: A controlled single case design with time series analysis. *Journal of Psychosomatic Research*, 34: 553–61.

Wang, H. H.; Chang, Y. H.; and Liu, D. M. (1992). A study of the effectiveness of acupuncture analgesia for colonoscopic examination compared with conventional premedication. *American Journal of Acupuncture*, 20: 217–21.

Wang, L.; Wang, A.; and Zhang, S. (1985). Clinical analysis and experimental observation on acupuncture and moxibustion treatment of patellar tendon terminal disease in athletes. *Journal of Traditional Chinese Medicine*, 5: 162–66.

Wyon, et al. (1995). Effects of acupuncture on climacteric vasomotor symptoms, quality of life, and urinary excretion of neuropeptides among postmenopausal women. *Menopause*, 2:3–12.

Yang, S.; et al. (1994). Clinical observation on needling extrachannel points in treating mental depression. *Journal of Traditional Chinese Medicine*, 14: 14–18.

Zhang, W.; et al. (1987). Acupuncture treatment of apoplectic hemiplegia. *Journal of Traditional Chinese Medicine*, 7: 157–60.

Chapter 6: WESTERN HERBAL MEDICINE

Arfeen, Z.; et al. (1995). A double-blind randomized controlled trial of ginger for the prevention of postoperative nausea and vomiting. *Anaesth. Intensive Care*, 23: 433–36.

Bach, D.; et al. (1997). Phytopharmaceutical and synthetic agents in the treatment of benign prostatic hyperplasia (BPH). *Phytomedicine*, 3(4): 309–13.

Bauer, R. (1996). Echinacea drugs—effects and active ingredients (Review). *Z Arztl. Fortbild Qualitatssich*, 90(2): 111–15.

Bauer, U. (1984). Six-month double-blind randomized clinical trial of Ginkgo Biloba extract versus placebo in two parallel groups of patients suffering from peripheral arterial insufficiency. *Arzneimittelforschung*, 34: 716–20.

Blumenthal, M., and Malone, D. (1997). Review of claims and supportive data from clinical studies on selected herbs and phytomedicines popular in the U.S. marketplace (unpublished, commissioned review).

Blumenthal, M.; et al., eds. (1998). Klein, S., and Rister, R. S., translators. *German Commission E. Monographs: Therapeutic Monographs on Medicinal Plants for Human Use.* Austin, Tex.: American Botanical Council.

Bone, M. E.; et al. (1990). Ginger root—A new antiemetic. The effect of ginger root on postoperative nausea and vomiting after major gynecological surgery. *Anaesthesia,* 48: 669–71.

Braechman, J. (1994). The extract of Serenoa repens in the treatment of benign prostatic hyperplasia: A multicenter open study. *Current Therapeutic Research,* 55: 776–85.

Braunig, B.; et al. (1992). Echinacea purpurea radix for strengthening the immune response in flu-like infections. *Z Phytotherapie,* 13: 7–13.

Carraro, J. C.; et al. (1996). Comparison of phytotherapy (Permixon) with finasteride in the treatment of benign prostate hyperplasia: A randomized international study of 1,098 patients. *Prostate,* 29(4): 231–40.

Champault, G.; et al. (1984). The medical treatment of prostatic adenoma—a controlled study: PA-109 versus placebo in 110 patients. *Ann. Urol. (Paris),* 6: 407–10.

Coeugniet, E., and Kuhnast, R. (1986). Recurrent candidiasis: Adjuvant immunotherapy with different formulations of Echinacin®. *Therapiewoche,* 36: 3352–58.

The Complete German Commission E Monographs: Therapeutic Guide to Herbal Medicines (1998). Austin, Tex.: American Botanical Council, and Boston: Integrative Medicine Communications.

Consumer Reports (1995). Herbal Roulette. November, 698–705.

Daiber, W. (1983). Climacteric complaints: Success without using hormones. *Arztliche Praxis,* 35: 1946–47.

De Weerdt, C. J.; et al. (1996). Herbal medicines in migraine prevention. Randomized double-blind placebo controlled crossover trial of a feverfew preparation. *Phytomedicine,* 3(3): 225–30.

Dorling, E. (1980). Do ginsenosides influence the performance? Results of a double-blind study. *Notabene medici,* 10(5): 241–46.

Duker, E-M.; et al. (1991). Effects of extracts from *Cimicifuga racemosa* on gonadotropin release in menopausal women and ovariectomized rats. *Planta Med.,* 57: 420–24.

Engels, H. J., and Wirth, J. C. (1997). No ergogenic effects of ginseng (*Panaz ginseng* C. A. Meyer) during graded maximal aerobic exercise. *Journal of American Dietary Association,* 97(10): 1110–15.

Engels, H. J.; et al. (1996). Failure of chronic ginseng supplementation to affect work performance and energy metabolism in healthy adult females. *Nutritional Research,* 16: 1295–1305.

Ernst, E. (1996). Ginkgo Biloba in treatment of intermittent claudication. A systematic research based on controlled studies in the literature. *Fortschr. Med.*, 114(8): 85–87.

Ferenci, P.; et al. (1989). Randomized controlled trial of silymarin treatment in patients with cirrhosis of the liver. *Journal of Hepatol.*, 9(1): 105–13.

Fintelmann, V., and Albert, A. (1980). The therapeutic activity of Legalon® in toxic hepatic disorders demonstrated in a double blind trial. *Therapiewoche*, 30: 5589–94.

Fischer-Rasmussen; et al. (1991). Ginger treatment of hyperemesis gravidarum. *European Journal of Obstet. Gynecol. Reprod. Biology*, 38: 19–24.

Floersheim, G. L.; et al. (1982). Poisoning by the deathcap fungus (*Amanita phalloides*): Prognostic factors and therapeutic measures. *Schweiz Med. Wochenschr.*, 112: 1164–77.

Forgo, I., and Kirchdorfer, A. M. (1982). The effect of different ginsenoside concentrations on physical work capacity. *Notabene Medici*, 12(9): 721–27.

Grontved, A.; et al. (1988). Ginger root against seasickness. A controlled trial on the open sea. *Acta Otolaryngol (Stockh)*, 105: 45–49.

Grunwald, J.; et al. (1992). Effects of garlic powder tablets on blood lipids and blood pressure. The Danish Multicenter Kwai Study. *European Journal of Clinical Research*, 3: 179–86.

Hanack, T., and Bruckel, M. H. (1983). The treatment of mild stable forms of angina pectoris using Crategutt® novo. *Therapiewoche*, 33: 4331–33.

Harrer, G.; and Sommer, H. (1994). Treatment of mild/moderate depressions with Hypericum. *Phytomedicine*, 1: 3–8.

Heptinstall, S.; et al. (1992). Parthenolide content and bioactivity of feverfew Tanacetum parthenium (L.) Schultz-Bip. Estimation of commercial and authenticated feverfew products. *Journal of Pharmacology*, 44: 391–95.

Heymsfield, Steven B.; et al. (1998). Garcinia cambogia (Hydroxycitric Acid) as a potential antiobesity agent. *JAMA*, November 11, 390(18): 1596–1600.

Hikino, H., and Kiso, Y. (1988). Natural Products for Liver Disease. In H. Wagner, et al., *Economic and Medicinal Plant Research*. Vol 2. New York: Academic Press, 39–72.

Holzgartner, H.; et al. (1992). Comparison of the efficacy and tolerance of a garlic preparation vs. bezafibrate. *Arzneimittelforschung*, 42(12): 1473–77.

Hruby, C. (1984). Silibinin in the Treatment of Deathcap Fungus Poisoning. *Forum*, 6: 23–26.

Johnson, E. S. (1983). Patients Who Chew Chrysanthemum Leaves. *MIMS Magazine*, May, 15: 32–35.

Johnson, E. S.; et al. (1985). Efficacy of feverfew as prophylactic treatment of migraine. *British Medical Journal*, 291: 569–73.

Johnston, B. (1997). One-third of nation's adults use herbal remedies: Market estimated at $3.24 billion. *HerbalGram*, 40: 49.

Kleijnen, J., and Knipschild, P. (1992a). Ginkgo Biloba for cerebral insufficiency. *British Journal of Clinical Pharmacology*, 34: 352–58.

———. (1992b). Ginkgo Biloba. *Lancet*, 340: 1136–39.

Koch, H. P., and Lawson, L. D., eds. (1996). *Garlic: The Science and Therapeutic Application of Allium Sativum L. and Related Species*. 2d ed. Baltimore: Williams & Wilkins Publishing Co.

Le Bars; et al. (1997). A placebo controlled, double-blind, randomized trial of an extract of Ginkgo Biloba for dementia. *JAMA*, 278(16): 3127–32.

Leathwood, P. D., and Chauffard, F. (1985). Aqueous extract of valerian reduces latency to fall asleep in man. *PlantaMed*, 51: 144–48.

Leathwood, P. D.; et al. (1982). Aqueous extract of valerian root (*Valeriana officinalis L.*) improves sleep quality in man. *Pharmacol. Biochem. Behavior*, 17: 65–71.

Leuchtgens, H. (1993). Crataegus special extract WS 1442 in NYHA II heart failure. A placebo controlled randomized double-blind study. *Forstschr. Med.*, 111(20–21): 352–54.

Litovitz, T. L.; et al. (1996). 1995 annual report of the American Association of Poison Control Centers Toxic Exposure Surveillance System. *American H. Emerg. Medicine*, 14(5): 487–537.

Loew, D.; Albrecht, M.; and Podzuweit, H. (1996). Efficacy and tolerability of a hawthorn preparation in patients with heart failure stage I and II according to NYHA—A surveillance study. Second International Congress on Phytomedicine, Munich.

Lowe, F. C., and Ku, J. C. (1996). Phytotherapy in treatment of benign prostate hyperplasia: A critical review. *Urology*, 48(1): 12–20.

Magliulo, E.; et al. (1978). Results of a double-blind study on the effect of silymarin in the treatment of acute viral hepatitis, carried out at two medical centres. *Med. Klinik*, 73(28–29): 1060–65.

Melchart, D.; et al. (1994). Immunomodulation with echinacea—A systematic review of controlled clinical trials. *Phytomedicine*, 1: 245–54.

Melchart, D.; et al. (1995). Results of five randomized studies on the immunomodulatory activity of preparations of echinacea. *Journal of Alternative Complementary Medicine*, 1(2): 145–60.

Mowrey, D. B., and Clayson, D. E. (1982). Motion sickness, ginger and psychophysics. *Lancet*, 1: 655–57.

Murphy, J. J.; et al. (1988). Randomized double-blind placebo controlled trial of feverfew in migraine prevention. *Lancet*, 8604: 189–92.

Murray, M. (1996). Understanding the benefits of standardized botanical extracts. *American Journal of Natural Medicine*, 3(8): 6–12.

———. (1997). Remifemin: Answers to some common questions. *American Journal of Natural Medicine*, 4(3): 3–5.

Palasciano, G.; et al. (1994). The effect of silymarin on plasma levels of malon-dialdehyde in patients receiving long term treatment with psychotropic drugs. *Curr. Therapeutic Research*, 55(5): 537–45.

Palevitch, D.; et al. (1997). Feverfew *(Tanacetum parthenium)* as a prophylac-tic treatment for migraine: A double-blind placebo controlled study. *Phytotherapy Research*, 11(7): 508–11.

Perharic, L.; et al. (1994). Toxicological problems resulting from exposure to tra-ditional remedies and food supplements. *Drug Safety*, 11: 284–94.

Petho, A. (1987). Menopausal complaints: Change-over of a hormone treatment to a herbal gynecological remedy practicable? *Arztliche Praxis*, 47: 1551–53.

Phillips, S.; et al. (1993). *Zingiber officinale* (ginger)—An antiemetic for day case surgery. *Anaesthesia*, 48(8): 715–19.

Poser, G. (1971). Experience in the treatment of chronic hepatitis with silymarin. *Arzneimittelforschung*, 21: 1209–12.

Reh, C., and Laux, P. (1992). Hypericum extrakt bei depressionen—eine wirk-same alternative. *Therapiewoche*, 42: 1576–81.

Reuter, H. D.; et al. (1996). Therapeutic effects and applications of garlic and its preparations. In H. P. Koch and L. D. Lawson, eds. *Garlic: The Science and Therapeutic Application of Allium Sativum L. and Related Species.* 2d ed. Baltimore: Williams & Wilkins Publishing Co.

Rosenfeld, M. S. (1989). Evaluation of the efficacy of a standardized ginseng extract in patients with psychophysical asthenia and neurological disorders. *La Semana Medica*, 173(9): 148–54.

Scaglione, F.; et al. (1990). Immunomodulatory effects of two extracts of *Panax ginseng* C.A. Meyer. *Drugs Under Experimental & Clinical Research*, 26: 537–42.

Scaglione, F.; et al. (1996). Efficacy and safety of the standardized ginseng extract G 115 for potentiating vaccination against common cold and/or influenza syn-drome. *Drugs Under Experimental & Clinical Research*, 22(2): 65–72.

Schmid, R.; et al. (1994). Comparison of seven commonly used agents for pro-phylaxis of seasickness. *Journal of Travel Medicine*, 1(4): 203–6.

Schmidt, U.; et al. (1994). Efficacy of the hawthorn (crataegus) preparation LI 132 in 78 patients with chronic congestive heart failure defined as NYHA functional class II. *Phytomedicine*, 1: 17–24.

Schmidt-Voigt, J. (1988). Treatment of nervous sleep disturbances and inner restlessness with a purely herbal sedative. *Therapiewoche*, 36: 663.

Schneider, B. (1992). Ginkgo Biloba extract in peripheral arterial diseases. Meta-analysis of controlled clinical studies. *Arzneimittelforschung*, 42: 428–36.

Schoneberger, D. (1992). The influence of immune-stimulating effects of pressed juice from Echinacea purpurea on the course and severity of colds. *Forum Immunol.*, 8: 2–12.

Seifert, T. (1988). Therapeutic effects of valerian in nervous disorders: A field study. *Therapeutikon,* 2: 94.

Siegel, R. K. (1979). Ginseng abuse syndrome: Problems with the panacea. *JAMA,* 241(15): 1614–15.

Silagy, C., and Neil, A. (1994). Garlic as a lipid lowering agent—A meta-analysis. *Journal R. Coll. Physicians Lond.,* 28: 39–45.

Sotaniemi, E. A.; et al. (1995). Ginseng therapy in non-insulin-dependent diabetic patients. *Diabetes Care,* 18: 1373–75.

Steiner, M.; et al. (1996). A double-blind crossover study in moderately hypercholesterolemic men that compared the effect of aged garlic extract and placebo administration on blood lipids. *American Journal of Clinical Nutrition,* 64: 866–70.

Stoll, W. (1987). Phytopharmacon influences atrophic vaginal epithelium: Double-blind study—cimicifuga vs. estrogenic substances. *Therapeuticum,* 1: 23–31.

Tauchert, M.; et al. (1994). Effectiveness of hawthorn extract LI 132 compared with the ACE inhibitor Captopril: Multicenter double-blind study with 132 NYHA stage II. *Muench Med. Wochenschr.* 136 Suppl: §27–§33.

UC Berkeley Wellness Letter (1997). The Wellness Guide to Herbal Medicines. September, 4–5.

Vesper, J., and Hangsen, K-D. (1994). Efficacy of Ginkgo Biloba in 90 outpatients with cerebral insufficiency caused by old age. *Phytomedicine,* 1: 9–16.

Vorbach, E. U.; et al. (1996). Therapie von insomnien, wirksamkeit, und vertraglichkeit eines baldrianpraparats. *Psychopharmakother,* 3: 109–15.

Vorberg, G. (1984). Treatment of menopause symptoms—Successful hormone-free therapy with Remifemin®. *ZFA,* 60: 626–29.

Wagner, H. (1997). Herbal immunostimulants for the prophylaxis and therapy of colds and influenza. *European Journal of Herbal Medicine,* 3(1).

Warnecke, G. (1985). Influencing menopausal symptoms with a phytotherapeutic agent: Successful therapy with Cimicifuga mono-extract. *Med. Welt,* 36: 871–74.

Warshafsky, S.; et al. (1993). Effect of garlic on total serum cholesterol. *Ann. Intern. Medicine,* 119: 599–605.

Weikl, A.; et al. (1996). Crataegus special extract WS 1442. Assessment of objective effectiveness in patients with heart failure. *Fortschr Med.,* 114(24): 291–96.

Weil, A. (1989). A New Look at Botanical Medicine. *Whole Earth Review,* Fall, 5–7.

WHO. *Radix Ginseng* (monograph). Geneva: World Health Organization. In press 1998.

Wilt, Timothy J.; et al. (1998). Saw Palmetto extracts for treatment of benign prostatic hyperplasia. *JAMA,* November 11, 280(18):1604–9.

Woelk, H.; et al. (1994). Benefits and risks of the hypericum extract LI 160; drug monitoring study with 3,250 patients. *Journal of Geriatric Psychiatry & Neurology*, October, 7 Suppl. 1: §34–§38.

Chapter 7: NATUROPATHIC MEDICINE

Aganoff, J. A., and Boyle, G. J. (1994). Aerobic exercise, mood states and menstrual cycle symptoms. *Journal of Psychosomatic Research*, 38(3): 183–92.

Alun Jones, V. A.; et al. (1982). Food intolerance: a major factor in the pathogenesis of irritable bowel syndrome. *Lancet*, 2: 1115–17.

Anah, C. O.; et al. (1982). High dose ascorbic acid in Nigerian asthmatics. The attenuation of exercise-induced bronchospasm by ascorbic acid. *Ann. Allergy*, 49(3): 146–51.

Antoun, M. D., and Taha, O. M. (1981). Studies on Sudanese medicinal plants. II. Evaluation of an extract of *Lupinus termis* seeds in chronic eczema. *Journal of Natural Products*, 44(2): 179–83.

Atani, J. A.; et al. (1990). Effect of Abana on ventricular function in ischemic heart disease. *Jpn Heart Journal*, 31(6): 829–35.

Atherton, D. J.; et al. (1978). A double-blind crossover trial of an antigen-avoidance diet in atopic eczema. *Lancet*, February, 25: 401–3.

Avery, D. H.; et al. (1993). Dawn simulation of winter depression: A controlled study. *American Journal of Psychiatry*, 150(1): 113–17.

Berges, R. R.; et al. (1995). Randomised, placebo controlled, double-blind clinical trial of beta-sitosterol in patients with benign prostatic hypertrophy. *Lancet*, 345: 1529–32.

Brigo, B., and Serpelloni, G. (1991). Homeopathic treatment of migraines: A randomized double-blind study of 60 cases (homeopathic remedy versus placebo). *Berlin Journal of Research in Homeopathy*, 1(2): 98–106.

Bruggermann, G.; et al. (1990). Results of a double-blind study of diclofenac + vitamin B1, B6, B12 vs diclofenac in patients with acute pain of the lumbar vertebrae: A multicenter study. *Klin Wochenschr*, 68(2): 116–20.

Buck, A. C.; et al. (1990). Treatment of outflow tract obstruction due to benign prostatic hypertrophy with the pollen extract, Cernilton: A double-blind, placebo controlled study. *British Journal of Urology*, 66(4): 398–404.

Burack, J. H.; et al. (1996). Pilot randomized controlled trial of Chinese herbal treatment for HIV-associated symptoms. *Journal of AIDS Hum. Retrovirology*, 12:386–93.

Calabrese, C. (1997). (Unpublished, commissioned review.)

Canner, P. L.; et al. (1986). Fifteen-year mortality in coronary drug project patients: Long-term benefit with niacin. *Journal of American Coll. Cardiology*, 8(6): 1245–55.

Capsaicin Study Group (1992). Effect of treatment with capsaicin on daily activities of patients with painful diabetic neuropathy. *DiabetesCare*, 15(2): 159–65.

Carpendale, M. T.; et al. (1993). Does ozone alleviate AIDS diarrhea? *Journal of Clinical Gastroenterology*, September, 17(2): 142–45.

Caruso, I., and Pietrogrande, V. (1987). Italian double-blind multicenter study comparing S-adenosylmethionine, naproxen, and placebo in the treatment of degenerative joint disease. *American Journal of Medicine*, 83(5A): 66–71.

Champault, G.; et al. (1984). A double-blind trial of an extract of the plant *Serenoa repens* in benign prostatic hypertrophy. *British Journal of Clinical Pharmacology*, 18: 461–62.

Chandra, R. K. (1992). Effect of vitamin and trace-element supplementation on immune responses and infection in elderly subjects. *Lancet*, 340: 1124–27.

Cherchi, A.; et al. (1985). Effects of L-carnitine on exercise tolerance in chronic stable angina: A multicenter, double-blind, randomized, placebo controlled crossover study. *Int. Journal of Clinical Pharm. Ther. Toxicology*, 23:569–72.

Collip, P. J.; et al. (1975). Pyridoxine treatment of childhood bronchial asthma. *Ann. Allergy*, 35: 93–97.

Coodley, G. O.; et al. (1993). Beta carotene in HIV infection. *Journal of AIDS*, 6: 272–76.

Damrau, F. (1962). Benign prostatic hyperplasia: amino acid therapy of symptomatic relief. *American Journal of Geriatrics*, 10: 426–30.

Deal, C. L.; et al. (1991). Treatment of arthritis with topical capsaicin: a double-blind trial. *Clinical Therapy*, 13(3): 383–95.

Duncan, B.; et al. (1993). Exclusive breast feeding for at least four months protects against otitis media. *Pediatrics*, 91(5): 867–72.

Eby, G. A.; et al. (1984). Reduction in duration of common colds by zinc gluconate lozenges in a double-blind study. *Antimicrob. Agents Chemo.*, 25(1): 20–24.

Egger, J.; et al. (1983). Is migraine food allergy? A double-blind controlled trial of oligoantigenic diet treatment. *Lancet*, 344: 865–69.

Ehlers, A.; et al. (1995). Treatment of atopic dermatitis: A comparison of psychological and dermatological approaches to relapse prevention. *Journal of Consulting & Clinical Psychology*, 63(4): 624–25.

Faccinetti, F.; et al. (1991). Magnesium prophylaxis of menstrual migraine: Effects on intracellular magnesium. *Headache*, 31: 298–304.

Fergusson, D. M., and Horwood, L. J. (1994). Early solid food diet and eczema in childhood: A ten-year longitudinal study. *Pedatr. Allergy Immunology*, 5(6 Suppl): 44–47.

Ferley, J. P.; et al. (1989). A controlled evaluation of a homeopathic preparation in the treatment of influenza-like syndromes. *British Journal of Pharmacology*, 27: 329–35.

Friese, K. H.; et al. (1996). Acute otitis media in children: Comparison between conventional and homeopathic therapy. *HNO*, 44(8): 462–66.

Frost, H.; et al. (1995). Randomised controlled trial for evaluation of fitness programme for patients with chronic low back pain. *BMJ*, 310: 151–54.

Girodo, M. E.; et al. (1992). Deep diaphragmatic breathing: Rehabilitation exercises for the asthmatic patient. *Arch Phys Med Rehabil*, 73(8): 717–20.

Gupta, S.; et al. (1979). *Tylophora indica* in bronchial asthma: A double-blind study. *Ind. Journal of Med. Research*, 69: 981–89.

Heller, B. (1978). Pharmacological and clinical effects of d-phenylalanine in depression and Parkinson's disease. In Mosnaim and Wolf, eds., *Noncatecholic Phenylethylamines, Part I*. New York: Marcel Dekker, 397–417.

Henry, M.; et al. (1993). Improvement of respiratory function in chronic asthmatic patients with autogenic therapy. *Journal of Psychosomatic Research*, 37(3): 265–70.

Hilton, E.; et al. (1992). Ingestion of yogurt containing *Lactobacillus acidophilus* as prophylaxis for candidal vaginitis. *Ann. Int. Med.*, 116: 353–57.

Hudson, T. (1991). Consecutive case study research of carcinoma in situ of cervix employing local escharotic treatment combined with nutritional therapy. *Journal of Naturopathic Medicine*, 2:6–10.

———. (1993). Escharotic treatment for cervical dysplasia and carcinoma. *Journal of Naturopathic Medicine*, 4(1): 23.

Hurst, D. S. (1990). Allergy management of refractory serous otitis media. *Otolaryngology Head Neck Surgery*, 102(6): 664–69.

Jones, D. Y. (1987). Influence of dietary fat on self-reported menstrual symptoms. *Physiology and Behavior*, 40(4): 483–87.

Kaiser, J. D. (1994). *Immune Power: Combining Holistic and Standard Medical Therapies into the Optimal Treatment Program for HIV*. New York: St. Martin's Press.

Kangasniemi, P.; et al. (1978). Levotryptophan treatment in migraine. *Headache*, 18: 161–66.

Kreitsch, K.; et al. (1988). Prevalence, presenting symptoms, and psychological characteristics of individuals experiencing a diet related mood disturbance. *Behavioral Therapy*, 19: 593–604.

Kulkarni, R. R.; et al. (1991). Treatment of osteoarthritis with a combination herbomineral formulation: A double-blind, placebo controlled, crossover study. *Journal of Ethnopharmacology*, 33(1–2): 91–95.

Linde, K.; et al. (1996). St. John's Wort for depression: An overview and meta-analysis of randomised clinical trials. *BMJ*, 313(7052): 253–58.

Linton, S. J.; et al. (1989). The secondary prevention of low back pain: A controlled study with follow-up. *Pain*, 36: 197–207.

London, R. S.; et al. (1987). Efficacy of alpha-tocopherol in the treatment of the premenstrual syndrome. *Journal of Reproducive Medicine*, 32(6): 400–404.

London, R. S.; et al. (1991). Effect of a nutritional supplement on premenstrual symptomatology in women with premenstrual syndrome: A double-blind longitudinal study. *Journal of Americal Coll. Nutrition*, 10(5): 494–99.

Maiwald, Von L.; et al. (1988). Therapy of common cold with a combination homeopathic preparation compared with acetylsalicylic acid. *Arzneim.-Forsch. (Drug Res)*, 38(1)4: 578–82.

McCarren, T.; et al. (1985). Amelioration of severe migraine by fish oil (w-3) fatty acids. *American Journal of Clinical Nutrition*, 41: 874a.

Meade, T. W.; et al. (1990). Low back pain of mechanical origin: Randomised comparison of chiropractic and hospital outpatient management. *British Medical Journal*, 300: 1431–37.

Moran, G.; et al. (1991). A controlled study of the psychoanalytic treatment of brittle diabetes. *Journal of American Acad. Child Adolescent Psychiatry*, 30(60): 926–35.

Mumcuoglu, M.; et al. (1994). Inhibition of several strains of influenza virus and beneficial effect of Sambucol in the treatment of naturally occurring influenza B in a double-blind preliminary study. *6th Int. Congr. Infect. Dis.*, April 26–30, 392.

Murphy, J.; Heptinstall, S.; and Mitchell, J. R. A. (1988). Randomised double-blind placebo controlled trial of feverfew in migraine prevention. *Lancet*, ii: 189–92.

Murray, Michael, and Pizzorno, Joseph (1998). *Encyclopedia of Natural Medicine*. Prima Publishing.

Neri, A.; Sabah, G.; and Samra, Z. (1993). Bacterial vaginosis in pregnancy treated with yogurt. *Acta Obstet. Gyn. Scand.*, 72: 17–19.

Nsouli, T. M.; et al. (1994). Role of food allergy in serous otitis media. *Ann. Allergy*, 73: 215–19.

Ogle, K. A., and Bullock, J. D. (1980). Children with allergic rhinitis and/or bronchial asthma treated with elimination diet: A five-year follow-up. *Ann. Allergy*, 44: 273–78.

Paolisso, G.; et al. (1993). Pharmacologic doses of vitamin E improve insulin action in healthy subjects and non-insulin-dependent diabetic patients. *American Journal of Clinical Nutrition*, 57: 650–56.

Pena, E. (1962). *Melaleuca alternifolia* oil: its use for trichomonal vaginitis and other vaginal infections. *Obstet. Gyn.*, 19(6): 793–95.

Pfister, R. (1981). Problems in the treatment and aftercare of chronic dermatoses. A clinical study on Hamatum ointment. *Fortschr Med.*, 99(31–32): 1264–68.

Pye, J. K.; et al. (1985). Clinical experience of drug treatments for mastalgia. *Lancet*, 2: 373–77

Rahlfs, V. W., and Mossinger, P. (1979). *Asa foetida* in irritable colon: double-blind trial. *Deutsche Med. Woch*, 104(4): 140–43.

Rastogi, D. P.; et al. (1993). Evaluation of homeopathic therapy in 129 asymptomatic HIV carriers. *British Homeopathy Journal*, 82:48.

Ravina, A.; et al. (1995). Clinical use of the trace element chromium (III) in the treatment of diabetes mellitus. *Journal of Trace Element Experimental Medicine*, 8: 183–90.

Reilly, D. T.; et al. (1994). Is evidence for homeopathy reproducible? *Lancet*, 344: 1601–6.

Rejholec, V. (1987). Long-term studies of antiosteoarthritic drugs: An assessment. *Semin Arthritis Rheum*, 17(2 Suppl I): 35–53.

Robbins, L. D. (1989). Cyrotherapy for headache. *Headache*, 29: 598–600.

Rovat, L. C. (1992). Clinical research in osteoarthritis design and results of short-term and long-term trials with disease modifying drugs. *Int. Journal of Tissue Reactions*, 14(5): 243–51.

Salmaggi, P.; et al. (1993). Double-blind, placebo controlled study of S-adenosyl-L-methionine in depressed post-menopausal women. *Psychother. Psychom.*, 59: 34–40.

Scafidi, F., and Field, T. (1996). Massage therapy improves behavior in neonates born to HIV positive mothers. *Journal Pediatric Psychology*, 21(6): 889–97.

Sharma, R. D.; et al. (1990). Effect of fenugreek seeds on blood glucose and serum lipids in type I diabetes. *European Journal of Clinical Nutrition*, 44(4): 301–6.

Shaw, G.; et al. (1991). Stress management for irritable bowel syndrome: a controlled trial. *Digestion*, 50: 36–42.

Sheehan, M. P.; et al. (1992). Efficacy of traditional Chinese herbal therapy in adult atopic dermatitis. *Lancet*, 340: 13–17.

Solomon, S., and Guglielmo, K. M. (1985). Treatment of headache by transcutaneous electrical stimulation. *Headache*, 25: 12–15.

Spence, D. W.; et al. (1990). Progressive resistance exercise: Effect on muscle function and anthropometry of a select AIDS population. *Arch. Phys. Med. Rehabil.*, 71(9): 644.

Standish, L.; et al. (1992). One year open trial of naturopathic treatment of HIV infection class IV-A in men. *Journal of Naturopathic Medicine*, 3(1): 42–64.

Tamborini, A. T.; et al. (1993). Value of standardized gingko biloba extract (Egb 761) in the management of congestive symptoms of premenstrual syndrome. *Rev. Fr. Gynecol. Obstet.*, 88(7–9): 447–57.

Tang, A. M.; et al. (1996). Effects of micronutrient intake on survival in human immunodeficiency virus type I infection. *American Journal of Epid.*, 143(12): 1244–56.

Tempeste, E.; et al. (1987). L-acetylcarnitine in depressed elderly subjects: A crossover study vs. placebo. *Drugs Exptl. Clin. Res.*, 13(7): 417–23.

Thys-Jacobs, S.; et al. (1989). Calcium supplementation in premenstrual syndrome: A randomized crossover trial. *Journal of Gen. Intern. Medicine*, 4(3): 183–89.

Trentham, D. (1993). Effects of oral administrations of type II collagen on rheumatoid arthritis. *Science*, 261(5129): 1727–29.

Trock, D.; et al. (1993). A double-blind trial of the clinical effects of pulsed electromagnetic fields in osteoarthritis. *Journal of Rheumatology*, 20(3): 456–60.

Turner, J. A., and Jensen, M. P. (1993). Efficacy of cognitive therapy for chronic low back pain. *Pain*, 52: 169–77.

Unge, G.; et al. (1983). Effect of dietary tryptophan restrictions on clinical symptoms in patients with endogenous asthma. *Allergy*, 38: 211–12.

Vague, P.; et al. (1987). Nicotinamide may extend remission phase in insulin-dependent diabetes. *Lancet*, 1: 619–20.

Wanke, C.; et al. (1996). A medium chain triglyceride-based diet in patients with HIV and chronic diarrhea reduces diarrhea and malabsorption: A prospective, controlled trial. *Nutrition*, 12(11/12): 766–71.

Weil, A. (1995). *Natural Health, Natural Medicine.* Boston: Houghton Mifflin.

Weng, W. L.; et al. (1984). Therapeutic effect of *Crataegus pinnatifida* on 46 cases of angina pectoris: A double-blind study. *Journal of Traditional Chinese Medicine*, 4(4): 293–97.

Werbach, M. (1993). *Healing Through Nutrition.* New York: HarperCollins.

Whorwell, P. J.; et al. (1984). Controlled trial of hypnotherapy in the treatment of severe refractory irritable-bowel syndrome. *Lancet*, ii: 1232–34.

Wolffers, I.; et al. (1994). Use of alternative treatments by HIV positive and AIDS patients in the Netherlands. International AIDS Conference.

Chapter 8: HOMEOPATHY

Abelson, M. B.; et al. (1995). An effective treatment for allergy sufferers. *Contact Lens Spectrum*, December, 18–32.

Andrade, L.; et al. (1991). A randomised controlled trial to evaluate the effectiveness of homeopathy in rheumatoid arthritis. *Scand. Journal Rheumatology*, 20: 204–8.

Benveniste, J.; et al. (1991). L'agitation de solutions hautement diluées n'induit pas d'activité biologique specifique. *C. R. Acad. Sci. Paris*, 312: 461.

Boyd, W. E. (1941). The action of microdoses of mercuric chloride on diastase. *British Homeopathic Journal*, 1:1–28, and (1942) 32: 106é11.

Brigo, B., and Serpelloni, G. (1991). Homeopathic treatment of migraine: A randomized double-blind study of sixty cases (homeopathic remedy versus placebo). *Berlin Journal on Research in Homeopathy,* 1: 98–106.

Consumer Reports (1994). Homeopathy: Much ado about nothing? March, 10–15.

Davenas, E.; Beauvais, F.; and Amara, J. (1988). Human basophil degranulation triggered by very dilute antiserum against IgE. *Nature,* 333: 816–18.

de Lange de Klerk, E. S. M.; et al. (1994). Effect of homeopathic medicines on daily burden of symptoms in children with recurrent upper respiratory tract infections. *British Medical Journal,* 6965: 1329–32.

Del Giudice, E., and Preparata, G. (1990). Superradiance: A new approach to coherent dynamical behaviors of condensed matter. *Frontier Perspectives,* 1(2). Philadelphia: Temple University, Center for Frontier Sciences.

Demangeat, J. L.; et al. (1992). Modifications des temps de relaxation RMN à 4 z des protons du solvant dans les très hautes dilutions salines de silice/ lactose. *Journal of Medical Nucl. Biophy.,* 16:35–45.

Dietz, Vance, and Jacobs, Jennifer (1997). Vaccination: Attitudes and Practices of Physicians Who Use Homeopathy. *Alternative and Complementary Therapies,* December, 414–18.

Dorfman, P.; Lasserre, M. N.; and Tetau, M. (1987). Préparation à l'accouchement par homéopathie-expérimentation en double insu versu placebo. *Cahiers de Biothérapie,* 94: 77–81.

Ferley, J. P.; Zmirou, D.; D'Adhemar, D.; and Balducci, F. (1989). A controlled evaluation of a homeopathic preparation in the treatment of influenza-like syndromes. *British Journal of Clinical Pharm.,* 27: 329–35.

Fisher, P.; et al. (1989). Effect of homeopathic treatment on fibrositis (primary fibromyalgia). *British Medical Journal,* 299: 365–66.

Friese, K. H.; Kruse, S.; and Moeller, H. (1996). Acute otitis media in children. Comparison between conventional and homeopathic therapy. *HNO,* 44: 462–66.

Gaus, W., Walach, H., and Haag, G. (1992). Die Wirksamkeit der Klassischen Homeopathischen Therapie bei chronischen Kopfschmerzen. *Der Schmerz (Pain),* 6: 134–140.

Gibson, R. G.; et al. (1980). Homeopathic therapy in rheumatoid arthritis: Evaluation by double-blind clinical therapeutical trial. *British Journal of Clinical Pharm.,* 9: 453–59.

Jacobs, J. (1997). Clinical research outcomes: A review of the literature in homeopathic medicine (unpublished, commissioned review).

Jacobs, J.; et al. (1993). Homeopathic treatment of acute childhood diarrhea. A randomized clinical trial in Nicaragua. *British Homeopathic Journal,* 82: 83–86.

Jacobs, J.; et al. (1994). Treatment of acute childhood diarrhea with homeopathic medicine: A randomized clinical trial in Nicaragua. *Pediatrics,* 92: 719–25.

Jonas, W., and Jacobs, J. (1996) *Healing with Homeopathy*. New York:.Warner Books.

Khuda-Bukhsh, A. R., and Banik, S. (1991). Assessment of cytogenetic damage in X-irradiated mice and its alteration by oral administration of potentized homeopathic drug, ginseng D200. *Berlin Journal of Research in Homeopathy*, 1, 4/5: 254.

Kleijnen, J.; Knipschild, P.; and Rieter, G. (1991). Clinical trials of homeopathy. *British Medical Journal*, 302: 316–23.

Kohler, T. (1991). Wirksamkeitsnachweis eines Homöopathikums bei chronischer Polyarthritis—eine randomisierte Doppelblindstudie bei niedergelassenen Ärzten. *Der Kassenarzt*, 13: 48–52.

Labrecque, M.; et al. (1992). Homeopathic treatment of plantar warts. *Canadian Medical Association Journal*, 146: 1749–53.

Lepaisant, C. (1994). *Essais thérapeutiques du syndrome prémenstruel—étude en double aveugle avec folliculinum*. Université de Caen (thesis).

Linde, K.; et al. (1994). Critical review and meta-analysis of serial agitated dilutions in experimental toxicology. *Human and Experimental Toxicology*, 13: 481–92.

Linde, Klaus; et al. (1997). Are the clinical effects of homeopathy placebo effects? A meta-analysis of placebo controlled trials. *Lancet*, September 20, 350: 834–43.

Lo, Shui-Yin (1996). Anomalous state of ice. *Modern Physics Letters B*, 10(19): 909–19.

Lo, Shui-Yin; et al. (1996). Physical properties of water with Ie structures. *Modern Physics Letters B*, 10(19): 921–30.

Maddox, J. (1988). When to believe the Unbelievable. *Nature*, 787.

Paterson, J. (1943). Report on the mustard gas experiments (Glasgow and London). *British Homeopathic Journal*, 33: 1–12.

Reilly, D.; et al. (1994). Is evidence for homeopathy reproducible? *Lancet*, 344: 1601–6.

Reilly, D. T., and Taylor, M. A. (1985). Potent placebo or potency? *British Homeopathy Journal*, 74: 65–75.

Reilly, D. T.; et al. (1986). Is homeopathy a placebo response? Controlled trial of homeopathic potency, with pollen in hayfever as model. *Lancet*, ii(8512): 881–85.

Shipley, M.; et al. (1983). Controlled trial of homeopathic treatment of osteoarthritis. *Lancet*, 1: 97–98.

Smith, R. B., and Boericke, G. W. (1968). Changes caused by succussion on N. M. R. patterns and bioassay of bradykinin triacetate (BKTA) succussions and dilution. *Journal of the American Institute of Homeopathy*, 61: 197–212.

Ullman, D. (1996). *The Consumer's Guide to Homeopathy*. Berkeley, Calif.: Homeopathic Educational Services.

Ustianowski, P. A. (1974). A clinical trial of Staphysagria in postcoital cystitis. *British Homeopathy Journal,* 63: 276–77.

Weisenauer, M., and Gaus, W. (1985). Double-blind trial comparing the effectiveness of the homeopathic preparation Galphimia potentisation D6, galphimia dilution 10^{-6} and placebo on pollinosis. *Arzneimittel Forschung/Drug Research,* 35: 1745–47.

―――. (1991). Wirksamkeitsnachweis eines Homöopathikums bei chronischer Polyarthritis—eine randomisierte Doppelblindstudie bei niedergelassenen Ärzten. *Aktuelle Rheumatologie,* 16: 1–9.

Weisenauer, M.; Gaus, W.; and Haussler, S. (1990). Behandlung der Pollinosis mit Galphimia glauca. Eine Doppelblindstudie unter Praxisbedingungen. *Allergologie,* 13: 359–63.

Weisenauer, M.; Hassler, S.; and Gaus, W. (1983). Pollinosis—Therapie mit Galphimia glauca. *Fortschritte der Medizin,* 101: 811–14.

Weisenauer, M., and Ludtke, R. (1995). The treatment of pollinosis with Galphimia glauca D4—a randomized placebo controlled clinical trial. *Phytomedicine,* 2: 3–6.

―――. (1996). A meta-analysis of homeopathic treatment of pollinosis with Galphimia glauca. *Forschung Komplementärmedizin,* 3: 230–34.

Weiser, M.; et al. (1998). Homeopathic vs conventional treatment of vertigo: a randomized double-blind controlled clinical study. *Archives of Otolaryngology, Head and Neck Surgery,* 124: 879–885.

Whitmarsh, T. E., Coleston-Shields, D.E., and Steiner, T.J. (1997). Double-blind randomized placebo-controlled study of the homeopathic prophylaxis of migraine. *Cephalgia,* 17: 600–604.

Chapter 9: CHIROPRACTIC

Adams, A. H., and Gatterman, M. (1997). The state of the art of research on chiropractic education. *Journal of Manipulative and Physiological Therapeutics,* 20(3): 179–84.

Aker, P.; et al. (1996). Conservative management of mechanical neck pain: Systematic overview and meta-analysis. *British Medical Journal,* 313: 1291–96.

Anderson, R.; et al. (1992). A meta-analysis of clinical trials of manipulation. *Journal of Manipulative and Physiological Therapeutics,* 15(3): 181–94.

Assendelft, W. J. J., and Bouter, L. M. (1993). Does the goose really lay golden eggs? A methodological review of workmen's compensation studies. *Journal of Manipulative and Physiological Therapeutics,* 16: 161–68.

Assendelft, W. J. J.; Bouter, L. M.; and Knipschild, P. G. (1996). Complications of spinal manipulation. A comprehensive review of the literature. *Journal of Family Practice,* 42: 475–80.

Assendelft, W. J. J.; et al. (1995). The relationship between methodological quality and conclusions in reviews of spinal manipulation. *JAMA*, 274: 1942–48.

Balon, Jeffrey; et al. (1998). A comparison of active and simulated chiropractic manipulation as adjunctive treatment for childhood asthma. *New England Journal of Medicine*, 339: 1013–20.

Berman, B. M.; et al. (1995). Physicians' attitudes toward complementary or alternative medicine: A regional survey. *Journal of American Board of Family Practice*, 8(36): 1–6.

Bigos, S.; et al. (1994). Acute low back problems in adults. *Clinical Practice Guideline*, No. 14. AHCPR Publication No. 95-0642. Rockville, Md.: Agency for Health Care Policy and Research, Public Health Service, U.S. Department of Health and Human Services, December.

Blunt, K. L.; Rajwani, M. H.; and Guerriero, R. C. (1997). The effectiveness of chiropractic management of fibromyalgia patients: A pilot study. *Journal of Manipulative and Physiological Therapeutics*, July/August, 20(6): 389–99.

Boline, P. D.; et al. (1995). Spinal manipulation versus amitriptyline for the treatment of chronic tension-type headaches: A randomized clinical trial. *Journal of Manipulative and Physiological Therapeutics*, 18: 148–54.

Bove, Geoffrey, and Nilsson, Niels (1998). Spinal manipulation in the treatment of episodic tension-type headache. *JAMA*, November 11, 280(18): 1576–79.

Brennan, P.; et al. (1991). Enhanced phagocytic cell respiratory burst induced by spinal manipulation: Potential role of substance P. *Journal of Manipulative and Physiological Therapeutics*, 14(7): 399–408.

Bronfort, G.; Assendelft, W. J. J.; and Bouter, L. (1996). Efficacy of spinal manipulative therapy conditions other than neck and back pain: A systematic review and best evidence synthesis. *Proceedings of the 1996 International Conference on Spinal Manipulation*, Bournemouth, England, October 18–19, 105–6.

Carette, S.; et al. (1991). A controlled trial of corticosteroid injections into facet joints for chronic low back pain. *New England Journal of Medicine*, October 3, 325(14): 1002–7.

Carey, T. S.; et al. (1995). The outcomes and costs of care for acute low back pain among patients seen by primary care practitioners, chiropractors, and orthopedic surgeons. *New England Journal of Medicine*, 333: 913–17.

Cassidy, J. D.; et al. (1995). Scientific monograph of the Quebec task force on whiplash-associated disorders. *Spine*, 20(8S): 1S–74S.

Cherkin, D. C., and McCormack, F. A. (1989). Patient evaluation of low back pain care from family physicians and chiropractors. *West. Journal of Medicine*, 150: 351–55.

Cherkin, D. C., and Mootz, R. D. (1998). *Chiropractic in the United States: Training, Practice, and Research*. Washington, D.C.: Agency for Health Care Policy and Research. Preprint of unpublished review (Grant HS07915).

Cherkin, Daniel C.; et al. (1998). A comparison of physical therapy, chiropractic manipulation, and provision of an educational booklet for the treatment of patients with low back pain. *New England Journal of Medicine*, 339: 1021–29.

Clinical Standards Advisory Group Report on Low Back Pain (1996). London: HMSO.

Collinge, William (1996). *The American Holistic Health Association Complete Guide to Alternative Medicine*. New York: Warner Books.

Consumer Reports (1994). Chiropractors. June, 16–23.

Coulter, I. D.; et al. (1995). *The Appropriateness of Spinal Manipulation and Mobilization of Cervical Spine: A Literature Review, Indications and Ratings by a Multi-Disciplinary Expert Panel*. Santa Monica, Calif.:RAND, MR-647-CCR.

Deyo, R. A. (1983). Conservative therapy for low back pain. *JAMA*, 250: 1057–62.

Deyo, R. A., and Diehl, A. K. (1986). Patient satisfaction with medical care for low back pain. *Spine*, 11: 28–30.

Deyo, R. A.; et al. (1990). A controlled trial of transcutaneous electrical nerve stimulation (TENS) and exercise for chronic low back pain. *New England Journal of Medicine*, June 7, 322(23): 627–34.

Donaldson, M.; Yordy, K.; and Vanselow, N. (1994). *Defining Primary Care: An Interim Report. Committee on the Future of Primary Care*. Division of Health Care Services, Institute of Medicine. Washington, D.C.: National Academy Press.

Goertz, C. (1996). Summary of the 1995 ACA annual statistical survey on chiropractic practice. *Journal of American Chiropractic Association*, 33(6): 35–41.

Harvard Health Letter (1999). Fact and fiction about chiropractic. January, 24(3): 1–3.

Hawk, C.; Meeker, W.; and Hansen, D. (1997). The national workshop to develop the chiropractic research agenda. *Journal of Manipulative and Physiological Therapeutics*, 20: 111–16.

Hernandez, R. (1997). Law requires health insurers to pay for chiropractic care. *New York Times*, August 22.

Hurwitz, E. L.; et al. (1996). Manipulation and mobilization of the cervical spine. A systematic review of the literature. *Spine*, 21: 1746–60.

Jarvis, K. B.; Phillips, R. B.; and Morris, E. H. (1991). Cost per case comparison of back injury of chiropractic versus medical management for conditions with identical diagnostic codes. *Journal of Occupational Medicine*, 33(8): 847–51.

Kane, R. L.; et al. (1974). Manipulating the patient: A comparison of the effectiveness of physician and chiropractor care. *Lancet*, 1: 1333–36.

Koes, B. S.; et al. (1996). Spinal manipulation for low back pain. An updated systematic review of randomized clinical trials. *Spine,* 21: 2860–73.

Koes, B. S.; et al. (1991). Spinal manipulation and mobilization for back and neck pain: A blinded review. *MBJ,* 303: 1298–1303.

Kokjohn, K.; et al. (1990). The effect of spinal manipulation on pain and prostaglandin levels in women with primary dysmenorrhea. *Journal of Manipulative and Physiological Therapeutics,* 13: 101–6.

Manga, P.; et al. (1993). *The effectiveness and cost-effectiveness of chiropractic management of low-back pain.* Report funded by the Ontario Ministry of Health. Ottawa, Ontario: Plan Manga and Associates, Inc.

Meade, T. W.; et al. (1995). Randomised comparison of chiropractic and outpatient management for low back pain: Results from extended follow up. *British Medical Journal,* 300: 1431–37.

Meade, T. W.; et al. (1990). Low back pain of mechanical origin: Randomized comparison of chiropractic and hospital outpatient treatment. *British Medical Journal,* 300: 1431–37.

Meeker, W.; et al. (1996). Chiropractic research capacity and infrastructure in North America: Results of four surveys. In S. Mulrouney, et al., eds., *Proceedings of the National Workshop to Develop the Chiropractic Research Agenda.* Washington, D.C.: U.S. Dept. of Health and Human Services Contract 240-95-0036, Health Resources and Services Administration Bureau of Health Professions.

Meeker, William C. (1997). An Overview of the Efficacy, Effectiveness, and Efficiency of Chiropractic Care. (Unpublished, commissioned review.)

Mootz, R. D. (1996). The impact of health policy on chiropractic. *Journal of Manipulative and Physiological Therapeutics,* 19(4): 257–64.

Mootz, R. D., and Meeker, W. C. (1994). Referral patterns of American Back Society attendees. *Chiropractic Technique,* 6(1): 1–4.

Mootz, R. D.; Coulter, I. D.; and Hansen, D. T. (1997). Health services research related to chiropractic: Review and recommendations for research prioritization by the chiropractic profession. *Journal of Manipulative and Physiological Therapeutics,* 20(3): 201–17.

Morgan, J. P.; et al. (1985). A controlled trial of spinal manipulation in the management of hypertension. *Journal of American Osteopathic Association,* 85: 308–13.

Mosley, C. D.; Cohen, I. G.; and Arnold, R. M. (1996). Cost-effectiveness of chiropractic care in a managed care setting. *American Journal of Managed Care,* 2(3): 280–82.

New England Journal of Medicine (1998). Editorial: What role for chiropractic in health care? October 8, 339(15): 1074–75.

Nielsen, N. H.; et al. (1995). Chronic asthma and chiropractic spinal manipulation: A randomized clinical trial. *Clinical and Experimental Allergy*, 25: 80–88.

Nilsson, N. (1995). A randomized controlled trial of the effect of spinal manipulation in the treatment of cervicogenic headache. *Journal of Manipulative and Physiological Therapeutics*, 18: 435–40.

Osterbauer, P. J. (1996). Technology assessment of the chiropractic subluxation. *Top Clinical Chiropractic*, 3(1): 1–9.

Parker, G. B.; Tupling, H.; and Pryor, D. S. (1978). A controlled trial of cervical manipulation for migraine. *Australian and NZ Journal of Medicine*, 8: 589–93.

Reed, W.; et al. (1994). Chiropractic management of primary nocturnal enuresis. *Journal of Manipulative and Physiological Therapeutics*, 17: 596–600.

Sawyer, C.; et al. (1997). Clinical research within the chiropractic profession: Status, needs and recommendations. *Journal of Manipulative and Physiological Therapeutics*, 20(3): 169–79.

Shekelle, P. G. (1994). *The Use and Costs of Chiropractic Care in the Health Insurance Experiment*. Santa Monica, Calif.: RAND.

Shekelle, P. G.; et al. (1991). *The Appropriateness of Spinal Manipulation for Low Back Pain: Indications and Ratings by a Multi-Disciplinary Expert Panel*. Santa Monica, Calif.: RAND, R-4025/2-CCR.

Shekelle, P. G.; et al. (1992). Spinal manipulation for low back pain. *American Intern. Medicine*, 117: 590–98.

Stano, M., and Smith, M. (1995). Chiropractic and medical costs of low back care. *Medical Care*, 34(3): 191–204.

Verhoef, M. J.; Page, S. A.; and Waddell, S. C. (1997). The chiropractic outcome study: Pain, functional ability and satisfaction with care. *Journal of Manipulative and Physiological Therapeutics*, 20: 235–40.

Yates, R. G.; et al. (1988). Effects of chiropractic treatment on blood pressure and anxiety: A randomized, controlled trial. *Journal of Manipulative and Physiological Therapeutics*, 11: 484–88.

Chapter 10: AYURVEDIC MEDICINE AND YOGA

Alexander, C. N.; et al. (1989). Transcendental meditation, mindfulness, and longevity: An experimental study with the elderly. *Journal of Pers. Soc. Psychology*, 57: 950–64.

Bharani, A.; et al. (1995). Salutary effect of *Terminalia Arjuna* in patients with severe refractory heart failure. *Int. Journal of Cardiology*, 49: 191–99.

Charles, V., and Charles, S. X. (1992). The use and efficacy of Azadirachta indica ADR ("Neem") and Cucurma longa ("Turmeric") in scabies. A pilot study. *Tropical and Geographical Medicine*, 44(1–2): 178–81.

Chopra, Deepak (1989). *Quantum Healing: Exploring the Frontiers of Mind-Body Medicine*. New York: Bantam Books.

————. (1992). Letter to the Editor. *JAMA*, March 11, 267(10): 1338.

Chopra, R. N.; et al. (1982). *Indigenous Drugs of India*. Calcutta: Academic Publishers.

Complementary Medicine for the Physician (1997). Ayurvedic therapy may provide plant-based treatment for Parkinson's disease. 2(6): 1, 47–48.

Dogra, J.; et al. (1994). Indigenous free radical scavenger MAK 4 and 5 in angina pectoris. Is it only a placebo? *Journal of the Association of Physicians of India*, 42(6): 466–67.

Dwivedi, S., and Agarwal, M. P. (1994). Antianginal and cardioprotective effects of Terminalia arjuna, an indigenous drug, in coronary artery disease. *Journal of the Association of Physicians of India*, 42(4): 287–89.

Etzel, R. (1996). Special extract of *Boswellia serrata* (H15) in the treatment of rheumatoid arthritis. *Phytomedicine*, 3(1): 91–94.

Faruqi, S.; et al. (1995). Herbal pharmacotherapy for the attenuation of electroconvulsive shock-induced anterograde and retrograde amnestic deficits. *Convuls. Ther.*, 11: 241–47.

Gelderloos, P.; et al. (1991). Effectiveness of the Transcendental Meditation program in preventing and treating substance misuse; a review. *International Journal of the Addictions*, March, 26(3): 293–325.

Glaser, J. L.; et al. (1991). Improvement in seasonal respiratory allergy with Maharishi Amrit Kalash 5, an Ayurvedic herb immunomodulator. *Proceedings of the American Association of Ayurvedic Medicine*, 7(1): 6.

Glaser, J. L.; et al. (1992). Elevated serum dehydroepiandrosterone sulfate levels in practitioners of the Transcendental Meditation (TM) and TM-Sidhi programs. *Journal of Behavioral Medicine*, August, 15(4): 327–41.

Jain, S. K. (1994). Ethnobotany and research on medicinal plants in India. *CIBA Found. Symp.*, 185: 153–64.

Janssen, G. W. H. M. (1989). The application of Maharishi Ayur-Veda in the treatment of ten chronic diseases: A pilot study. *Ned Tijdschr Geneeskd*, 5: 586–94.

Kulkarni, R. R.; et al. (1991). Treatment of osteoarthritis with a herbomineral formulation: A double-blind, placebo-controlled, cross-over study. *Journal of Ethnopharmacology*, 33(1–2): 91–96.

Lad, V. (1995). An introduction to Ayurveda. *Alternative Therapy*, 1(3): 57–63.

Madanmohan, D.; et al. (1992). Effect of yoga training on reaction time, respiratory endurance and muscle strength. *Indian Journal of Physiology and Pharmacology*, 36(4): 229–33.

Manyam, B. V. (1996). Method of Evaluating Ayurvedic Drugs in Parkinsonism. (Unpublished pilot study.)

Manyam, B. V.; et al. (1995). An Alternative Medicine Treatment for Parkinson's Disease: Results of a Multicenter Clinical Trial. *The Journal of Alternative and Complementary Medicine*, 1(3): 249–55.

Mishra, S. K. (1997). An overview of Ayurvedic medicine and yoga. (Unpublished, commissioned review.)

Niwa, Y. (1991). Effect of Maharishi-4 and Maharishi-5 on inflammatory mediators with special reference to their free radical scavenging effect. *Indian Journal of Clinical Practice*, 1: 23–27.

Orme-Johnson, D. (1987). Medical care utilization and the transcendental meditation program. *Psychosomatic Medicine*, 49: 493–507.

Paranjpe, P.; and Kulkarni, P. H. (1995). Comparative efficacy of four Ayurvedic formulations in the treatment of acne vulgaris: A double-blind randomised placebo-controlled clinical evaluation. *Journal of Ethnopharmacology*, 49: 127–32.

Patel, C. (1973). Yoga and bio-feedback in the management of hypertension. *Lancet*, 1053–55.

Prasad, M. L.; et al. (1992). Idiopathic inflammatory myopathy: Clinicopathological observations in the Indian population. *British Journal of Rheumatology*, December, 31(12): 855–59.

Riegel, Barbara; et al. (1998). Teaching ayurvedic and western health promotion strategies to healthy adults. *American Journal of Health Promotion*, 12(4): 258–62.

Sadhukhan, B.; et al. (1994). Clinical evaluation of a herbal antidiabetic product. *Journal of Indian Medical Association*, 92: 115–17.

Saraf, M. N.; et al. (1989). Studies on the mechanism of action of *Semicarpus anacardium* in rheumatoid arthritis. *Journal of Ethnopharmacology*, 25(2): 159–64.

Schell, F. J.; et al. (1994). Physiological and psychological effects of Hatha-Yoga exercise in healthy women. *International Journal of Psychosomatics*, 41(1–4): 46–52.

Schneider, R. H.; et al. (1990). Health promotion with a traditional system of natural health care: Maharishi Ayur-Ved. *Journal of Social Behavior and Personality*, 5(3): 1–27.

Shaffer, H.; et al. (1997). Comparing hatha yoga with dynamic group psychotherapy for enhancing methadone maintenance treatment: A randomized clinical trial. *Alternative Therapies*, 3(4): 57–67.

Shanbhag, V. (1988). The role of *sankha-bhasma* (an Ayurvedic medicine) in the treatment of acne vulgaris. M.D. thesis, University of Poona, February.

Sharma; et al. (1993). Improvement in cardiovascular (CV) risk factors through Maharishi panchakarma (PK) purification procedure (abstract). *Federation of American Societies of Experimental Biology*, 7(4): A801.

Sharma, H. M.; Feng, Y.; and Panganamala, R. V. (1989). Maharishi Amrit Kalash (MAK) prevents human platelet aggregation. *Clin Ter Cardiovasc*, 8: 227–30.

Sharma, H. M.; Krieger, J.; and Dwivedi, C. (1990). Antineoplastic properties of dietary Maharishi-4 and Maharishi Amrit Kalash Ayurvedic food
supplements. *European Journal of Pharmacology*, 183: 193.

Sharma, H. M.; et al. (1990). Antineoplastic properties of Maharishi-4 against
DMBA-induced mammary tumors in rats. *Pharmacol Biochem Behavior*, 35:
767–73.

Smit, H. F.; Woerdenbag, H. J.; and Singh, R. H. (1995). Ayurvedic herbal
drugs with possible cytostatic activity. *Journal of Ethnopharmacology*, 47:
75–84.

Srivastava, K. C. (1989). Extracts from two frequently consumed spices—cumin
(Cuminum ciminum) and turmeric (Curcuma longa)—inhibit platelet aggre-
gation and alter eicosanoid biosynthesis in human blood platelets.
Prostaglandins Leukot Essent Fatty Acids, 37: 57–64.

Srivastava, K. C.; et al. (1992). Ginger (Zingiber oficinale) in rheumatism and
musculoskeletal disorders. *Medical Hypotheses*, 39(4): 3422–48.

Telles, S.; et al. (1993). Physiological changes in sports teachers following 3
months of training in Yoga. *Indian Journal of Medical Sciences*, 47(10):
235–38.

Thyagarajan, S. P.; et al. (1988). Effect of *Phyllanthus amarus* on chronic carriers of hepatitis B virus. *Lancet*, 2: 764–66.

Verma, S. K.; et al. (1988). Effect of Commiphora mukul (gum guggulu) in
patients of hyperlipidemia with special reference to HDL-cholesterol. *Indian
Journal of Medical Research*, April, 87: 356–60.

Wallace, R. K. (1970). Physiological effects of transcendental meditation. *Science*, 167: 1751–54.

Chapter 11: SPIRITUALITY AND HEALING

Achterberg, J.; et al. (1993). *Report of the Panel on Mind/Body Interventions*.
Prepared for the National Institutes of Health, Office of Alternative Medicine, February 1.

Allen, K., and Blascovich, J. (1996). The value of service dogs for people with
severe ambulatory disabilities: A randomized controlled trial. *JAMA*, 275:
1001–6.

Amoateng, A. Y., and Bahr, S. J. (1986). Religion, family, and adolescent drug
use. *Sociological Perspectives*, 29(1): 53–76.

Armstrong, B.; et al. (1977). Blood pressure in Seventh-Day Adventist vegetarians. *American Journal of Epidemiology*, 105: 444–49.

Ash, C. R. (1997). Therapeutic touch: Healing through the hands. *Complementary Medicine*, 2(1): 1, 6–7.

Benor, D. J. (1990). Survey of spiritual healing research. *Complementary Medical Research*, 4(3): 9–33.

Benson, H. (1987). *Your Maximum Mind*. New York: Times Books/Random House.

Berkel, J., and de Waard, F. (1983). Mortality pattern and life expectancy of Seventh-Day Adventists in the Netherlands. *International Journal of Epidemiology*, 12(4): 455–59.

Berkeley Wellness Letter (1992). Where there is hope there is life. March, 2–3.

Berkman, L., and Syme, S. (1979). Social networks, host resistance, and mortality: a 9 year follow-up study of Alameda County residents. *American Journal of Epidemiology*, 109: 186–92.

Beston, H. (1928). *The Outermost House*. New York: Penguin Books.

Block, K. I. (1997). The role of the self in healthy cancer survivorship: A view from the front lines of treating cancer. *Advances*, 13(1): 6–26.

Bower, B. (1991). Stress goes to the dogs. *Science News*, 140: 285.

Brown, D. R.; et al. (1990). Religiosity and psychological distress among blacks. *Journal of Religion and Health*, 29(1): 55–68.

Bruhn, J.; et al. (1966). Social aspects of coronary heart disease in two adjacent ethnically different communities. *American Journal of Public Health*, 56: 2493–2506.

Bruhn, J., and Wolf, S. (1978). Update on Roseto, Pennsylvania: Testing a prediction. *Psychosomatic Medicine*, 40: 86.

Buchholz, W. (1990). Hope (generic). *JAMA*, 263(17): 2357–5238.

Byrd, R. (1988). Positive therapeutic effects of intercessory prayer in a coronary care unit population. *Southern Medical Journal*, 81: 826–29.

Clay, R. (1996). Psychologists' faith in religion begins to grow. *APA Monitor*, 27(8): 1, 48.

Cohen, S.; et al. (1997). Social ties and susceptibility to the common cold. *JAMA*, June, 25: 1940–45.

Collipp, P. H. (1969). The efficacy of prayer: A triple blind study. *Medical Times*, 97: 201–4.

Comstock, G. W., and Partridge, K. B. (1972). Church attendance and health. *Journal of Chronic Disease*, 25: 665–72.

Connelly, J. E.; et al. (1989). Health perceptions of primary care patients and the influence on health care utilization. *Medical Care*, 27(S): 99–109.

Cummings, N. A., and VandenBos, G. R. (1981). The twenty years Kaiser-Permanente experience with psychotherapy and medical utilization: implications for national health policy and national health insurance. *Health Policy Quarterly*, 1(2): 159–75.

Desmond, D. P., and Maddux, J. F. (1981). Religious programs and careers of chronic heroin users. *American Journal of Drug and Alcohol Abuse* (1): 71–83.

Dossey, L. (1993). *Healing Words: The Power of Prayer and the Practice of Medicine.* San Francisco: Harper.

———. (1997a). *Be Careful What You Pray For.* New York; HarperCollins.

———. (1997b). The healing power of pets; A look at animal-assisted therapy. *Alternative Therapies,* 3(4): 8–16.

Elgin, D., and LeDrew, C. Global consciousness change. (Unpublished manuscript, 1997.)

Enstrom, J. E. (1989). Health practices and cancer mortality among active California Mormons. *Journal of the National Cancer Institute,* 81: 1807–14.

Fitzgibbons, R. P. (1986). The cognitive and emotive uses of forgiveness in the treatment of anger. *Psychotherapy,* 23: 629–33.

Forbes, S. (1994). Hope: An essential human need in the elderly. *Journal of Gerontol. Nursing,* 20(6): 5–10.

Fox, A., and Fox, B. (1988). *Wake Up! You're Alive.* Deerfield Beach, Fla.: Health Communications, Inc., 85.

Friedmann, E.; et al. (1980). Animal companions and one-year survival of patients after discharge from a coronary care unit. *Public Health Rep.,* 95(4): 307–12.

Galton, F. (1872). Statistical inquiries into the efficacy of prayer. *Fortnightly Review,* 12: 125–35.

Gardner, J. W., and Lyon, J. L. (1982a). Cancer in Utah Mormon men by church activity level. *American Journal of Epidemiology,* 116: 243–57.

———. (1982b). Cancer in Utah Mormon women by church activity level. *American Journal of Epidemiology,* 116: 258–65.

Gartner, J.; et al. (1991). Religious commitment and mental health: A review of the empirical literature. *Journal of Psychology and Theology,* 19: 6–25.

Goleman, D., and Gurin, J. (1993). *Mind Body Medicine.* New York: Consumer Reports Books, 11.

Grad, B. (1965). Some biological effects of the "laying on of hands": A review of experiments with animals and plants. *Journal of American Society of Psychical Research,* 59: 95–127.

Hadaway, C. K.; et al. (1984). Religious involvement and drug use among urban adolescents. *Journal for the Scientific Study of Religion,* 23(2): 109–28.

Harvard Health Letter (1998). Faith and healing: Making a place for spirituality. February, 23(4): 1–3.

Heidt, P. (1981). Effects of therapeutic touch on anxiety level of hospitalized patients. *Nursing Research,* 1: 32–37.

Hertsgaard, D., and Light, H. (1984). Anxiety, depression, and hostility in rural women. *Psychological Reports,* 55: 673–74.

House, J. S.; et al. (1982). The association of social relationship and activities with morality: Prospective evidence from the Tecumseh community health study. *American Journal of Epidemiology,* 116: 123–40.

Kaczorowski, J. M. (1989). Spiritual well-being and anxiety in adults diagnosed with cancer. *Hospice Journal*, 5: 105–16.

Kass, J. D.; et al. (1991). Health outcomes and a new index of spiritual experience. *Journal for the Scientific Study of Religion*, 30: 203–11.

Katcher, A. H., and Friedmann, E. (1980). Potential health value of pet ownership. *Continuing Education*, 2(2): 117–21.

Kiecolt-Glaser, J.; et al. (1987). Marital quality, marital disruption, and immune function. *Psychosomatic Medicine*, 49: 13–34.

King, D., and Bushwick, B. (1994). Beliefs and attitudes of hospital inpatients about faith healing and prayer. *Journal of Family Practice*, 39(4): 349–52.

Koenig, H. G. (1998). Intrinsic religiosity and depression. *American Journal of Psychiatry*, 110–14.

Koenig, Harold G. (1995). *Research on Religion and Aging.* Westport, Conn.: Greenwood Press, 153.

Koenig, Harold G.; et al. (1994). Religious practices and alcoholism in southern adult population. *Hospitals and Community Psychiatry*, 45(3): 225–31.

Koenig, Harold G.; et al. (1997). Attendance at Religious Services, Interleukin-6, and Other Biological Parameters of Immune Function in Older Adults. *International Journal of Psychiatry in Medicine*, 27(3): 233–50.

Krause, N. (1992). Providing support to others and well-being in later life. *Journal of Gerontology*, 47: 300–311.

Krieger, D. (1979). *Therapeutic Touch: How to Use Your Hands to Help or Heal.* Englewood Cliffs, N.J.: Prentice-Hall.

Larson, D. B.; et al. (1989). The impact of religion on men's blood pressure. *Journal of Religion and Health*, 28: 265–78.

Levin, J. S., and Vanderpool, H. Y. (1987). Is frequent religious attendance really conducive to better health? Toward an epidemiology of religion. *Social Science and Medicine*, 24: 589–600.

———. (1991). Religious factors in physical health and the prevention of illness. *Prevention in Human Services*, 9(2): 41–64.

Lynn, J. (1997). Perceptions by family members of the dying experience of older and seriously ill patients. *Ann. Intern. Med.*, January 15, 126: 97–106.

Matthews, D. A., and Larson, D. B. (1995). The faith factor: An annotated bibliography of clinical research on spiritual subjects. *National Institute for Healthcare Research*, 3.

Maunsell, E.; et al. (1995). Social support and survival among women with breast cancer. *Cancer*, 76: 631–37.

McClelland, D. C. (1985). *Human Motivation.* Glenview, Ill.: Scott, Foresman and Co.

McCullough, M. E. (1997). How religious commitment may promote longer life. *Faith and Medicine Connection*, 1(3): 3.

McSherry, E.; et al. (1986). Pastoral care departments: More necessary in the DRG era? *HCMR Review*, 11(1): 47–59.

MD (1986). Does prayer help patients? December: 35.

Moore, N. (1996). Spirituality in Medicine. *Alternative Therapies*, 2(6): 24–26, 103–5.

Myers, D. G., and Diener, E. (1997). The new scientific pursuit of happiness. *Harvard Mental Health Letter*, August, 4–7.

Nerem, R. M.; et al. (1980). *Science*, 208: 1475.

Oleckno, W. A., and Blacconiere, M. J. (1991). Relationship of religiosity to well-ness and other health-related behaviors and outcomes. *Psychol. Rep.*, 68: 819–26.

Oxman, T. E.; et al. (1995). Lack of social participation or religious strength and comfort as risk factors for death after cardiac surgery in the elderly. *Psychosomatic Medicine*, 57: 5–15.

Pelletier, K. R. (1981). *Longevity: Fulfilling Our Biological Potential*. New York: Delta, 322–24.

———. (1994). *Sound Mind, Sound Body*. New York: Fireside.

Peterson, C. (1988). Explanatory style as a risk factor for illness. *Cognitive Therapy and Research*, 12: 117–30.

Petrie, K. J.; et al. (1996). Role of patients' view of their illness in predicting return to work and functioning after myocardial infarction: longitudinal study. *British Medical Journal*, 312: 1191–94.

Poloma, M. M., and Pendleton, B. F. (1991). The effects of prayer and prayer experiences on measures of general well-being. *Journal of Psychology and Theology*, 19(1): 71–83.

Pressman, P.; et al. (1990). Religious belief, depression, and ambulation status in elderly women with broken hips. *American Journal of Psychiatry*, 147: 758–60.

Quinn, J. F. (1989). Therapeutic touch as energy exchange: Replication and extension. *Nursing Science Quarterly*, 12: 78–87.

Reynolds, P., and Kaplan, G. A. (1990). Social connections and risk for cancer: Prospective evidence from the Alameda County study. *Behavioral Medicine*, Fall: 101–10.

Russek, L. G., and Schwartz, G. E. (1996). Narrative descriptions of parental love and caring predict health status in midlife: A 35-year follow-up of the Harvard Mastery of Stress Study. *Alternative Therapies*, 2(6): 55–62.

Scheier, M., and Carver, C. (1985). Optimism, coping, and health: Assessment and implications of generalized outcome expectancies. *Health Psychol.*, 4(3): 219–47.

Schlitz, M., and Braud, W. (1997). Distant intentionality: Assessing the evidence. *Alternative Therapies*, 3(6): 62–73.

Science (1982). Tumor rejection in rats after inescapable or escapable shock. 216: 437–39.

Sleek, S. (1994). Spiritual problems included in DSM-IV. *APA Monitor,* June, 8.

Sosa, R.; et al. (1980). The effect of a supportive companion on prenatal problems, length of labor and mother-infant interactions. *New England Journal of Medicine,* 303: 597–600.

Spiegel, D.; et al. (1989). Effect of psycho-social treatment on survival of patients with metastatic breast cancer. *Lancet,* 2(8668): 888–91.

Strawbridge, W.; et al. (1997). Frequent attendance at religious services and mortality over 28 years. *American Journal of Public Health,* 87(6): 957–61.

Tibbits, D. (1997). Spirituality and healing in medicine. (Unpublished, commissioned review.)

Uchino, B. N.; et al. (1992). Age-related changes in cardiovascular response as a function of a chronic stressor and social support. *Journal of Personal Soc. Psychology,* 63(5): 839–46.

Voorhees, C.; et al. (1996). Heart, body, and soul: Impact of church-based smoking cessation interventions on readiness to quit. *Preventive Medicine,* 25: 277–85.

Walker, S. R.; et al. (1997). Intercessory prayer in the treatment of alcohol abuse and dependence: A plot investigation. *Alternative Therapies,* 3(6): 79–86.

Williams, R. B.; et al. (1992). Prognostic importance of social and economic resources among medically treated patients with angiographically documented coronary artery disease. *JAMA,* 276: 520–24.

Williams, R., and Williams, V. (1993). *Anger Kills.* New York: HarperCollins.

Wirth, D. (1990). The effect of non-contact therapeutic touch on the healing rate of full-thickness surgical wounds. *Subtle Energies,* 1: 1–20.

Chapter 12: CAM INSURANCE

American Academy of Actuaries (1995). *Medical Savings Accounts.* Washington, D.C.: AAA.

Aragon Consulting Group (1996). What Americans Think About Health Insurance Reform. *Medical Benefits,* April 30, 7.

Aubry, W. (1996). Clinical effectiveness, scientific evidence, and cost. An agenda for complementary and alternative therapies. Presented at NIH/AHCPR Workshop, University of Arizona, Tucson, Ariz. October 9.

Beauregard, K. (1993). Private Health Insurance: Persons Denied Coverage Due to Poor Health. *National Medical Expenditure Survey.* Washington, D.C.: U.S. Department of Health and Human Services.

Berss, Marcia (1993). Our System Is Just Overwhelmed. *Forbes,* May 24, 40.

Burner, Sally T., and Waldo, Daniel R. (1995). National Health Expenditure Projections, 1994–2005. *Health Care Financing Review*, Summer, 16: 238.

Ciba-Geigy Corporation (1996). 1996 Trends and Forecasts: CibaGeneva Pharmacy Benefit Report. *Medical Benefits*, July 30, 3.

Coughlin, Kenneth M. (1993). Pay-Related Health Care Plans Bring Equity to Cost Sharing. *Business and Health*, February, 39.

Donelan, Karen; et al. (1996). All Payer, Single Payer, Managed Care, No Payer: Patients' Perspectives in Three Nations. *Health Affairs*, Summer, 15(2): 254–65.

Eisenberg, D. M. (1997). Advising patients who seek alternative medical therapies. *Ann. Intern. Med.*, 128(1): 78–82.

Eisenberg, D. M., et al. (1993). Unconventional medicine in the United States. *New England Journal of Medicine*, 328: 246–52.

Employee Benefit Research Institute (1994). Public Attitudes on Flexible Benefits, 1994. *Medical Benefits*, July 30, 1.

Farley Short, Pamela, and Lair, Tamra J. (1996). Health Insurance and Health Status. *Medical Benefits*, February 28, 8.

Fuchs, Victor R., and Hahn, James S. (1990). How does Canada do it? *New England Journal of Medicine*, 323(13): 884–90.

Geisel, Jerry (1996). New Employer Duties Under Health Reforms. *Business Insurance*, August 19, 1.

Goodwin, N. (1997). A health insurance revolution. *New Age Journal*, March/April, 95–99.

Hahn, Beth, and Flood, Ann Barry (1995). No insurance, public insurance, and private insurance. *Journal of Health Care for the Poor and Uninsured*, 6(1): 41–59.

Health Insurance Association of America (1994). *Long-Term Care Insurance in 1994.* Washington, D.C.: HIAA, 9.

Herzlinger, R. (1997). *Market Driven Health Care.* Reading, Mass.: Addison-Wesley Publishing Company.

———. (1994). The Quiet Health Care Revolution. *Public Interest*, Spring, 115: 72–90.

Katz, Steven J., and Hofer, Timothy P. (1994). Socio-economic disparities in preventive care persist despite universal coverage. *JAMA*, 272(7): 530–34.

Keeler, Emmett B. (1996). Can medical savings accounts for the nonelderly reduce health care costs? *JAMA*, 275(21): 1666–71.

Kellerman, Vivien (1993). Growing Numbers Seek Out Alternative Medicine. *New York Times*, April 4, Section 13L1, 1.

Landmark Healthcare (1996). *Health Maintenance Organizations and Alternative Medicine: A Closer Look.* Sacramento, Calif.

Lehrman, S. (1996). Alternative medicine: Insurers cover new ground. *Harvard Health Letter*, 22(2): 1.

Manning, William G., et al. (1987). Health insurance and the demand for medical care: Evidence from a randomized experiment. *American Economic Review*, June, 77(3): 251–77.

Marie, Ariane; Pelletier, Kenneth R.; Astin, John A.; and Hansen, Erik. A Review of the Incorporation of Complementary Alternative Medicine by Mainstream Physicians. Submitted for publication.

Medalia Healthcare PCP Strategy (1997). Alternative Medicine Integration and Coverage, July, 6.

Padgug, R. (1995). Alternative medicine and health insurance. *The Mt. Sinai Journal of Medicine*, 62(2): 152–58.

Pell, C. (1996). Alternative medicine: A worldview. *Alternative Therapies*, 2(6): 95.

Pelletier, K.; et al. (1997). Current trends in the integration and reimbursement of complementary and alternative medicine by managed care, insurance carriers, and hospital providers. *American Journal of Health Promotion*, 12(2): 112–22.

Ready, Tinker (1994). Did More Cardiac Care in U.S. Produce Better Outcomes than in Canada? *Medical Benefits*, January 15, 7–8.

ReliaStar (1997). *State Health Rankings.* Minneapolis, October 7.

Relman, Arnold S. (1986). The United States and Canada: Different approaches to health care. *New England Journal of Medicine*, 315(25): 1608–10.

St. Anthony's Alternative Medicine Integration & Coverage (1997). Alternative link develops CAM coding system. September, 6.

Studdert, David M.; et al. (1998). Medical malpractice implications of alternative medicine. *JAMA*, November 11, 280(18): 1610–15.

U.S. Bureau of the Census (1994). *Statistical Abstract of the United States, 1994.* Washington, D.C.: Government Printing Office, 460, table 703.

Warden, Chris (1993). Other Paths to Health Reform. *Investor's Business Daily*, May 4, 1.

Weeks, J. (1997a). CAM Integration into Insurance and Managed Care and the Role of the Consumer. (Unpublished; commissioned review.)

———. (1997b). "Alternative," "complementary" or "integrative": Problems with language. *St. Anthony's Business Report on Alternative & Complementary Medicine*, May, 1–3.

Welch, W. Pete; et al. (1997). A detailed comparison of physician services for the elderly in the United States and Canada. *JAMA*, 275(18): 1410–16.

Chapter 13: INTEGRATIVE MEDICINE

Banks, Dwayne A., and Fossel, Michael (1997). Telomeres, cancer, and aging: Altering the human life span. *JAMA*, October 22/29, 278(16): 1345–48.

Barsky, Arthur. (1988) *Worried Sick: Our Troubled Quest for Wellness.* Boston: Little Brown.

Bennett, William I.; Goldfinger, Stephen E.; and Johnson, Timothy (1987). *Your Good Health: How to Stay Well, and What to Do When You're Not.* Cambridge, Mass.: Harvard University Press.

Bucholz, William M. (1990). Hope (generic). *JAMA*, 263(17): 2357–58.

Chopra, Deepak (1989). *Quantum Healing: Exploring the Frontiers of Mind/Body Medicine.* New York: Bantam Books.

Cousins, Norman (1988). Intangibles in medicine: An attempt at a balancing perspective. *JAMA*, 260(11): 1610–12.

Cowen, Emory L. (1991). In pursuit of wellness. *American Psychologist*, 46(4): 404–8.

DeAngelis, Tori (1991). When going gets tough, "the hopeful keep going." *APA Monitor*, July 18–19.

Engel, George L. (1960). A unified concept of health and disease. *Perspectives in Biology and Medicine,* 3: 459–85.

Fries, James S., and Crapo, L. M. (1981). *Vitality and Aging.* San Francisco: W. H. Freeman.

Gordon, James (1996). *Manifesto for a New Medicine.* Reading, Mass: Addison-Wesley Publishing Company.

Harvard Health Letter (1992). The seven best tests. Special supplement, July, 9–12.

Herzlinger, Regina E., and Calkins, David (1985). How companies tackle health care costs. *Harvard Business Review,* November–December, 70–80.

Herzlinger, Regina E., and Schwartz, Jeffrey (1985). How companies tackle health care costs: Part 1. *Harvard Business Review,* July-August, 69–81.

Holman, Halsted (1991). Psychosocial support and the management of chronic illness. *Advances,* 7(3): 8–9.

JAMA (1998). Editorial: Alternative medicine meets science. November 11, 280(18): 1618–19.

Kent, J.; Coates, T. J.; Pelletier, K. R.; and O'Regan, B. (1989). Unexpected recoveries: Spontaneous remission and immune functioning. *Advances: Journal of the Institute for the Advancement of Health,* 6(2): 66–73.

Murphy, Michael (1992). *The Future of the Body: Explorations into the Further Evolution of Human Nature.* Los Angeles: J. P. Tarcher.

Ober, K. Patrick (1997). The Pre-Flexnerian Reports: Mark Twain's Criticism of Medicine in the United States. *Ann. Intern. Med.,* 126: 157–63.

Ornstein, Robert, and Sobel, David (1987). The Healing Brain. *Psychology Today,* March, 48–52.

Pennisi, Elizabeth, and Williams, Nigel (1997). Will Dolly Send in the Clones? *Science,* March 7, 275: 1415–16.

Popkin, B. M., and Patterson, R. E. (1987). Older Americans are uncertain about diet guidelines. *American Journal of Clinical Nutrition,* April, 55: 823–30.

Quick, J. C.; et al. (1990). Health promotion: Education and treatment. In *Work and Well Being: An Agenda for the 90's.* Washington, D.C.: American Psychological Association and National Institute of Occupational Health and Safety position paper.

Rivlin, Richard S. (1992). Nutrition. *JAMA,* 268(3): 382–83.

Rothberg, Joseph M.; Bartone, Paul T.; Holloway, Harry C.; and Marlowe, David H. (1990). Life and death in the U.S. Army. *JAMA,* 264(7): 2241–44.

Rowe, John W., and Kahn, Robert L. (1987). Human Aging: Usual and Successful. *Science,* July 10, 237: 143–49.

Thomas, Patricia (1997). Scientific Progress: Top Ten Medical Advances of 1996. *Harvard Health Letter,* March, 22(5): 1–3.

Ullmann, Daniel; et al. (1991). Cause-specific mortality among physicians with differing life-styles. *JAMA,* 265(18): 2352–57.

Walsh, Diana Chapman (1990). The private side of public health. *Journal of Public Health,* Winter, 405–11.

Williams, Redford (1989). The Trusting Heart. *Psychology Today,* 23(5): 36–42.

Winkleby, Marilyn A.; Jatulis, Darius E.; Frank, Erica; and Fortmann, Stephen P. (1992). Socioeconomic status and health: How education, income, and occupation contribute to risk factors for cardiovascular disease. *American Journal of Public Health,* 82(6): 816–20.

INDEX